Advances in Periprosthetic Joint Infection

E. Carlos Rodríguez-Merchán
Editor

Advances in Periprosthetic Joint Infection

Springer

Editor
E. Carlos Rodríguez-Merchán
Department of Orthopedic Surgery
Hospital Universitario La Paz
Madrid, Madrid, Spain

ISBN 978-3-032-02944-7 ISBN 978-3-032-02945-4 (eBook)
https://doi.org/10.1007/978-3-032-02945-4

This Springer imprint is published by the registered company Springer Nature Switzerland AG
The registered company address is: Gewerbestrasse 11, 6330 Cham, Switzerland

Preface

As the editor of this book, I have tried to bring together the most recent advances in periprosthetic joint infection (PJI) in a single volume. The book has 17 chapters, which have been written by experts in joint arthroplasty of the shoulder, elbow, hip, knee, and ankle. In the first chapter, the most relevant information on general concepts related to PJI has been reviewed. In Chap. 2, the most recent advances in the diagnosis of PJI have been analyzed. Then, in the next four chapters, an update of recent information on shoulder arthroplasty has been carried out: diagnosis; risk factors; open debridement, antibiotics, and implant retention (DAIR); and revision shoulder arthroplasty. The most recent information on total elbow arthroplasty has been analyzed in Chap. 7. Chapters 8 and 9 have been devoted to total hip arthroplasty (THA): diagnosis of PJI and revision THA. Then, Chaps. 10, 11, 12, 13, 14, and 15 have been devoted to PJI in total knee arthroplasty (TKA): risk factors; prevention; antibiotic prophylaxis; DAIR; revision TKA; and knee arthrodesis after failure of TKA due to infection. Current data on PJI in total ankle arthroplasty have been analyzed in Chap. 16. Finally, in Chap. 17, flap coverage in patients with PJI has been reviewed. As the editor of the book, I thank all the authors for their generous participation, and I hope that the contents of the book will be useful to colleagues involved in the diagnosis and treatment of PJI.

Madrid, Spain E. Carlos Rodríguez-Merchán

Contents

General Concepts on Periprosthetic Joint Infection: A Review of Current Relevant Data

1

E. Carlos Rodríguez-Merchán, Hortensia De la Corte-Rodríguez, and Juan M. Román-Belmonte

1.1 Introduction

Periprosthetic joint infection (PJI) is a serious adverse event of total joint arthroplasty (TJA). Even with contemporary treatments, failure rates are unacceptably elevated with a 5-year mortality rate of 26% [1]. PJI is a unique clinical entity, notably different from infections entailing native bones or joints. PJI is characterized by an intricate interaction between microbes, mainly bacteria but once in a while fungi, and the host immune reaction. Only a negligible microbial burden is needed to start a PJI; etiologic organisms can stick to the surfaces of arthroplasty components and create biofilms [2].

Biofilms notably show a considerable resistance to a broad array of antimicrobial drugs and are adept at averting innate immune defenses. The offending microorganisms in PJI typically begin in the skin microbiome and might be introduced throughout the perioperative stage of the implantation procedure. On other occasions, these microorganisms can seed the implant in the postoperative stage via hematogenous dissemination or direct inoculation from adjacent infected tissues [2].

There is no universally established definition for PJI. The clinical display of PJI differs; the classical characteristics of infection, such as fever, leukocytosis, and signs of sepsis, are frequently absent. A prosthesis is a foreign body, and its mere existence is a risk factor for infection. The microbial load required to cause an infection in a prosthetic joint is much less than that for a natural joint. The strongest compelling factor of a PJI is a joint aspirate or surgically attained periprosthetic material that generates a microorganism when cultured. Other findings compelling a PJI comprise a sinus tract communicating with the joint space, wound dehiscence, flagrant purulence, prosthetic loosening, synovial fluid leukocytosis with neutrophilia, and raised serum inflammatory markers. Nevertheless, failure to identify an etiologic pathogen does not exclude the existence of PJI. PJIs are a substantial clinical problem. PJIs substantially raise morbidity and mortality and have exceeded polyethylene (PE) wear as the main indication for revision arthroplasty [2]. The purpose of this chapter is to review the most relevant recent information on PJI.

E. C. Rodríguez-Merchán (✉)
Department of Orthopedic Surgery, Hospital Universitario La Paz, Madrid, Madrid, Spain

H. De la Corte-Rodríguez
Department of Physical and Rehabilitation Medicine, Hospital Universitario La Paz, Madrid, Spain

J. M. Román-Belmonte
Department of Physical and Rehabilitation Medicine, Hospital Universitario Cruz Roja San José y Santa Adela, Madrid, Spain

E. C. Rodríguez-Merchán (ed.), *Advances in Periprosthetic Joint Infection*,
https://doi.org/10.1007/978-3-032-02945-4_1

1.2 PJI and Immunity

Most publications on PJI have concentrated on development of better biomarkers for diagnostics and management approaches entailing new antibiotic delivery methods, antibiofilm drugs, and bacteriophages. However, the function of the immune system, our first line of defense during PJI, is not well comprehended. Evidence of infection in individuals with PJI is encountered within circulation, synovial fluid, and tissue and entails numerous metabolites, antimicrobial peptides, and soluble receptors that are part of the PJI diagnosis workup. Macrophages, neutrophils, and myeloid-derived suppressor cells (MDSCs) are first recruited into the joint by chemokines and cytokines created by immune cells and bacteria and are triggered by pathogen-associated molecular patterns. Although these cells are effective killers of planktonic bacteria by phagocytosis, opsonization, degranulation, and recruitment of adaptive immune cells, biofilm-associated bacteria are disturbing. Biofilm is not only a physical obstacle for the immune system but also prompts effector functions. Besides, bacteria have built up mechanisms to dodge the immune system by inactivating effector molecules, promoting killing or anti-inflammatory effector cell phenotypes, and intracellular persistence and dissemination. Comprehending these faults and the mechanisms by which bacteria can undermine the immune system might reveal novel strategies to better prepare our own immune system to fight against PJI. Moreover, preoperative immune system evaluation and screening for dysregulation might help in creating preventative methods to diminish PJI prevalence [1].

1.3 The Influence of Gut Microbiome on Early PJI

Early PJI represents one of the most serious adverse events of TJA. Recently, some data have highlighted the possible connection between dysregulation of the gut microbiota and degenerative illnesses of joints. It has been hypothesized that microbiome dysbiosis might raise the risk of PJI by promoting bacterial translocation from these areas to the bloodstream or by weakening local or systemic immune reactions. Although the ways binding the gut microbiome to infection susceptibility are not yet known, new studies suggest that the presurgical gut microbiota—a prior unconsidered component—might impact the patient's ability to withstand infection. Consequently, studying the possible influence of the microbiome on PJI might bring new knowledge into the pathogenesis and treatment of these diseases. For a successful treatment, a correct surgical technique in conjunction with an antibacterial concept is paramount. Regarding surgical treatment, diverse strategies include surgical irrigation, Debridement, Antibiotics, and Implant Retention (DAIR) with or without PE exchange. Other options could be one-stage or two-stage revision arthroplasty. Interventions that either directly aim at gut microbes as well as interventions that change the composition and/or function of the commensal microbes represent an innovative and potentially successful field to be studied. In recent times, innovative therapeutic approaches have appeared in the field of microbiome restoration and the treatment of gut-related diseases. If dysbiosis is shown to be a substantial contributor, developing therapies for dysbiosis might represent a new frontier in the control of PJIs [3]. Dysbiosis is an imbalance in bacterial composition, changes in bacterial metabolic activities, or changes in bacterial distribution within the gut. The three types of dysbiosis are: (1) loss of beneficial bacteria; (2) overgrowth of potentially pathogenic bacteria; and (3) loss of overall bacterial diversity [4].

1.4 Organism Profile and C-Reactive Protein (CRP) Response Are Different in PJI in Patients with Hepatitis

According to Akkaya et al. (2024), hepatitis B and C are relevant and relatively frequent health issues. It is known that many individuals who underwent total knee and hip arthroplasty were also diagnosed with hepatitis. These individuals are at higher risk of PJI [5]. In a retrospective case-controlled single-center study, Akkaya et al. aimed to study the differences in PJI cases in hepatitis B and C patients. A total of 270 individuals with hepatitis and nonhepatitis (control group) who underwent one-stage septic exchange to the hip and knee joints were analyzed. The mean CRP levels of hepatitis B- and C-positive individuals, who underwent one-stage septic exchange in the knee joint, were 23.6 mg/L. In the control group, this value was 43.1 mg/L and a statistically significant difference was found between the groups. Gram-negative organisms were identified in a larger proportion of individuals with hepatitis who developed PJI in both hip and knee joints and underwent one-stage septic exchange. PJIs caused by Gram-negative bacteria were found more frequently in individuals with hepatitis than in the control group. Besides, the CRP rise was less in individuals with hepatitis compared to PJI cases in the control group. The conclusion was that patient-specific assessment is needed in cases of PJI in patient groups with coexisting hepatitis [5].

1.5 The PJI-TNM Classification for PJIs

In 2024, Baertl et al. assessed the clinical application of the PJI-TNM classification for PJI by determining intraobserver and interobserver reliability. To facilitate its utilization in clinical practice, an educational app was subsequently developed and assessed. A total of 10 orthopedic surgeons classified 20 cases of PJI based on the PJI-TNM (T = tissue and implant conditions, N = nonhuman cells (bacteria and fungi), M = morbidity of the patient) classification (Table 1.1) [6]. Subsequently, the classification was reassessed utilizing the PJI-TNM app. Classification accuracy was estimated separately

Table 1.1 PJI-TNM classification

Tissue and implant conditions		
T	**T0**	**a** (stable standard implant without important soft tissue defect)
		b (stable revision implant without important soft tissue defect)
	T1	**a** (loosened standard implant without important soft tissue defect)
		b (loosened revision implant without important soft tissue defect)
	T2	**a** (severe soft tissue defect with standard implant)
		b (severe soft tissue defect with revision implant)
Nonhuman cells (bacteria and fungi)		
N	**N0**	**a** [no mature biofilm formation (*former*: acute), directly postoperatively]
		b [no mature biofilm formation (*former*: acute), late hematogenous]
	N1	**a** [mature biofilm formation (*former*: chronic), without “difficult to treat bacteria”]
		b [mature biofilm formation (*former*: chronic), with culture-negative infection]
	N2	**a** [mature biofilm formation (*former*: chronic), with “difficult to treat bacteria”]
		b [mature biofilm formation (*former*: chronic), with polymicrobial infection]
		c [mature biofilm formation (*former*: chronic), with fungi]
Morbidity of the patient		
M	**M0**	Not or only mildly compromised (Charlson Comorbidity Index: 0–1)
	M1	Moderately compromised patient (Charlson Comorbidity Index: 2–3)
	M2	Severely compromised patient (Charlson Comorbidity Index: 4–5)
	M3	**a** (patient refuses surgical treatment)
		b (patient does not benefit from surgical treatment)
		c (patient does not survive surgical treatment)

r = Reinfection (if the infection involves a previously infected implant, the situation is considered as “reinfection” and an “r” is put in front of the classification, e.g., rT1aN1aM2)

PJI = Periprosthetic joint infection; TNM [T = tissue and implant conditions, N = nonhuman cells (bacteria and fungi), M = morbidity of the patient] for each subcategory (reinfection, tissue and implant condition, nonhuman cells, and morbidity of the individual). Overall, interobserver and intraobserver agreements were substantial across the 20 classified cases. Analyses for the variable "reinfection" showed an almost perfect interobserver and intraobserver agreement with a classification accuracy of 94.8%. The category "tissue and implant conditions" revealed moderate interobserver and substantial intraobserver reliability, while the classification accuracy was 70.8%. For "nonhuman cells," accuracy was 81% and interobserver agreement was moderate with an almost perfect intraobserver reliability. The classification accuracy of the variable "morbidity of the patient" reached 73.5% with a moderate interobserver agreement, but the intraobserver agreement was significant. The application of the app generated comparable outcomes across all subgroups. The PJI-TNM classification system captured the heterogeneity of PJI and can be applied with significant inter- and intraobserver reliability. The PJI-TNM educational app was intended to facilitate application in clinical practice. An important limitation was the correct evaluation of the implant situation. To address this, a reassessment according to intraoperative findings was strongly advised by Baertl et al. [6].

1.6 Gloves Contamination During Revision Surgery for PJI

According to Ludwick et al. (2024), the utilization of double gloving has become a standard practice for joint replacement surgeons. However, since there is limited information on how gloves are contaminated during both primary and revision arthroplasty, no precise protocol exists to direct surgeons on when, or if, to change their gloves [7]. In their study, they assessed the contamination of gloves during TJAs. The study included 25 infected cases and 10 primaries, which were carried out at the same institution utilizing the same surgical protocol from three fellowship-trained surgeons. Samples were taken every 20 min from the beginning of the surgery until the joint was irrigated. To evaluate cross-contamination during infected cases, Ludwick et al. sampled gloves utilizing blood agar plates. In primary cases, culture swabs of anterior chamfer cuts and sterile instruments on the back table were utilized as negative controls. Next-generation sequencing (NGS) was utilized as an adjunct to recognize low-virulence bacteria. In the primary cases, all samples were found to be culture negative but 3 (8.1%) of the 37 samples were found to have a low, unidentifiable bacterial mass via NGS testing. In the infected cases, 41 (59.4%) of the 69 samples generated positive microbial results. The positivity rate was higher in the samples collected after the arthrotomy was carried out (70%) compared to samples collected before the arthrotomy was carried out (40%), when the surgeon was only dissecting superficial layers. Gloves appeared to be a frequent source of cross-contamination in the intraoperative field during revision TJA. Due to the higher percentage of positive samples following the opening of the joint, Ludwick et al. hypothesized that the arthrotomy allowed for the spread of bacteria across the operative area. It was concluded that while further research is needed to formulate a precise protocol for the changing of gloves during TJA, it might be beneficial to carry out a thorough irrigation of the joint and change of the gloves immediately following arthrotomy [7].

1.7 Application of the New Irrigation Protocol to Reduce Recurrence Rate in the Management of PJI

In 2024, Wu et al. stated that irrigation was a customary treatment for acute and chronic PJI. However, there had been no unified standard for irrigation during surgery for PJI in the past, and its effectiveness is dubious. In their study, Wu et al. created a new irrigation protocol to improve the infection control rate and diminish the postoperative recurrence rate of individuals with PJI [8]. Wu et al. performed a single-institution retrospective review with a total of 56 individuals who underwent revision total hip or knee arthroplasties due to PJI. Conventional irrigation (CI) was utilized in 32 individuals, and standard operating procedure of irrigation (SOPI) was utilized in 24. The CI protocol carried out an empirical irrigation after debridement, which was quite random. The SOPI protocol clearly stipulates the soaking concentration and time of hydrogen peroxide and povidone-iodine. The irrigation was performed three times, and tissue samples were taken from multiple parts prior to and after irrigation, which were sent for microbial culture. The important statistical indicators were the rate of positive microbiological culture and postoperative recurrence rate with a mean follow-up of 24 months. The drainage volume was lower in the SOPI cohort than in the CI cohort on postoperative days 3 and 7. Additionally, the percentage of positive microbiological cultures after the third irrigation was lower than that before and after the first irrigation. The most frequent causative organism was *Staphylococcus aureus*, which was detected in 25% and 12.5% of the SOPI and CI cohorts, respectively. The failure rate at the final follow-up was 8.3% and 31.3% for the SOPI and CI cohorts, respectively. Compared with the traditional CI method, SOPI almost completely removed microorganisms. Therefore, SOPI has the potential to become a standardized irrigation process worthy of promotion, effectively diminishing the postoperative recurrence rate of individuals with PJI [8].

1.8 Outcomes of Culture-Negative or Culture-Positive PJIs

Lai et al. (2024) performed a systematic review and meta-analysis on PJIs to compare results and antibiotic side effects in culture-negative or culture-positive PJIs and evaluate treatment options for culture-negative PJIs [9]. The two types of PJIs did not differ substantially in infection control rates (culture-negative PJI 79% vs. culture-positive PJI 77%), either after all types of surgical treatment or after two-stage revision arthroplasty, single-stage revision arthroplasty, or DAIR. Similarly, Lai et al. did not find differences in periprosthetic or spacer fracture and hip joint or spacer dislocation. For culture-negative PJIs, the infection control rate was 85% after two-stage revision arthroplasty, 91% after single-stage revision arthroplasty, and 70% after DAIR. The study showed higher incidence of antibiotic side effects for culture-negative PJIs. The clinical results of one-stage revision and two-stage revision were comparable. Therefore, both of them can be considered in surgical treatment for culture-negative PJIs [9].

1.9 PJI in Patients with Multiple Joint Arthroplasties

According to Mansour et al. (2024), the number of TJAs performed in the United States is rising every year. Owing to the aging population and excellent long-run prosthesis survival, 45% of individuals who experience TJA will receive two or more joint arthroplasties during their lifetimes. PJI is among the most frequent complications after TJA. Assessment and management of PJI in individuals with multiple TJAs is challenging, and no consensus exists for the optimal treatment. Multiple PJI can occur simultaneously (synchronous) or be separated by extended time (metachronous). Patient risk factors for both scenarios have been published and might guide assessment and long-run treatment. Whether to carry out joint aspiration for asymptomatic prostheses in the presence of suspected PJI in individuals with multiple TJAs is controversial. Moreover, no consensus exists regarding whether individuals who have multiple TJAs and develop PJI in a single joint should be considered for prolonged antibiotic prophylaxis to diminish the risk of future infections. Finally, the optimal treatment of synchronous joint infections, whether by DAIR, one-stage, or two-stage revision, has not been determined [10].

1.10 Increased Risk of PJI After Traumatic Injury in Joint Revision Patients

In 2024, Li et al. stated that PJI is a serious adverse event after TJA. Although some risk factors of PJI were well studied, the relationship between trauma and PJI remained unknown in revision individuals [11]. In the study of Li et al, a total of 71 individuals with trauma history prior to revisions (trauma group) were propensity score matched (PSM) at a 1:5 ratio with a control group of revision individuals without a history of trauma. Then, the cumulative incidence rate of PJI within 3 years after operation between the two cohorts was compared. The secondary endpoints were aseptic revisions within 3 postoperative years, complications up to 30 postoperative days, and readmission up to 90 days. During a minimum 3-year follow-up, survival was comparatively analyzed between the trauma group and the control group. The cumulative incidence of PJI was 41% in individuals with trauma history against 27% in the controls. Correspondingly, the cumulative incidence of aseptic re-revisions was 13% in individuals with trauma history compared with 5% in the control group (Fig. 1.1). Cox regression showed that trauma history was a risk factor of PJI and aseptic re-revisions. The study of Li et al. showed that revision individuals with trauma history carried a higher risk of PJI compared to those without trauma history. Furthermore, after revisions, the trauma individuals were still at higher risk for management failure due to PJI, periprosthetic joint fracture, and mechanical complications. Figure 1.2 shows the Trojan Horse hypothesis of trauma-associated PJI (schematic representation of the mechanisms by which pathogens from other sites cause PJI) [11].

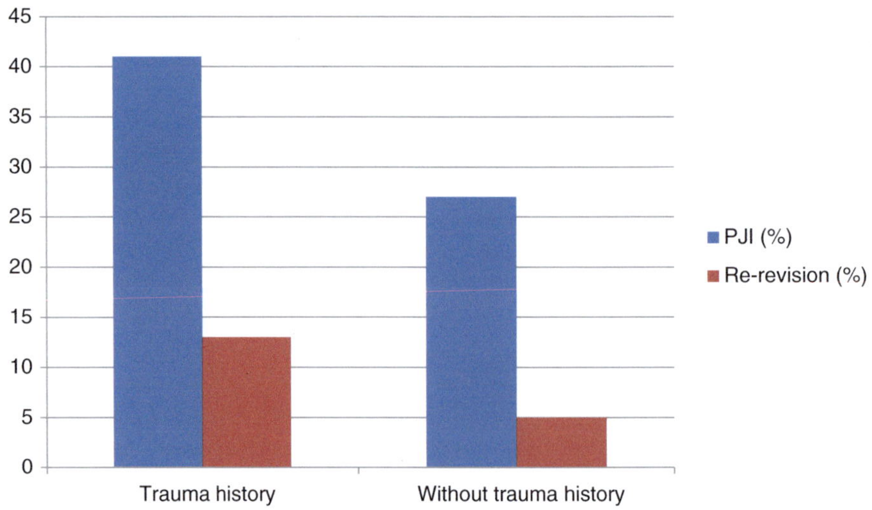

Fig. 1.1 Individuals with trauma history versus individuals without trauma history: cumulative incidence of periprosthetic joint infection (PJI): 41% vs. 27%; cumulative incidence of aseptic re-revision: 13% vs. 5%

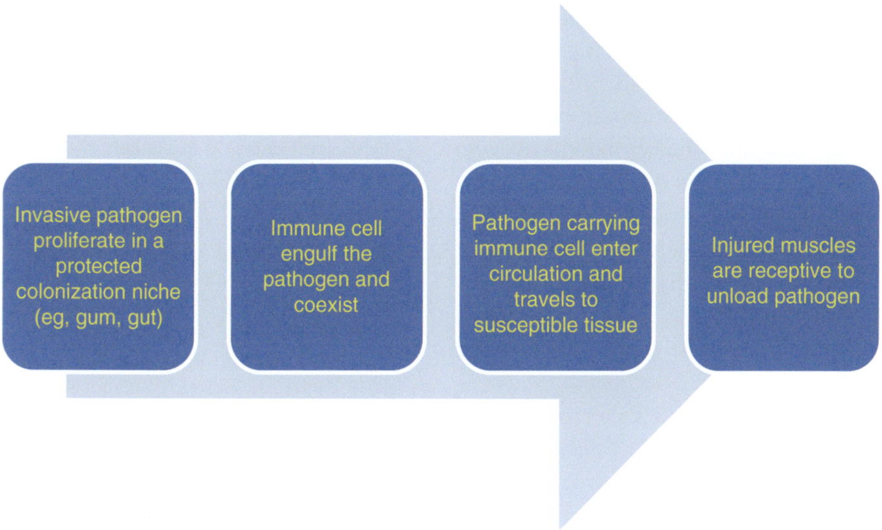

Fig. 1.2 Trojan Horse hypothesis of trauma-associated periprosthetic joint infection (PJI). Schematic representation of the mechanisms by which pathogens from other sites cause PJI

1.11 Conclusions

The review of the current relevant data concerning PJI has led to the following conclusions:

1. PJI is a serious adverse event of TJA. Even with contemporary treatments, failure rates are unacceptably elevated with a 5-year mortality rate of 26%.
2. Comprehending the mechanisms by which bacteria can undermine the immune system might reveal novel strategies to better prepare our own immune system to fight against PJI. Moreover, preoperative immune system evaluation and screening for dysregulation might help in creating preventative methods to reduce PJI prevalence.
3. If dysbiosis is shown to be a substantial contributor, developing therapies for dysbiosis might represent a new frontier in the control of PJIs.
4. PJIs caused by Gram-negative bacteria were found more frequently in individuals with hepatitis than in the control group. Besides, the CRP rise was less in individuals with hepatitis compared to PJI cases in the control group. Therefore, patient-specific assessment is needed in cases of PJI in patient groups with coexisting hepatitis.
5. The PJI-TNM classification system can be applied with significant inter- and intraobserver reliability.
6. While further research is needed to formulate a precise protocol for the changing of gloves during TJA, it might be beneficial to carry out a thorough irrigation of the joint and change of the gloves immediately following arthrotomy.
7. Compared with the traditional CI method, SOPI almost completely removed microorganisms. Therefore, SOPI has the potential to become a standardized irrigation process worthy of promotion, effectively diminishing the postoperative recurrence rate of individuals with PJI.
8. A systematic review and meta-analysis on PJIs compared results and antibiotic side effects in culture-negative or culture-positive PJIs and evaluated treatment options for culture-negative PJIs. The two types of PJIs did not differ substantially in infection control rates (culture-negative PJI 79% vs. culture-positive PJI 77%), either after all types of surgical treatment or after two-stage revision arthroplasty, single-stage revision arthroplasty, or DAIR.

9. Whether to carry out joint aspiration for asymptomatic prosthesis in the presence of suspected PJI in individuals with multiple TJAs is controversial. Moreover, no consensus exists regarding whether individuals who have multiple TJAs and develop PJI in a single joint should be considered for prolonged antibiotic prophylaxis to diminish the risk of future infections. Finally, the optimal treatment of synchronous joint infections, whether by DAIR, one-stage, or two-stage revision, has not been determined.
10. Trauma history is a risk factor of PJI and aseptic re-revisions.

References

1. Piuzzi NS, Klika AK, Lu Q, Higuera-Rueda CA, Stappenbeck T, Visperas A. Periprosthetic joint infection and immunity: current understanding of host-microbe interplay. J Orthop Res. 2024;42(1):7–20. https://doi.org/10.1002/jor.25723.
2. Ayoade F, Li DD, Mabrouk A, Todd JR. Periprosthetic joint infection. In: StatPearls [Internet]. Treasure Island: StatPearls Publishing; 2024.
3. Longo UG, Lalli A, Bandini B, Angeletti S, Lustig S, Budhiparama NC. The influence of gut microbiome on periprosthetic joint infections: state of the art. J ISAKOS. 2024;9(3):353–61. https://doi.org/10.1016/j.jisako.2024.01.011.
4. DeGruttola AK, Low D, Mizoguchi A, Mizoguchi E. Current understanding of dysbiosis in disease in human and animal models. Inflamm Bowel Dis. 2016;22(5):1137–50. https://doi.org/10.1097/MIB.0000000000000750.
5. Akkaya M, Akcaalan S, Perrone FL, Sandiford N, Gehrke T, Citak M. Organism profile and C-reactive protein (CRP) response are different in periprosthetic joint infection in patients with hepatitis. Arch Orthop Trauma Surg. 2024;144(1):341–6. https://doi.org/10.1007/s00402-023-05059-7.
6. Baertl S, Rupp M, Kerschbaum M, Morgenstern M, Baumann F, Pfeifer C, et al. The PJI-TNM classification for periprosthetic joint infections. Bone Joint Res. 2024;13(1):19–27. https://doi.org/10.1302/2046-3758.131.BJR-2023-0012.R2.
7. Ludwick L, Chisari E, Ong C, Krueger C, Courtney PM, Parvizi J. Gloves contamination during revision surgery for periprosthetic joint infection. J Arthroplasty. 2024;39(2):480–2. https://doi.org/10.1016/j.arth.2023.07.007.
8. Wu X, Chen W, Rong R, Pan B, Hu X, Zheng L, et al. Application of the new irrigation protocol to reduce recurrence rate in the management of periprosthetic joint infection. Orthop Surg. 2024;16(3):577–84. https://doi.org/10.1111/os.13948.
9. Lai YH, Xu H, Li XY, Zhao WX, Lv N, Zhou ZK. Outcomes of culture-negative or -positive periprosthetic joint infections: a systematic review and meta-analysis. Jt Dis Relat Surg. 2024;35(1):231–41. https://doi.org/10.52312/jdrs.2023.1437.
10. Mansour E, Clarke HD, Spangehl MJ, Bingham JS. Periprosthetic infection in patients with multiple joint arthroplasties. J Am Acad Orthop Surg. 2024;32(3):e106–14. https://doi.org/10.5435/JAAOS-D-23-00120.
11. Li H, Zheng Q, Niu E, Xu J, Chai W, Xu C, et al. Increased risk of periprosthetic joint infection after traumatic injury in joint revision patients. Arthroplasty. 2024;6(1):8. https://doi.org/10.1186/s42836-024-00235-5.

Diagnosis of Periprosthetic Joint Infection

2

E. Carlos Rodríguez-Merchán,
Hortensia De la Corte-Rodríguez,
and Juan M. Román-Belmonte

2.1 Introduction

Periprosthetic joint infection (PJI) is an unusual yet disastrous complication following total joint arthroplasty (TJA) [1]. TJA aims to reestablish patients' quality of life by alleviating pain and improving joint function. While PJI affects a small percentage of individuals, with an estimated incidence of 1–9% after primary TJA, this postoperative complication requires a long hospitalization, lengthy antibiotic treatment, and additional surgery [2]. Technological and implant design breakthroughs have helped diminish the frequency of aseptic TJA failure, but PJI remains a clinically significant problem with high patient morbidity [3].

PJI can be difficult to diagnose. Investigations have demonstrated that many infections are undiagnosed, possibly due to poor diagnostic workup and the existence of culture-negative infection. PJI diagnosis needs a methodical plan and a standardized set of criteria [4]. Early and accurate diagnosis of PJI is crucial to maximizing the chances of successful management. However, we are yet to determine a single "gold standard" test for the diagnosis of PJI. Consequently, the diagnosis of PJI is frequently challenging [1].

Establishing the correct diagnosis of PJI is paramount to avert unnecessary treatments in individuals with aseptic failure. Besides, the PJI diagnosis could not entirely rely upon clinical findings due to the heterogeneity in host factors (e.g., age and comorbidities), variability in infection stage, differences in anatomical location of the implicated joint, and differences in pathogenicity/virulence of the causative organisms, which may confound the clinical picture. Moreover, intraoperative contamination is deemed to be the principal culprit that can lead to early or delayed infection, with the hematogenous spread being the most frequent manner. On the other hand, early and hematogenous infections frequently begin unexpectedly, while chronic late infections are caused by less virulent bacteria and tend to exhibit a more quiescent mode [2].

Misinterpreting PJI as aseptic mechanical loosening frequently leads to unsatisfactory revision TJA, persistent infection, and poor long-term outcomes [3]. The purpose of this chapter is to review the most relevant recent information on the diagnosis of PJI.

E. C. Rodríguez-Merchán (✉)
Department of Orthopedic Surgery, Hospital Universitario La Paz, Madrid, Madrid, Spain

H. De la Corte-Rodríguez
Department of Physical and Rehabilitation Medicine, Hospital Universitario La Paz, Madrid, Spain

J. M. Román-Belmonte
Department of Physical and Rehabilitation Medicine, Hospital Universitario Cruz Roja San José y Santa Adela, Madrid, Spain

E. C. Rodríguez-Merchán (ed.), *Advances in Periprosthetic Joint Infection*,
https://doi.org/10.1007/978-3-032-02945-4_2

2.2 The New EBJIS Definition of PJI

The new European Bone and Joint Infection Society (EBJIS) definition has some advantages in clinical practice [4]. It recognizes more clinically significant infections and precisely establishes those with the highest risk of management failure. It diminishes the number of individuals with dubious diagnoses. Therefore, the EBJIS classification of PJIs might offer a better comprehension of management results and risk factors for failure.

2.3 Pathology and Laboratory Medicine

According to Mazzella et al. (2024), pathologists hold an essential role in assisting with PJI diagnosis, maintaining laboratory test quality, and interpreting test results. Collaboration between clinicians and pathologists is crucial to render optimal patient care and diminish the burden of PJI. A "scoring-based" definition of PJI has been reported by Mazzella et al. [3].

2.4 Current Relevance of Biomarkers

According to Tripathi et al. (2023), novel biomarkers like calprotectin, lipocalcin, monocyte to lymphocyte ratio, neutrophil to lymphocyte ratio, platelet to lymphocyte ratio (PLR), and platelet count to mean platelet volume ratio (PC/mPV) have shown potential as diagnostic biomarkers for PJI. Precise preoperative diagnosis of PJI presents a challenge for clinicians, especially in cases of low-virulence organisms. The serum parameters, in general, have insufficient accuracy for diagnosing PJI due to false positivity in individuals with systemic inflammatory conditions and autoimmune illnesses. Lower sensitivities can be explained by an improper immune response in individuals with encapsulated joint infection (forming biofilms) and those being administered systemic antibiotics [5].

Currently, serum CRP, interleukin 6 (IL-6), and fibrinogen appear to perform best in terms of accuracy among biomarkers. Although the accuracy is limited, Tripathi et al. recommend these three parameters in the preoperative diagnosis of PJI as suggestive criteria. However, results should be interpreted with caution in the clinical practice. On the other hand, synovial biomarkers are much more specific and sensitive than their serum counterparts. Alpha defensin and leukocyte esterase have demonstrated their accuracy in many studies in establishing the presence of infection. Tripathi et al. stated that C-reactive protein (CRP), erythrocyte sedimentation rate (ESR), and synovial CRP were all good predictors of PJI, and that alpha defensin and leukocyte esterase were also useful diagnostic tests with good applicability [5]. The most important serum and synovial biomarkers used in the diagnosis of PJI are summarized in Table 2.1 [1].

2.4.1 Synovial Biomarkers

In 2023, Diniz et al. evaluated the utility of different simple synovial biomarkers in the diagnosis of PJI as defined by the EBJIS. They retrospectively identified all individuals experiencing revision hip or knee arthroplasty from 2013 to 2019 on a prospectively maintained database [6]. Only individuals with a minimum required infection diagnostic workup were included in the study. Individuals with comorbidities that might affect the accuracy of synovial biomarkers were excluded. Receiver operating characteristic (ROC) curves were used to evaluate the diagnostic utility of synovial fluid white blood cell (WBC) count, polymorphonuclear leukocyte percentage (PMN%), CRP, adenosine deaminase (ADA), and alpha-2-microglobulin (A2M). In total, 102 individuals met the inclusion criteria. Of these, 58 were classified as infection unlikely, 8 as infection likely, and 36 as infection confirmed. Synovial WBC count demonstrated the best utility for the diagnosis of PJI, followed by PMN%, synovial CRP, ADA, and A2M. They encountered added value in the combined interpretation of different biomarkers. They calcu-

Table 2.1 European Bone and Joint Infection Society (EBJIS) criteria for the diagnosis of clinically suspected prosthetic joint infection (PJI)

	Infection unlikely (all findings negative)	Infection likely (two positive findings)[a]	Infection confirmed (any positive finding)
Clinical and blood workup			
Clinical features	Clear alternative reason for implant dysfunction (e.g., fracture, implant breakage, malposition, tumor)	(1) Radiological signs of loosening within the first 5 years after implantation (2) Previous wound healing problems (3) History of recent fever or bacteremia (4) Purulence around the prosthesis[b]	Sinus tract with evidence of communication to the joint or visualization of the prosthesis
C-reactive protein (CRP)		>10 mg/L (1 mg/dL)[c]	
Synovial fluid cytological analysis[d]			
Leukocyte count (cells/μL)[c]	< / = 1,500	>1,500	>3,000
Polymorphonuclear (PMN) leukocytes (%)[c]	< /= 65%	>65%	>80%
Synovial fluid biomarkers			
Alpha-defensin[e]			Positive immunoassay or lateral-flow assay[e]
Microbiology[f]			
Aspiration fluid		Positive culture	
Intraoperative (fluid and tissue)	All cultures negative	Single positive culture[g]	>2 positive samples with the same microorganism
Sonication (Colony-forming units—CFU/mL)[h]	No growth	>1 CFU/mL or any organism[g]	>50 CFU/mL of any organism
Histology[c]			
High-power field - HPF (400× magnification)	Negative	Presence of >5 neutrophils in a single HPF	Presence of >/= 5 neutrophils in >/= 5 HPF
			Presence of visible microorganisms
Others			
Nuclear imaging	Negative 3-phase isotope bone scan[c]	Positive white blood cell count (WBC) scintigraphy[i]	

[a]Infection is only likely if there is a positive clinical feature or raised serum CRP together with another positive test (synovial fluid, microbiology, histology, or nuclear imaging)

[b]Except in adverse local tissue reaction (ALTR) and crystal arthropathy cases

[c]Should be interpreted with caution when other possible causes of inflammation are present: gout or other crystal arthropathy, metallosis, active inflammatory joint disease (e.g., rheumatoid arthritis), periprosthetic fracture, or the early postoperative period

[d]These values are valid for hips and knee PJI. Parameters are only valid when clear fluid is obtained and no lavage has been performed. Volume for the analysis should be >250 L, ideally 1 mL, collected in an EDTA-containing tube and analyzed in <1 h, preferentially using automated techniques. For viscous samples, pretreatment with hyaluronidase improves the accuracy of optical or automated techniques. In case of bloody samples, the adjusted synovial WBC = synovial WBC observed – [WBC blood/RBC (red blood cells) blood × RBC synovial fluid] should be used

[e]Not valid in cases of adverse local tissue reaction (ALTR), hematomas, or acute inflammatory arthritis or gout

[f]If antibiotic treatment has been given (not simple prophylaxis), the results of microbiological analysis may be compromised. In these cases, molecular techniques may have a place

[g]Interpretation of single positive culture (or <50 CFU/mL in sonication fluid) must be cautious and taken together with other evidence. If a preoperative aspiration identified the same microorganism, they should be considered as two positive confirmatory samples. Uncommon contaminants or virulent organisms (e.g., *S. aureus* or Gram-negative rods) are more likely to represent infection than common contaminants (such as coagulase-negative staphylococci, micrococci, or *Cutibacterium acnes*)

[h]If centrifugation is applied, then the suggested cutoff is 200 CFU/mL to confirm infection. If other variations to the protocol are used, the published cut-offs for each protocol must be applied

[i]WBC scintigraphy is regarded as positive if the uptake is increased at the 20-h scan, compared to the earlier scans (especially when combined with complementary bone marrow scan)

lated high sensitivity and negative predictive value if at least two of them were negative and high specificity and positive predictive value if at least two were elevated [6].

2.5 Platelet to Volume Ratio

According to Denyer et al. (2023), recent studies have suggested utilizing blood cell ratios, such as platelet to volume ratio (PVR) and PLR, to improve diagnostic accuracy of chronic PJI [7]. A retrospective review was performed to evaluate the accuracy of different marker combinations for diagnosing chronic PJI. A total of 573 individuals were included in the study, of which 124 had total knee arthroplasties (TKAs) and 122 had total hip arthroplasties (THAs) had a diagnosis of chronic PJI. Complete blood count and synovial fluid analysis were collected. The area under the curve (AUC), sensitivity, specificity, and positive and negative predictive values were estimated. The results of the analysis demonstrated that the combination of ESR, CRP, synovial WBC count, PMN%, and PVR had the highest AUC of 0.99 for knees, with sensitivity of 98% and specificity of 100%. Similarly, for hips, this combination had an AUC of 0.98, sensitivity of 96%, and specificity of 100% (Fig. 2.1). Denyer et al. supported the utilization of PVR estimated from readily available complete blood counts, combined with established markers, to improve the accuracy in diagnosing chronic PJI in both TKAs and THAs [7].

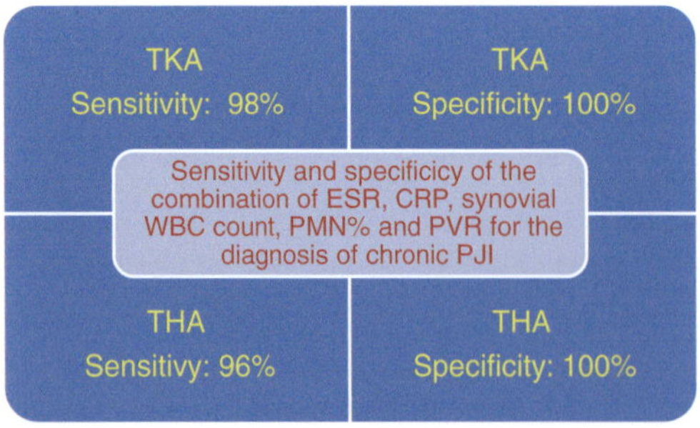

Fig. 2.1 Sensitivity and specificity of the combination of erythrocyte sedimentation rate (ESR), C-reactive protein (CRP), synovial white blood cell (WBC) count, polymorphonuclear leukocyte percentage (PMN%), and platelet volume ratio (PVR) for the diagnosis of chronic periprosthetic joint infection (PJI) of total knee arthroplasty (TKA) and total hip arthroplasty (THA)

2.6 The Absolute Synovial Polymorphonuclear Neutrophil Cell Count

In a study with level 3 evidence, Karlidag et al. (2023) hypothesized that synovial absolute neutrophil count (ANC) would improve the diagnostic accuracy of chronic PJI of TKA and THA [8]. The study included 260 individuals (134 men and 126 women, mean age of 70 years [range, 26 to 89]) who experienced aspiration during preoperative workup. Of these, 109 individuals (41.9%) were diagnosed with chronic PJI (50 TKAs, 59 THAs), and 151 individuals (58.1%) were diagnosed as aseptic (94 TKAs, 57 THAs). Data obtained from all individuals included age, sex, procedure type (THA or TKA), operation side, synovial WBC (cells/μL), synovial PMN%, and synovial alpha defensin immunoassay value at the admission were retrieved from the electronic medical record. The estimated optimal threshold for synovial ANC of 1415.5 cells/μL was associated with an AUC of 0.930 for chronic knee PJI diagnosis. The estimated optimal threshold for synovial ANC of 2247 cells/μL was associated with an AUC of 0.905 for chronic hip PJI diagnosis. This study showed that the synovial ANC served as a valuable marker in the diagnosis of PJI. This highly effective and efficient approach should be used for obtaining further information through standard tests, thereby ruling out the possibility of PJI [8].

2.7 Platelet-Related Markers

In 2024, Song et al. evaluated the diagnostic values of serum platelet count (PC), mean platelet volume ratio (MPV), PVR, PLR, platelet to neutrophil ratio (PNR), PC/albumin-globulin ratio (PC/AGR), and PC/CRP in the diagnosis of PJI. Medical records from 158 individuals who had undergone hip or knee revisions were retrospectively analyzed [9]. Of these, 79 cases were diagnosed with PJI and 79 with aseptic loosening (AL). PJI was defined using the Musculoskeletal Infection Society (MSIS) criteria [10] (Table 2.2). The plasma levels of CRP, ESR, PC, MPV, PVR, PLR, PNR, PC/AGR, and PC/CRP in the two cohorts were recorded and analyzed. In addition, tests were performed according to different joint types. The receiver operating characteristic curve was utilized to estimate the sensitivity and specificity of each indicator. The diagnostic value for each indicator was estimated according to the AUC. The PC, PVR, PLR, and PC/AGR levels in the PJI cohort were substantially higher than in the AL cohort, while PC/CRP levels were substantially lower. The AUC for PC/CRP and PC/AGR was 0.804 and 0.802, respectively, which were slightly lower than that of CRP (0.826) and ESR (0.846). ROC analysis for PC/CRP and PC/AGR showed cut-off values of 37.80 and 160.63, respectively, which yielded sensitivities of 73.42% and 84.81% and specificities of 75.95% and 65.82% for PJI. The AUCs of PLR and PC were 0.738 and 0.702. The AUC values for PVR, PNR, and MPV were 0.672, 0.553, and 0.544, respectively. The results of this study suggested that PC, PLR, PC/CRP, and PC/AGR values did not offer substantial advantages over ESR or CRP values when used for the diagnosis of PJI. Besides, PVR, PNR, and MPV were not reliable in the diagnosis of PJI [9].

Table 2.2 A "scoring-based" definition of periprosthetic joint infection (PJI)

Major criteria (at least one of the following)		**Decision**
Two positive cultures of the same organism		Infected
Sinus tract with evidence of communication to the joint		Infected
Preoperative diagnosis		
Minor criteria	**Score**	**Decision**
Elevated serum CRP >1 mg/dL or D-dimer >860 ng/mL	2	>6 infected
Serum ESR >30 mm/h	1	
Synovial WBC count >3000 cells/μL or leukocyte esterase ++	3	
Synovial alpha-defensin +	3	2–5 possibly infected
Synovial PMN% >80%	2	
Synovial CRP >6.9 mg/L	1	0–1 not infected
Intraoperative diagnosis		
Inconclusive preoperative score or dry tap	**Score**	**Decision**
Preoperative score		
Positive histology[a]	3	>6 infected
Positive purulence	3	4–5 inconclusive
Single positive culture	2	≤3 not Infected

CRP C-reactive protein, *ESR* erythrocyte sedimentation rate, *WBC* white blood cell count, *PMN%* polymorphonuclear leukocyte percentage

[a]5 or more neutrophils in each of 5 or more high power fields (HPF)

2.8 The Albumin to Globulin Ratio

In 2024, Dong et al. assessed the value of AGR and globulin (GLB) for diagnosing PJI. A total of 182 individuals experiencing revision after arthroplasty were included and divided into 2 cohorts; 61 in the knee cohort (PJI: 38; non-PJI: 23) and 121 in the hip cohort (PJI: 26; non-PJI: 95) [11]. They utilized receiver operating characteristic curves to determine the diagnostic value of AGR, GLB, and inflammatory markers (ESR and CRP). The receiver operating characteristic curves showed that the AUCs of AGR, GLB, ESR, and CRP in the knee cohort were 0.940, 0.928, 0.867, and 0.848, respectively, and they were 0.855, 0.831, 0.886, and 0.912 in the hip cohort. The optimal predictive cut-off values for AGR in knee and hip cohorts were 1.375 and 1.295, respectively. The sensitivity and specificity of AGR, respectively, were 94.7% and 87% (knee cohort) and 84.6% and 75.8% (hip cohort) for diagnosing PJI. The sensitivity of "AGR or ESR" and specificity of "AGR and GLB" in the knee cohort were 99.6% and 98.9%, respectively. Therefore, for knee or hip cohorts, AGR showed good value for the diagnosis of PJI, comparable with ESR and CRP. The AGR and GLB, together with CRP and ESR, should be utilized as the preferred indicators for diagnosing PJI. The "AGR or ESR" and "AGR and GLB" in the knee cohort had an excellent diagnostic value in sensitivity and specificity, respectively [11].

2.9 Synovial Fluid C-Reactive Protein

Maimidian et al. (2024) conducted a formal single clinical laboratory validation to establish the optimal clinical decision limit of synovial fluid (SF)-CRP (SF-CRP) for the diagnosis of PJI. A retrospective analysis of prospectively collected data was carried out utilizing ROC and AUC analyses. Synovial fluid samples from THAs and TKAs, received from over 2600 institutions, underwent clinical testing for PJI at a single clinical laboratory (CD Laboratories, Zimmer Biomet, Towson, MD). The optimal CRP cutoff (4.45 mg/L) for PJI, which yielded a sensitivity of 86.1% and a specificity of 87.1%, was specific to the assay methodology and laboratory performing the assay. Miamidian et al. proposed that an SF-CRP test with a laboratory-validated optimal clinical decision limit for PJI might be preferable, in a clinical diagnostic setting, to serum CRP tests that do not have laboratory-validated clinical decision limits for PJI [12].

2.10 Drain Fluid Cultures

In 2024, Ritcher et al. evaluated the diagnostic performance of drain fluid cultures in diagnosing infection persistence [13]. Drain samples were taken after every revision surgery for microbiological testing. Afterward, the results were assigned to the infection status according to the diagnostic criteria of the MSIS definition of PJI [10]. A total of 1084 revision surgeries in 183 individuals were included, resulting in a total sample size of 1552 drain fluid cultures. Overall sensitivity was 36%, specificity was 90.7%, and ROC-AUC was 0.63. Due to a high specificity and a low sensitivity, drain fluid cultures can rule in but cannot rule out infection persistence in PJI [13].

2.11 Next-Generation Sequencing (NGS)

In a systematic review and meta-analysis with level 4 evidence published in 2024, Su et al. stated that next-generation sequencing (NGS) is becoming a promising diagnostic tool for PJI, but its diagnostic value for PJI remains dubious. In their study, they assessed the diagnostic value of NGS compared to culture [14]. The pooled sensitivity, specificity, and diagnostic odds ratio of NGS were 87%, 94%, and 111, respectively. However, the pooled sensitivity, specificity, and diagnostic odds ratio of culture were 63%, 98%, and 93, respectively. The summary receiver operating characteristic (SROC) curve for NGS and culture showed that the areas under the curve (AUCs) were 0.96 and 0.82, respectively (Table 2.3). NGS had higher sensitivity and diagnostic accuracy but slightly lower specificity than culture. Su et al. suggested that NGS might have the potential to be a new tool for the diagnosis of PJI [14].

In 2024, Mahnic et al. compared amplicon metagenomic sequencing (16S AS) with traditional culture techniques for enhanced clinical decision-making in PJI [15]. They analyzed sonicate fluid from 27 individuals experiencing revision arthroplasty utilizing both methods, emphasizing the distinction between contami-

Table 2.3 Diagnosing periprosthetic joint infection (PJI)

Serum and plasma markers	Synovial markers
ESR and CRP	WBC count and PMN%
WBC	CRP
Percentage of neutrophils (%N)	Alpha defensin
Neutrophils to lymphocytes ratio (NLR)	Leukocyte esterase
Platelet count to mean platelet volume	IL-6
PC/mPV ratio	Calprotectin
Procalcitonin	
D-dimer	
Fibrinogen	
IL-6	
Albumin/globulin ratio	

From Ref. [1]

ESR erythrocyte sedimentation rate, *CRP* C-reactive protein, *WBC* white blood cell count, *PC/mPV* platelet count to mean platelet volume ratio, *IL-6* interleukin 6, *PMN%* polymorphonuclear leukocyte percentage

Table 2.4 Musculoskeletal Infection Society (MSIS) criteria for diagnosis of periprosthetic joint infection (PJI)

Major criteria[a]	Minor criteria[b]
Communicating sinus tract	Elevated ESR/CRP
Isolated organism in two different tissue/ fluid cultures	Elevated synovial leukocyte count
	Elevated synovial PMN%
	Purulent material
	Isolated organism in one tissue/fluid culture
	>5 neutrophils per HPF in 5 HPF histologic tissue analysis × 400 magnification

CRP C-reactive protein, *ESR* erythrocyte sedimentation rate, *HPF* high-power field, *PMN%* polymorphonuclear neutrophil percentage
[a]1 criterion is needed to establish diagnosis of PJI
[b]4 out of 6 minor criteria are needed to establish diagnosis of PJI

nants and true positives. Their findings showed moderate agreement between the two methods. The sensitivity of 16S AS compared to culture was 81%. Sequencing revealed greater microbial diversity, including anaerobic genera like *Anaerococcus* and *Citrobacter*. Interestingly, several culture-negative PJI samples showed diverse bacteria via 16S AS. The conclusion was that in spite of rigorous controls and algorithms to eliminate contaminants, confirming bacteria presence with 16S AS remained a challenge. This indicated the limitations of NGS as a clinical diagnostic tool [15] (Table 2.4).

Hao et al. (2024) performed a prospective trial among individuals who experienced knee or hip surgery due to PJI to compare the positivity rate of culture and metagenomic next-generation sequencing (mNGS) between cases with and without previous antimicrobial therapy, and the positivity rates between cases with different antimicrobial-free intervals [16]. Among 131 included PJIs, 91 (69.5%) had positive cultures and 115 (87.8%) had positive mNGS results. There was no substantial difference in the positivity rate of deep-tissue culture and synovial fluid mNGS between cases with and without previous antimicrobial therapy. The positivity rate of synovial fluid culture was higher in cases with previous antimicrobial therapy. The positivity rates of mNGS in synovial fluid diminished as the antimicrobial-free interval ranged from 4 to 14 days to 0 to 3 days. Therefore, mNGS was more advantageous than culture with a higher pathogen detection rate. However, this study suggested that antimicrobial drugs might need to be discontinued more than 3 days before sampling to further increase the positivity rate of mNGS for PJIs [16].

In 2024, Tan et al. evaluated the diagnostic value of mNGS across synovial fluid, prosthetic sonicate fluid, and periprosthetic tissues among individuals with PJI, intending to optimize specimen selection for mNGS in these individuals [17]. They analyzed 43 individuals diagnosed as PJI based on the MSIS criteria. Preoperative or intraoperative synovial fluid, periprosthetic tissues, and prosthetic sonicate fluid were collected, each divided into two portions for mNGS and culture. Comparative analyses were performed between the microbiological results and diagnostic efficacy derived from mNGS and culture tests. Moreover, the variability in mNGS diagnostic efficacy for PJI across different specimen types was evaluated. The sensitivity and specificity of mNGS diagnosis were 93% and 94.4% for all types of PJI specimens; the sensitivity and specificity of culture diagnosis were 72.1% and 100%, respectively. The diagnostic sensitivity of mNGS was substantially higher than that of culture, with no statistically significant difference in specificity. The sensitivity of the synovial fluid was 83.7% and the specificity was 94.4%; the sensitivity of the prosthetic sonicate fluid was 90.7% and the specificity was 94.4%; and the sensitivity of the periprosthetic tissue was 81.4% and the specificity was 100%. Remarkably, the mNGS of prosthetic sonicate fluid displayed a superior pathogen detection rate compared to other specimen types. It was concluded that NGS can function as an accurate diagnostic tool for identifying pathogens in PJI individuals utilizing three types of specimens. Due to its superior capacity in pathogen identification, prosthetic sonicate fluid can replace synovial fluid and periprosthetic tissue as the optimal sample choice for NGS [17] (Table 2.5).

Table 2.5 Periprosthetic joint infection (PJI): diagnostic value of next-generation sequencing (NGS) compared to culture

Parameter	NGS	Culture
Sensitivity	87%	63%
Specificity	94%	98%
Diagnostic odds ratio	111	93
Area under the curve (AUC)	0.96	0.92

In 2024, Shi et al. evaluated the application of mNGS technology to identify pathogens in PJI [18]. A retrospective analysis was performed on 65 individuals suspected of having PJI. The individuals were categorized into PJI (46 individuals) and non-PJI (19 individuals) cohorts based on the 2018 International Consensus Meeting criteria. Clinical information was collected, and both conventional bacterial culture and mNGS were carried out. The diagnostic performance of the two methods was compared and analyzed. mNGS showed a sensitivity of 89.13%, a specificity of 94.74%, a positive predictive value of 97.62%, a negative predictive value of 78.26%, and an overall diagnostic accuracy of 90.77%. Compared to microbial culture, mNGS showed superior diagnostic sensitivity while maintaining similar specificity. A total of 48 pathogens were successfully identified utilizing mNGS, with coagulase-negative staphylococci, streptococci, *Staphylococcus aureus*, and *Cutibacterium acnes* being the most frequent infectious agents. Notably, mNGS was utilized to identify 17 potential pathogens in 14 culture-negative PJI samples, highlighting its capacity to detect rare infectious agents, including *C. acnes* ($N = 5$), *Granulicatella adiacens* ($N = 1$), *Mycobacterium tuberculosis* complex ($N = 1$), and *Coxiella burnetii* ($N = 1$), among others, which are not detectable by routine culture methods. However, mNGS failed to detect the pathogen in four culture-positive PJI individuals, indicating its limitations. Among the 46 PJI individuals, 27 had positive culture and mNGS results. The results of mNGS were concordant with those of culture at the genus level in 6 individuals with PJI and at the species level in 18 individuals. Moreover, the study revealed a substantially greater proportion of *S. aureus* in the sinus tract cohort (45.45%) than in the non-sinus tract cohort (14.29%), indicating the association of this pathogen with sinus formation in PJI. Besides, there was no substantial difference in the occurrence of polymicrobial infections between the sinus tract cohort (27.27%) and the non-sinus tract cohort (33.33%). It was concluded that mNGS can serve as a valuable screening tool in addition to traditional culture methods to improve diagnostic accuracy through optimized culture strategies [18].

2.12 Conclusions

PJI can be difficult to diagnose. Early and accurate diagnosis of PJI is crucial to maximizing the chances of successful management. The new EBJIS definition has some advantages in clinical practice. It recognizes more clinically significant infections and precisely establishes those with the highest risk of management failure. It diminishes the number of individuals with dubious diagnoses.

The combination of ESR, CRP, synovial WBC count, and PMN% with PVR had the highest AUC of 0.99 for knees, with sensitivity of 98% and specificity of 100%. Similarly, for hips, this combination had an AUC of 0.98, sensitivity of 96%, and specificity of 100%. Drain fluid cultures can rule in but cannot rule out infection persistence in PJI.

NGS can function as an accurate diagnostic tool for identifying pathogens in PJI individuals utilizing three types of specimens. Due to its superior capacity in pathogen identification, prosthetic sonicate fluid can replace synovial fluid and periprosthetic tissue as the optimal sample choice for NGS.

References

1. Yilmaz MK, Abbaszadeh A, Tarabichi S, Azboy I, Parvizi J. Diagnosis of periprosthetic joint infection: the utility of biomarkers in 2023. Antibiotics (Basel). 2023;12(6):1054. https://doi.org/10.3390/antibiotics12061054.

2. Tsikopoulos K, Meroni G. Periprosthetic joint infection diagnosis: a narrative review. Antibiotics (Basel). 2023;12(10):1485. https://doi.org/10.3390/antibiotics12101485.
3. Mazzella FM, Zhang Y, Bauer TW. Update on the role of pathology and laboratory medicine in diagnosing periprosthetic infection. Hum Pathol. 2024;147:5–14. https://doi.org/10.1016/j.humpath.2024.01.009.
4. McNally M, Sigmund I, Hotchen A, Sousa R. Making the diagnosis in prosthetic joint infection: a European view. EFORT Open Rev. 2023;8(5):253–63. https://doi.org/10.1530/EOR-23-0044.
5. Tripathi S, Tarabichi S, Parvizi J, Rajgopal A. Current relevance of biomarkers in diagnosis of periprosthetic joint infection: an update. Arthroplasty. 2023;5(1):41. https://doi.org/10.1186/s42836-023-00192-5.
6. Diniz SE, Ribau A, Vinha A, Oliveira JC, Abreu MA, Sousa R. Simple and inexpensive synovial fluid biomarkers for the diagnosis of prosthetic joint infection according to the new EBJIS definition. J Bone Jt Infect. 2023;8(2):109–18. https://doi.org/10.5194/jbji-8-109-2023.
7. Denyer S, Eikani C, Sheth M, Schmitt D, Brown N. Diagnosing periprosthetic joint infection. Bone Jt Open. 2023;4(11):881–8. https://doi.org/10.1302/2633-1462.411.BJO-2023-0094.R1.
8. Karlidag T, Luo TD, Gehrke T, Citak M. How reliable is the absolute synovial polymorphonuclear neutrophil cell count in diagnosing periprosthetic joint infection? J Arthroplasty. 2024;39(4):1060–8. https://doi.org/10.1016/j.arth.2023.10.038.
9. Song ZY, Huang JC, Wang DH, Wang QK, Feng JW, Cao QQ, et al. Limited value of platelet-related markers in diagnosing periprosthetic joint infection. BMC Musculoskelet Disord. 2024;25(1):24. https://doi.org/10.1186/s12891-023-07142-x.
10. Parvizi J, Tan TL, Gaswami K, Higuera C, Della Valle C, Chen AF, et al. The 2018 definition of periprosthetic hip and knee infection: an evidence-based and validated criteria. J Arthroplasty. 2018;33(5):1309–1314.e2. https://doi.org/10.1016/j.arth.2018.02.078.
11. Dong M, Wang Y, Fan H, Yang D, Wang R, Feng Y. The albumin to globulin ratio performs well for diagnosing periprosthetic joint infection: a single-center retrospective study. J Arthroplasty. 2024;39(1):229–235.e4. https://doi.org/10.1016/j.arth.2023.08.002.
12. Miamidian JL, Toler K, McLaren A, Deirmengian C. Synovial fluid C-reactive protein clinical decision limit and diagnostic accuracy for periprosthetic joint infection. Cureus. 2024;16(1):e52749. https://doi.org/10.7759/cureus.52749.
13. Richter A, Altemeier A, Hold M, Lenhof S, Stauss R, Ettinger M, et al. Drain fluid cultures can rule in but cannot rule out infection persistence after surgical treatment of periprosthetic joint infections. J Orthop Sci. 2024;29(1):177–82. https://doi.org/10.1016/j.jos.2022.11.014.
14. Su S, Wang R, Zhou R, Bai J, Chen Z, Zhou F. Higher diagnostic value of next-generation sequencing versus culture in periprosthetic joint infection: a systematic review and meta-analysis. Knee Surg Sports Traumatol Arthrosc. 2024;32(9):2277–89. https://doi.org/10.1002/ksa.12227.
15. Mahnic A, Rak M, Trebše R, Rupnik M, Cőr A. Identification of prosthetic joint infections with 16S amplicon metagenomic sequencing – comparison with standard cultivation approach. Diagn Microbiol Infect Dis. 2024;109(1):116188. https://doi.org/10.1016/j.diagmicrobio.2024.116188.
16. Hao L, Bian W, Qing Z, Ma T, Li H, Xu P, et al. Will previous antimicrobial therapy reduce the positivity rate of metagenomic next-generation sequencing in periprosthetic joint infections? A clinical study. Front Cell Infect Microbiol. 2024;13:1295962. https://doi.org/10.3389/fcimb.2023.1295962.
17. Tan J, Wu L, Zhan L, Sheng M, Tang Z, Xu J, et al. Optimal selection of specimens for metagenomic next-generation sequencing in diagnosing periprosthetic joint infections. Front Cell Infect Microbiol. 2024;14:1356804. https://doi.org/10.3389/fcimb.2024.1356804.
18. Shi T, Chen H, Liu Y, Wu Y, Lin F. Clinical applications of metagenomic next-generation sequencing in the identification of pathogens in periprosthetic joint infections: a retrospective study. J Orthop Surg Res. 2024;19(1):301. https://doi.org/10.1186/s13018-024-04745-5.

3 Periprosthetic Joint Infection in Total Shoulder Arthroplasty: Diagnosis

E. Carlos Rodríguez-Merchán, Christian Carulli, and Gianluigi Pasta

3.1 Introduction

Periprosthetic joint infection (PJI) of the shoulder is a devastating complication with a reported incidence of 1–15.4% and is difficult to assess by contemporary diagnostic tools including serologic tests and arthrocentesis [1] (Fig. 3.1). In fact, substantial uncertainty endures about our contemporary methods of diagnosing shoulder PJI [2]. Besides, the diagnosis of PJI in total shoulder arthroplasty (TSA) remains a challenge. Conventional methods for assessing PJIs are poorly useful because of lower-virulence organisms affecting the shoulder [3]. The purpose of this chapter is to review the most recent literature on the diagnosis of PJI in TSA.

E. C. Rodríguez-Merchán (✉)
Department of Orthopedic Surgery, Hospital Universitario La Paz, Madrid, Madrid, Spain

C. Carulli
Orthopedic Clinic, University of Florence, Florence, Italy

G. Pasta
Department of Orthopedics and Traumatology, Fondazione Policlinico IRCCS San Matteo, University of Pavia, Pavia, Italy

E. C. Rodríguez-Merchán (ed.), *Advances in Periprosthetic Joint Infection*,
https://doi.org/10.1007/978-3-032-02945-4_3

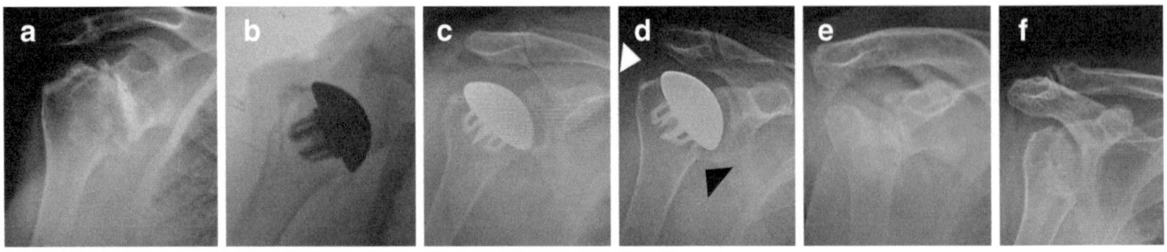

Fig. 3.1 (**a**–**f**) Right shoulder of a 81-year-old female patient with persistent symptomatic eccentric osteoarthritis and severe functional limitation (**a**); one month after, patient satisfied (**b**); image after 6 months (**c**); pain and effusion with subacromial space reduction (white arrow) and loosening with bone resorption on the medial aspect (black arrow) related to a late infection (**d**); due to persistent sinus tracts, implant removal and Girdlestone procedure were performed (**e**); and the patient did not want to undergo a further revision with a new implant once resolved the infection (**f**)

3.2 WBC/BM [Combined Labeled Leukocyte (WBC) and Technetium 99m Sulfur Colloid Bone Marrow Imaging Single-Photon Emission Computed Tomography] Diagnostic Performance

In 2019, Falstie-Jensen et al. investigated labeled white blood cell (WBC)/bone marrow (BM) single-photon emission computed tomography with computed tomography in diagnosing chronic PJI of the shoulder [4]. All individuals with a failed arthroplasty were scheduled for a diagnostic program including a WBC/BM. If an arthroplasty was revised, biopsy specimens were obtained and cultured for 2 weeks. The diagnostic performance of WBC/BM imaging was established utilizing biopsy specimens as a reference. Of the 49 individuals who experienced a WBC/BM scan, 29 (59%) were revised. Infection was present in 11 individuals, in whom 2 WBC/BM scans were true positives. The WBC/BM scan in 9 individuals was false negative. The remaining 18 individuals all had a true negative WBC/BM scan. WBC/BM demonstrated a sensitivity of 0.18 and specificity of 1 in detecting shoulder PJI. The positive predictive value was 1, and negative predictive value was 0.67. No individuals infected with *Cutibacterium acnes* resulted in a positive WBC/BM, nor had they preoperative or perioperative signs of infection. A positive WBC/BM was encountered only in individuals with obvious PJI. Therefore, the scan added nothing to the preoperative diagnosis. The WBC/BM single-photon emission computed tomography-computed tomography scan cannot be advised as a screening procedure when assessing failed shoulder arthroplasties for possible infection [4].

3.3 Serum C-Reactive Protein (CRP)

In a study with level 3 of evidence, Akgün et al. (2022) tried to establish cut-off values for diagnosing shoulder PJI and assessed the impact of the type of infecting microorganism and the classification subgroups according to the latest proposed International Consensus Meeting (ICM) criteria on the CRP level [5]. A retrospective analysis of all 136 individuals who experienced septic or aseptic revision shoulder arthroplasty was carried out. Shoulder PJI was defined according to the latest proposed definition criteria of the ICM. Serum CRP levels were compared between infected and noninfected cases, between infection subgroups, as well as between different species of infecting microorganisms. A receiver-operating characteristic (ROC) analysis was carried out to display the sensitivity and specificity of serum CRP level for shoulder PJI. A total of 52 individuals (38%) were classified as infected, 18 meeting the criteria for definitive infection, 26 for probable infection, and 8 for possible infection. According to the ROC curve, an optimized serum CRP threshold of 7.2 mg/L had a sensitivity of 69% and specificity of 74% (area under the curve = 0.72). Individuals with definitive infection cohort showed significantly higher median serum CRP levels (24.3 mg/L), when compared with probable, possible infection cohorts, and PJI unlikely cohort (8 mg/L, 8.3 mg/L, 3.6 mg/L, respectively). The most frequent isolated microorganism was *Cutibacterium acnes* in 25 individuals (48%) followed by coagulase-negative staphylococci (CNS) in 20 individuals (39%). Individuals with a PJI caused by highly virulent microorganisms had a significantly higher median serum CRP level compared to individuals with PJI caused by low-virulent microorganisms (48 mg/L vs. 11.3 mg/L). Serum CRP demonstrated a low sensitivity and specificity for the diagnosis of shoulder PJI, even applying cut-offs optimized by receiver-operating curve analysis. Low-virulent microorganisms and individuals with probable and possible infections were associated with lower CRP levels compared to individuals with definitive infection and infections caused by highly virulent microorganisms [5].

3.4 Serum D-Dimer

In a study with level 2 of evidence, Akgun et al. (2023) tried to validate the sensitivity and specificity of D-dimer in detecting shoulder PJI. All individuals who experienced septic or aseptic revision shoulder arthroplasty were analyzed [6]. The study group consisted of 30 individuals, of that 14 (47%) had a shoulder PJI according to the last proposed criteria of the ICM. The diagnostic validity of serum D-dimer regarding the detection of PJI was studied. The mean D-Dimer level was significantly higher for the individuals with shoulder PJI compared to individuals with aseptic failure (1.44 mg/L vs. 0.76 mg/L). Coagulase-negative staphylococci were the most frequently isolated pathogens, in 9/14 individuals (64%), followed by *Cutibacterium acnes* in 5/14 individuals (36%). According to the ROC analysis, a serum D-dimer threshold of 0.75 mg/L had a sensitivity of 86% and a specificity of 56% for detection of a shoulder PJI. The area under the curve was 0.74. A serum CRP cut-off of 10 mg/L demonstrated a sensitivity of 69% and a specificity of 88%. When both serum D-dimer and CRP above the thresholds of 0.75 mg/L and 10 mg/L, respectively, were utilized to identify a PJI, the sensitivity and specificity were 57% and 100%, respectively. Serum D-dimer demonstrated a good sensitivity but a poor specificity for the diagnosis of shoulder PJI. Combination of D-dimer and CRP led to an improvement in the specificity, however, at the cost of sensitivity. Thus, combination of both methods might be utilized as a confirmatory test in the diagnosis of shoulder PJI but not to rule out infection [6].

3.5 Arthroscopic Biopsy

A systematic review and meta-analysis published in 2023 by Karimi et al. analyzed the reliability and validity of arthroscopic biopsy for the diagnosis of shoulder PJI. After exclusion, the meta-analysis consisted of 7 articles with a total of 112 individuals. The calculated pooled sensitivity and specificity of arthroscopic biopsy for confirmation of shoulder PJI were 0.87 and 0.79. The pooled positive likelihood ratio and negative likelihood ratio were 4.15 and 0.17, respectively. The aggregate positive predictive value was 73.58%, and the aggregate negative predictive value was 89.83%. The diagnostic odds ratio of arthroscopic biopsy was 19.92. Arthroscopic biopsy in individuals suspected of shoulder PJI has good diagnostic accuracy, with high sensitivity and specificity. However, taking into account the various biopsy protocols (such as devices, numbers, and locations), further prospective studies are required to define the future role of arthroscopic biopsy in the diagnosis of shoulder PJI [2].

In 2022, Mederake et al. assessed the diagnostic value of the synovial biopsy in the diagnostic workup of low-grade PJI of the shoulder [7]. A retrospective evaluation was performed on 56 individuals experiencing revision surgery on their shoulder arthroplasty. A standardized preoperative workup was carried out comprising CRP value, leukocyte blood count, synovial fluid microbiological analyses and leukocyte count from joint aspiration, and five synovial biopsy samples for bacteriologic and histologic analyses obtained through an arthroscopic approach. During revision surgery, five samples of periprosthetic tissue were taken for bacteriologic and histologic analyses. The Musculoskeletal Infection Society (MSIS) criteria of 2014 were utilized to assess the diagnostic results. In total, 15 of 56 revised prostheses turned out as PJI (27%). When applying the aforementioned diagnostic workup, Mederake et al. obtained a sensitivity of 67% with a specificity of 95%. When carrying out a subgroup analysis on those individuals that had experienced a diagnostic biopsy, a sensitivity of 100% and a specificity of 83% was accomplished. With a sensitivity and specificity of 90% and 83%, respectively, the biopsy was the single method with the highest diagnostic value. The sensitivity of only 67% of the reported standard workup emphasized the difficulty in appropriately diagnosing low-grade infections after shoulder arthroplasty. The excellent specificity of 95% ensured, however, that noninfected prostheses were not incorrectly explanted. This study highlighted that synovial biopsy had a high diagnostic value and should be performed before complex revision surgeries to raise sensitivity in diagnosing a PJI [7].

3.6 Implant Sonication

In 2023, Mannaerts et al. tried to establish the value of implant sonication in the diagnosis of PJI in TSA. A retrospective analysis of individuals who experienced removal of their TSA combined with sonication of the implant for suspicion of PJI was carried out [8]. The diagnosis of PJI was based on the major criteria described by Parvizi. Mannaerts et al. estimated sensitivity, specificity, predictive values, likelihood ratios, and diagnostic accuracy for sonication cultures in comparison with periprosthetic tissue cultures. Data from 41 individuals were analyzed. Standard synovial fluid cultures combined with intraoperative periprosthetic tissue cultures had a sensitivity of 95%, specificity of 95% and total accuracy of 95%. Sonication cultures had a sensitivity of 91%, specificity of 68% and total accuracy of 80%. Six individuals had negative standard cultures but positive sonication cultures. In individuals with only one positive standard culture, the pathogen of the sonication culture corresponded to the pathogen of the positive soft tissue culture. This study encountered a possible added value of sonication of TSA in the diagnosis of PJI in conjunction with standard intraoperative cultures. In some individuals with suspicion of low-grade TSA infection, sonication could identify a possible causal microorganism in spite of negative standard cultures [8].

Table 3.1 summarizes the rates of sensitivity and specificity of the diagnostic methods used in the diagnosis of shoulder PJI.

Table 3.1 Rates of sensitivity, specificity, and total accuracy of different contemporary methods used to detect shoulder periprosthetic joint infection (PJI)

Method	Sensitivity	Specificity	Total accuracy
WBC/BM (combined labeled white blood cells [WBC] and technetium 99 m sulfur colloid bone marrow [BM] imaging single-photon emission computed tomography)	18%	100%	NA
Serum C-reactive protein (CRP) threshold of 7.2 mg/L	69%	74%	NA
Serum D-dimer threshold of 0.75 mg/L	86%	56%	NA
Serum D-dimer combined with CRP above the thresholds of 0.75 mg/L and 10 mg/L, respectively	57%	100%	NA
Arthroscopic biopsy	87–90%	79–83%	
Standard synovial fluid cultures combined with intraoperative periprosthetic tissue cultures	95%	95%	95%
Sonication cultures	91%	68%	80%

NA not available

3.7 Implant Sonication Fluid Cultures Versus Tissue Culture

In 2020, Akgün et al. studied the validity of implant sonication fluid cultures in the diagnosis of shoulder PJI compared with tissue culture [9]. This was a retrospective case-control study analyzing all individuals who experienced a revision surgery for any kind of suspected septic or aseptic event due to failed shoulder arthroplasty at their hospital. The diagnostic validity of implant sonication was analyzed on the basis of the last proposed definition criteria of the ICM and compared with standard tissue cultures. Of the 72 individuals, a total of 28 (38.9%) were classified as infected. Of the 28 infected individuals, 20 (71.4%) had an identified organism by tissue cultures, and *Cutibacterium acnes* was the most frequently isolated pathogen. The sensitivities of sonicate fluid [≥50 (colony-forming unit CFU)/mL)] and periprosthetic tissue culture for the diagnosis of periprosthetic shoulder infection were 36% and 61%, and the specificities were 97.7% and 100%, respectively. If no cut-off value was utilized in sonication culture, the sensitivity increased to 75% whereas the specificity dropped to 82%. Although there was no significant difference in sensitivity between tissue culture and the no cut-off sonication fluid culture (61% vs. 75%), the specificity of tissue culture was significantly higher (100% vs. 82%). Tissue culture demonstrated a higher sensitivity and specificity than implant sonication in the diagnosis of shoulder PJI and should remain the gold standard for microbiological diagnosis of shoulder PJI [9].

In 2021, Padolino et al. compared the results of sonication with intraoperative tissue sample cultures [10]. They analyzed 65 revision TSAs for suspected PJI. In each case, periprosthetic specimens were taken and explanted prostheses were put inside sterile fluid, sonicated, and then cultured. Among the 65 individuals, 36 were considered as possible, probable, or certain infection. Tissue cultures were positive for infection in 32 cases (52.3%) and in 19 cases, the positivity for *Cutibacterium acnes* was found. Sonication fluid cultures were positive in 40 cases (61.5%), with a positivity for *Cutibacterium acnes* in 27 cases. The sensitivities of sonication and tissue cultures for the diagnosis of shoulder PJI were 83.3% and 88.9%; the specificities were 65.5% and 93.1%, respectively. Therefore, the sonication technique did not show a clear advantage in postoperative shoulder PJI diagnosis, but it was a true aid in detecting *Cutibacterium acnes*. In any case, sensitivity and mostly specificity were higher with tissue cultures [10].

3.8 Concordance Between Preoperative Positive Aspiration Culture Results and Intraoperative Tissue Cultures

Hutchinson et al. (2023) analyzed the diagnostic accuracy of positive synovial fluid culture results in early pathogen identification for shoulder PJI [11]. A total of 35 individuals who met the MSIS criteria for PJI following primary anatomic or reverse arthroplasty were analyzed. The inclusion criteria required a positive preoperative intraarticular synovial fluid sample within 90 days and intraoperative tissue cultures at the time of arthrotomy. Concordance was established when the organism(s) identified from the aspirate correlated with the intraoperative specimens. Overall concordance was identified in 28 of 35 individuals (80%), with similar concordance for anatomic (21 of 24, 88%) and reverse (7 of 11, 64%) shoulder arthroplasties. Culture discordance happened in 7 of 35 individuals (20%): of these, 5 (14%) had no corresponding intraoperative culture growth, whereas 2 (6%) had polymicrobial intraoperative cultures. Monomicrobial *Cutibacterium acnes* PJI cases were the most frequent (24 of 35, 69%) and had an overall concordance rate of 79%. Of the five discordant *Cutibacterium acnes* individuals, two had polymicrobial intraoperative cultures and three had negative intraoperative culture results; all individuals with negative intraoperative culture results had received antibiotics between the time of aspiration and surgery. Considered separately, concordance in individuals who had a positive aspirate finding for *Cutibacterium acnes* and did not receive antibiotics prior to surgery was 19 of 21 (90%), with a sensitivity of 100% and a corresponding positive predictive value of 0.91. Preoperative positive aspiration culture results demonstrated favorable sensitivity and specificity when compared with intraoperative tissue cultures in identifying pathogenic microorganisms in individuals with shoulder PJI [11].

3.9 Concordance Between Preoperative Synovial Fluid Culture Results and Intraoperative Tissue Culture Results

Zanna et al. (2023) assessed the utility of preoperative culture data for early pathogen identification for shoulder PJI and determined the concordance between preoperative synovial fluid culture results and intraoperative tissue culture results [12]. Fifty individuals who met the 2014 MSIS criteria for shoulder PJI were retrospectively reviewed for clinical and demographic data. This group of individuals was divided into two cohorts based on the concordance between preoperative and intraoperative culture results. The pathogens identified on preoperative and intraoperative cultures were classified as high virulence or low virulence. Concordance between preoperative aspiration and intraoperative tissue culture was identified in 28 of 50 individuals (56%). Preoperative cultures positive for Gram-positive species were more likely to be concordant than discordant. Preoperative cultures positive for *Cutibacterium acnes* were more likely to be concordant with intraoperative cultures. There were more individuals with polymicrobial infection in the discordant cohort compared with the concordant cohort. No statistically significant correlation between the preoperative serum CRP level and the intraoperative category of bacteria was found. *Staphylococcus aureus* and coagulase-negative staphylococci were associated with high specificity and negative predictive value. Preoperative cultures positive for *Cutibacterium acnes* showed sensitivity, specificity, positive predictive value, and negative predictive value lower than 0.8. Gram-negative pathogens showed the highest sensitivity and specificity, whereas polymicrobial infections demonstrated the lowest sensitivity and positive predictive value. Preoperative synovial fluid aspiration for shoulder PJI poorly predicted intraoperative culture results, with a discordance of 44%. More favorable concordance was found for monomicrobial preoperative cultures, particularly for Gram-negative organisms and methicillin-sensitive *Staphylococcus aureus*. The overall high rate of discordance between preoperative and intraoperative culture might prompt surgeons to base medical and surgical management on patient history and other factors and avoid relying solely on preoperative synovial fluid culture data [12].

3.10 Preoperative Arthroscopic Tissue Cultures Compared with Tissue Biopsy Samples Obtained at the Time of Revision Surgery

In a systematic review of seven studies, Tat et al. (2023) assessed the diagnostic accuracy of preoperative arthroscopic tissue cultures compared with tissue biopsy samples obtained at the time of revision surgery. The studies represented a balance of shoulder arthroplasty types, including anatomic TSA (N = 75, 38%), reverse TSA (N = 60, 30%), and hemiarthroplasty (N = 64, 32%) [3]. There were 56 of 120 arthroscopic procedures that returned positive tissue culture findings compared with 64 of 157 positive open biopsy culture findings obtained from revision surgery. The meta-analysis total for sensitivity and specificity for all studies combined indicated that arthroscopic tissue cultures (0.76 and 0.91, respectively) were superior to both aspiration (0.15 and 0.93, respectively) and a positive erythrocyte sedimentation rate (ESR) or CRP level (0.14 and 0.83, respectively) in diagnosing PJI. This systematic review showed that preoperative arthroscopic tissue biopsy utilized for microbiology cultures accurately foretells intra-

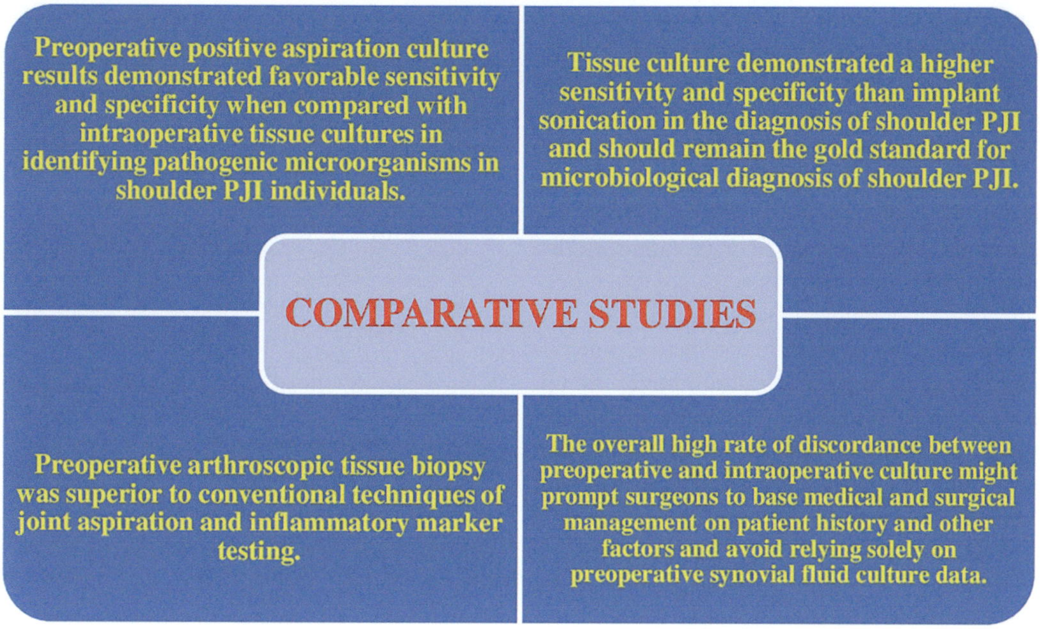

Fig. 3.2 Comparative results between different shoulder periprosthetic joint infection (PJI) diagnostic methods

operative culture findings obtained during revision surgery with high sensitivity and specificity. Besides, arthroscopy seems to be superior to conventional techniques of joint aspiration and inflammatory marker testing. Therefore, arthroscopic tissue cultures might be an emerging useful tool to help guide the management of PJI of the shoulder [3]. Figure 3.2 shows the comparative results between different shoulder PJI diagnostic methods.

3.11 Conclusions

Serum CRP has demonstrated a low sensitivity and specificity for the diagnosis of shoulder PJI. Serum D-dimer has demonstrated a good sensitivity but a poor specificity for the diagnosis of shoulder PJI. The combination of D-dimer and CRP improves the specificity, but at the cost of sensitivity. Thus, the combination of both methods might be utilized as a confirmatory test in the diagnosis of shoulder PJI, but not to rule out infection.

Arthroscopic biopsy in individuals suspected of shoulder PJI has good diagnostic accuracy, with high sensitivity and specificity. However, taking into account the various biopsy protocols (such as devices, numbers, and locations), further prospective studies are required to define the future role of arthroscopic biopsy in the diagnosis of shoulder PJI. Synovial biopsy had a high diagnostic value and should be performed before complex revision surgeries to increase sensitivity for diagnosing a PJI. Preoperative arthroscopic tissue biopsy utilized for microbiology cultures accurately foretells intraoperative culture findings obtained during revision surgery with high sensitivity and specificity. Besides, arthroscopy seems to be superior to conventional techniques of joint aspiration and inflammatory marker testing. Therefore, arthroscopic tissue cultures might be an emerging useful tool to help guide the management of PJI of the shoulder.

In some individuals with suspicion of low-grade TSA infection, sonication could identify a possible causal microorganism despite negative standard cultures. The sonication technique did not show a clear advantage in postoperative shoulder PJI diagnosis, but it was a true aid in detecting *Cutibacterium acnes*. In any case, sensitivity and mostly specificity were higher with tissue cultures. Tissue culture demonstrated a higher sensitivity and specificity than implant sonication in the diagnosis of shoulder PJI and should remain the gold standard for microbiological diagnosis of shoulder PJI.

Preoperative positive aspiration culture results demonstrated favorable sensitivity and specificity when compared with intraoperative tissue cultures in identifying pathogenic microorganisms in individuals with shoulder PJI. The overall high rate of discordance between preoperative and intraoperative culture might prompt surgeons to base medical and surgical management on patient history and other factors and avoid relying solely on preoperative synovial fluid culture data.

References

1. Namdari S, Nicholson T, Abboud J, Lazarus M, Ramsey ML, Williams G, et al. Comparative study of cultures and next-generation sequencing in the diagnosis of shoulder prosthetic joint infections. J Shoulder Elbow Surg. 2019;28(1):1–8. https://doi.org/10.1016/j.jse.2018.08.048.
2. Karimi A, Jalalpour P, Reddy RP, Sabzevari S, Keeling LE, Lin A. Diagnostic arthroscopy for periprosthetic shoulder arthroplasty infections: a systematic review and meta-analysis. JSES Int. 2023;7(5):835–41. https://doi.org/10.1016/j.jseint.2023.05.004.
3. Tat J, Tat J, Faber K. Arthroscopic tissue biopsy as a preoperative diagnostic test for periprosthetic shoulder arthroplasty infections: a systematic review and meta-analysis. J Shoulder Elbow Surg. 2023;32(7):1545–54. https://doi.org/10.1016/j.jse.2023.02.135.
4. Falstie-Jensen T, Daugaard H, Søballe K, Ovesen J, Arveschoug AK, Lange J, ROSA Study Group. Labeled white blood cell/bone marrow single-photon emission computed tomography with computed tomography fails in diagnosing chronic periprosthetic shoulder joint infection. J Shoulder Elbow Surg. 2019;28(6):1040–8. https://doi.org/10.1016/j.jse.2018.10.024.
5. Akgün D, Wiethölter M, Siegert P, Danzinger V, Minkus M, Braun KF, et al. The role of serum C-reactive protein in the diagnosis of periprosthetic shoulder infection. Arch Orthop Trauma Surg. 2022;142(8):1715–21. https://doi.org/10.1007/s00402-021-03779-2.
6. Akgün D, Al-Muhtaresh F, Paksoy A, Lacheta L, Minkus M, Karczewski D, Moroder P. The role of serum D-Dimer for the diagnosis of periprosthetic shoulder infection. Arch Orthop Trauma Surg. 2023;143(4):1855–60. https://doi.org/10.1007/s00402-022-04385-6.
7. Mederake M, Hofmann UK, Fink B. The significance of synovial biopsy in the diagnostic workup of the low-grade periprosthetic joint infection of shoulder arthroplasty. Arch Orthop Trauma Surg. 2022;142(11):3157–64. https://doi.org/10.1007/s00402-021-03932-x.
8. Mannaerts J, Wijnen V, Depypere M, Verhaegen F, Debeer P. The role of sonication in the diagnosis of periprosthetic joint infection in total shoulder arthroplasty. Acta Orthop Belg. 2023;89(2):201–6. https://doi.org/10.52628/89.2.10875.
9. Akgün D, Maziak N, Plachel F, Siegert P, Minkus M, Thiele K, et al. The role of implant sonication in the diagnosis of periprosthetic shoulder infection. J Shoulder Elbow Surg. 2020;29(6):e222–8. https://doi.org/10.1016/j.jse.2019.10.011.
10. Padolino A, Cataldo G, Tarallo L, Fabbri E, Merolla G, Micheloni GM, et al. Implant sonication versus intraoperative tissue sample cultures for periprosthetic joint infection (PJI) of shoulder arthroplasty. Acta Biomed. 2021;92(S3):e2021009. https://doi.org/10.23750/abm.v92iS3.11693.
11. Hutchinson ID, Mathew JI, Taylor SA, Fu MC, Dines DM, Carli AV, et al. How accurate are positive preoperative aspiration culture results in shoulder periprosthetic joint infection? A concordance study. J Shoulder Elbow Surg. 2023;32(6S):S17–22. https://doi.org/10.1016/j.jse.2023.02.013.
12. Zanna L, Sangaletti R, Akkaya M, Shen T, Abuljadail S, Gehrke T, et al. What is the concordance rate of preoperative synovial fluid aspiration and intraoperative biopsy in detecting periprosthetic joint infection of the shoulder? J Shoulder Elbow Surg. 2023;32(3):492–9. https://doi.org/10.1016/j.jse.2022.10.008.

4 Risk Factors of Periprosthetic Joint Infection in Shoulder Arthroplasty

E. Carlos Rodríguez-Merchán and Eloy Tabeayo

4.1 Introduction

Identifying the risk factors for shoulder periprosthetic joint infection (PJI) is crucial, as it enables us to prevent or mitigate complications following total shoulder arthroplasty (TSA). Infections can lead to loosening of the humeral component, potentially causing stem subsidence or loosening of the glenoid component. If left untreated, these issues can result in catastrophic component failure accompanied by severe osteolysis (Fig. 4.1). This topic has been extensively explored, with numerous systematic reviews and meta-analyses conducted to uncover potential associations between shoulder infections and various risk factors. These factors include male sex, age under 75, prior shoulder surgery, reverse shoulder arthroplasty, rotator cuff arthropathy as the primary diagnosis, inpatient shoulder arthroplasty, revision surgery, liver disease, alcohol overuse, iron-deficiency anemia, rheumatoid arthritis, and diabetes mellitus [1, 2] (Fig. 4.2).

The study by Walocha et al. (2024) investigated risk factors for the development of PJI within two years following primary reverse shoulder arthroplasty (RSA) for glenohumeral osteoarthritis (GHOA) [3]. Using a nationwide database, the study included 51,824 patients, of whom 879 (1.69%) developed a PJI. The study found that male sex, pathologic weight loss, iron deficiency anemia, obesity, rheumatoid arthritis, arrhythmias, and depressive disorders were significant risk factors for PJI within two years of RSA. The research highlighted that modifiable factors, such as obesity and anemia, could be targeted to reduce the risk of infections in high-risk patients. This study emphasized the importance of preoperative screening to identify these factors and adjust patient management accordingly to minimize PJI incidence.

The aim of this chapter is to review the most current evidence on the primary risk factors for shoulder PJI.

E. C. Rodríguez-Merchán (✉)
Department of Orthopedic Surgery, Hospital Universitario La Paz, Madrid, Madrid, Spain

E. Tabeayo
Department of Orthopedic Surgery, Albert Einstein College of Medicine, Montefiore Medical Center, New York, NY, USA
e-mail: etabeayo@montefiore.org

E. C. Rodríguez-Merchán (ed.), *Advances in Periprosthetic Joint Infection*,
https://doi.org/10.1007/978-3-032-02945-4_4

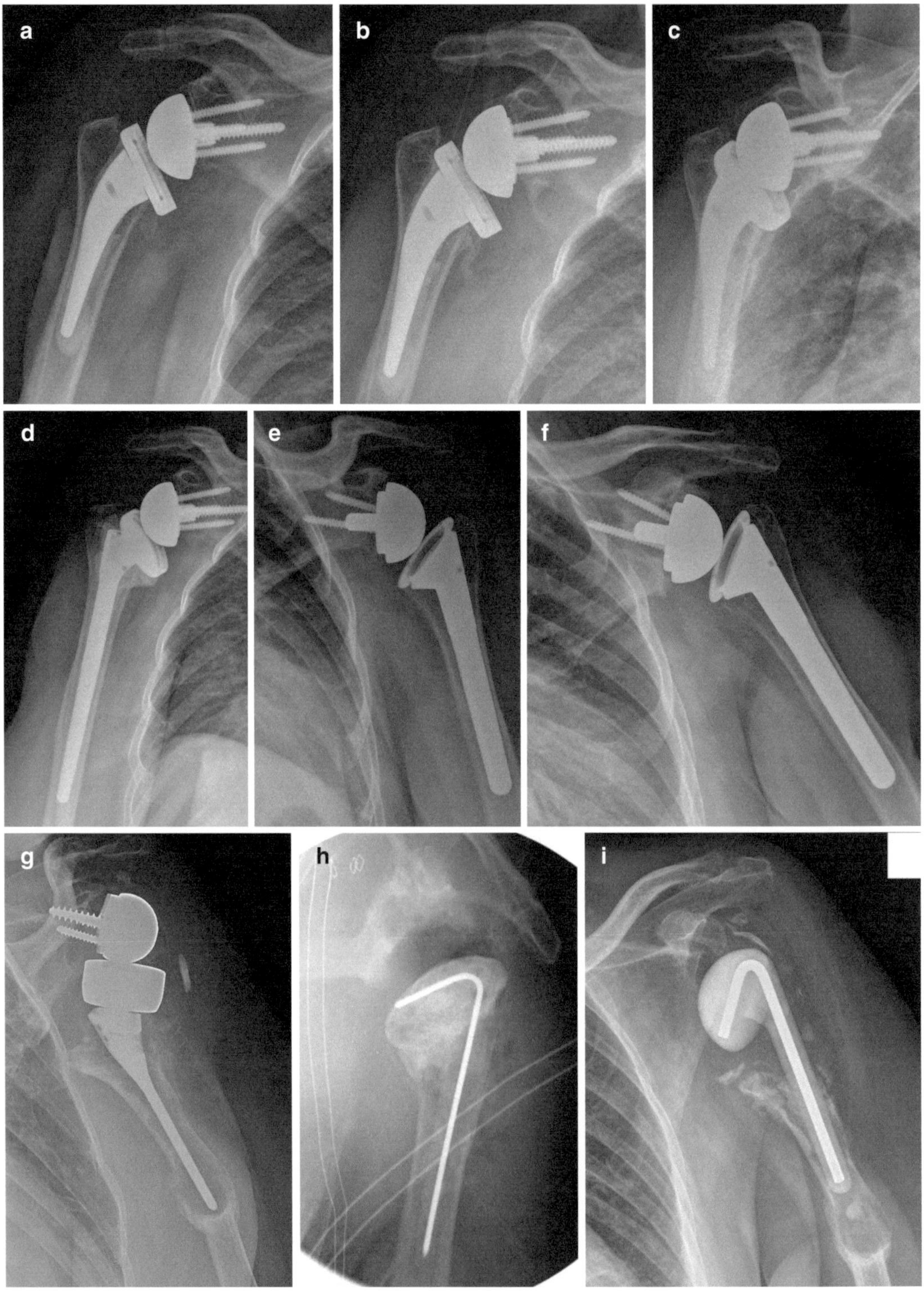

Fig. 4.1 Periprosthetic joint infection (PJI) of total shoulder arthroplasty (TSA): note the loosening of the humeral and glenoid components (**a**–**g**). In this case a two-stage revision arthroplasty was indicated. Images (**h**–**i**) show the articulated spacer implanted in the first stage of revision arthroplasty

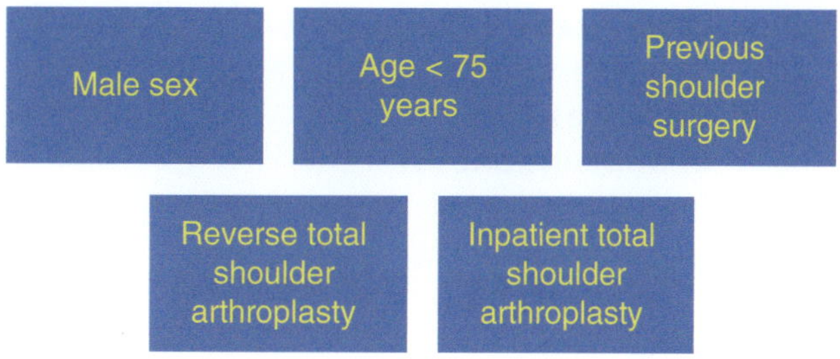

Fig. 4.2 Facts that increase the risk of shoulder periprosthetic joint infection (PJI)

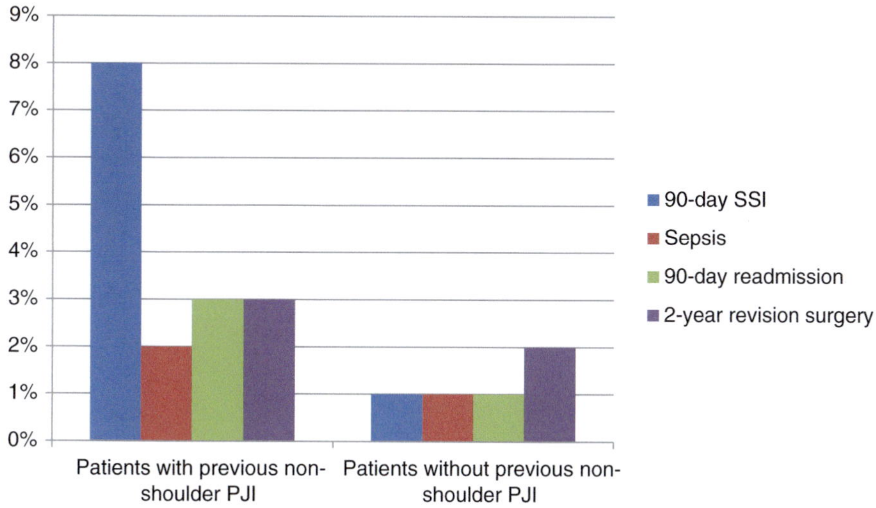

Fig. 4.3 Rates of surgical site infection (SSI), sepsis, 90-day readmission, and 2-year revision surgery in patients with previous non-shoulder periprosthetic joint infection (PJI) versus patients without previous non-shoulder PJI

4.2 Prior Non-shoulder PJI Contributes to the Increased Risk of Infectious Complications

Studies have indicated that prior non-shoulder PJI contributes to an increased risk of infectious complications in subsequent joint surgeries. Specifically, prior PJI in any joint, not just the shoulder, has been associated with higher risks of infection after shoulder arthroplasty. This is due to the potential for systemic immune system alterations, biofilm formation, or a chronic low-grade infection that can predispose to further complications. These findings suggest that such patients require more careful preoperative management to minimize infection risks [2].

The study by Agarwal et al. (2022) in the *Journal of the American Academy of Orthopaedic Surgeons* highlighted a significant finding: prior non-shoulder PJI increases the risk of infectious complications, healthcare utilization, and revision surgery after primary TSA. Their retrospective cohort study demonstrated that patients with a history of PJI in joints other than the shoulder had a notably higher risk of developing surgical site infections (SSI) and sepsis within 90 days of TSA, as well as a higher risk of requiring revision surgery within two years. Specifically, the risk of surgical site infection was 8% in the prior PJI group, compared with only 1% in the control group, and the rate of sepsis was also significantly elevated in the PJI group. Furthermore, these patients experienced more readmissions and longer hospital stays. This reinforces the importance of careful preoperative risk stratification and management for patients with a history of PJI, particularly when they are undergoing TSA [4] (Fig. 4.3).

4.3 Early Aseptic Reoperation After Shoulder Arthroplasty Increases Risk of Subsequent PJI

Early aseptic reoperation after shoulder arthroplasty has been identified as a significant risk factor for subsequent PJI. According to a study by Wickman et al. (2021), patients who underwent an aseptic reoperation within 90 days of their primary TSA or RSA had a markedly increased risk of developing PJI within the first year [5]. Specifically, the risk of PJI in patients who had an early aseptic reoperation was found to be 3.54% for TSA and 3.08% for RSA, compared with significantly lower rates in patients without early reoperations (0.75% and 0.73%, respectively).

This elevated risk was even more pronounced on multivariate analysis, where the odds of subsequent PJI were 14.19 times higher for TSA and 8.38 times higher for RSA patients who had an early aseptic reoperation. The most common indications for these early reoperations were prosthetic dislocation and rotator cuff tears, and the study highlights that minimizing postoperative complications in the acute period following shoulder arthroplasty is crucial for reducing the risk of infection.

Thus, avoiding unnecessary early reoperations and ensuring careful management during the initial postoperative period are key strategies in reducing the risk of subsequent infectious complications after shoulder arthroplasty [5] (Fig. 4.4).

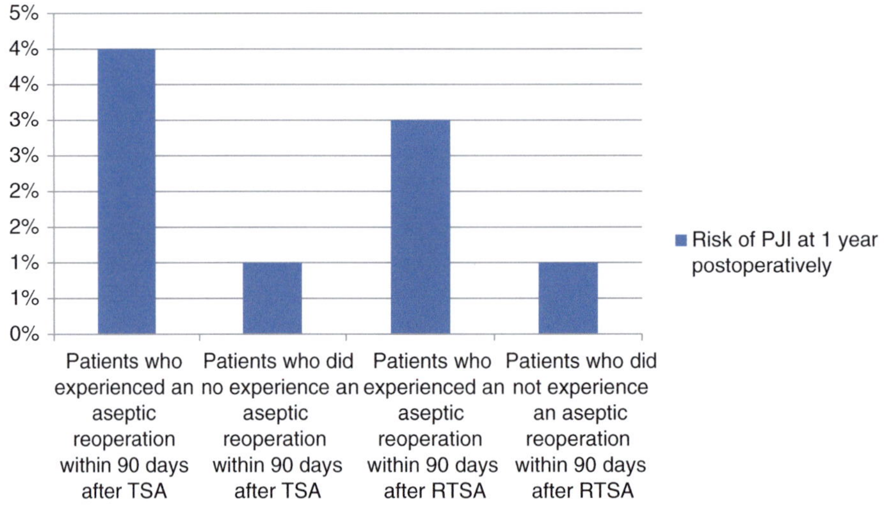

Fig. 4.4 Risk of periprosthetic joint infection (PJI) at 1 year postoperatively: patients who experienced an aseptic reoperation within 90 days after total shoulder arthroplasty (TSA) and reverse TSA (RTSA) versus patients who did not experience an aseptic reoperation within 90 days after TSA and RTSA

4.4 Preoperative Corticosteroid Injection Within 1 Month of TSA and RTSA Is Associated with Increased Risk of PJI

In their 2023 studies, Baksh et al. examined the relationship between preoperative corticosteroid injections and the risk of PJI following shoulder arthroplasty [6, 7]. Their findings indicated that corticosteroid injections given within 1 month prior to surgery were significantly associated with an increased risk of developing PJI. Specifically, patients who received corticosteroid injections within 6 weeks of reverse total shoulder arthroplasty (RTSA) had a notably higher incidence of infection, with an odds ratio (OR) of 2.1, suggesting more than double the risk of PJI compared with those who did not receive the injections.

However, the study also found that injections administered more than 1 month prior to surgery did not show a significant association with increased infection risk. This suggests that the timing of corticosteroid injections plays a crucial role in influencing infection outcomes, with injections closer to the surgery date presenting a higher risk due to their potential to suppress the immune system and impair wound healing. The authors emphasized that while corticosteroids are effective for managing pain and inflammation, their use within a month of surgery should be carefully managed, particularly in high-risk patients with comorbidities like diabetes or obesity.

4.5 Previous Rotator Cuff Repair Increases the Risk of Revision Surgery for PJI After RTSA

Several studies have examined the relationship between prior rotator cuff repair and an increased risk of complications, including revision surgery and PJI, following shoulder arthroplasty. These findings emphasize the impact of previous shoulder surgeries on postoperative outcomes, particularly the risk of infection and the need for revision surgery.

Morris et al. (2015), in the *Journal of Shoulder and Elbow Surgery*, found that previous rotator cuff surgery significantly increased the risk of infection following RSA. They noted that patients with a history of rotator cuff repairs had altered shoulder mechanics, which predisposed them to complications, including infection. Additionally, the increased risk of revision surgery for these patients was highlighted, as infection after RSA was often more challenging to treat in those with previous shoulder surgeries [8].

Jensen et al. (2017), in a study published in *Clinical Orthopaedics and Related Research*, also examined the effects of prior rotator cuff repair on the outcomes of TSA and found that such a history could increase the risk of complications like infection and the likelihood of needing revision surgery. They suggested that patients who had undergone previous rotator cuff surgeries might face compromised tissue integrity, which complicates healing and increases vulnerability to infection following TSA [9].

Boileau et al. (2016), in *The Journal of Bone and Joint Surgery*, found similar findings, reporting that patients who had rotator cuff repairs prior to undergoing RSA were at a higher risk for infection and revision surgery. The study suggested that structural changes after rotator cuff surgery, such as altered tendon function and shoulder biomechanics, contributed to poor healing and greater susceptibility to infection following shoulder arthroplasty [10].

These studies collectively emphasize that previous rotator cuff surgery is an important factor in predicting the risk of complications following shoulder arthroplasty, particularly the increased likelihood of PJI and the need for revision surgery (Fig. 4.5). These patients may require more intensive perioperative management to minimize infection risks.

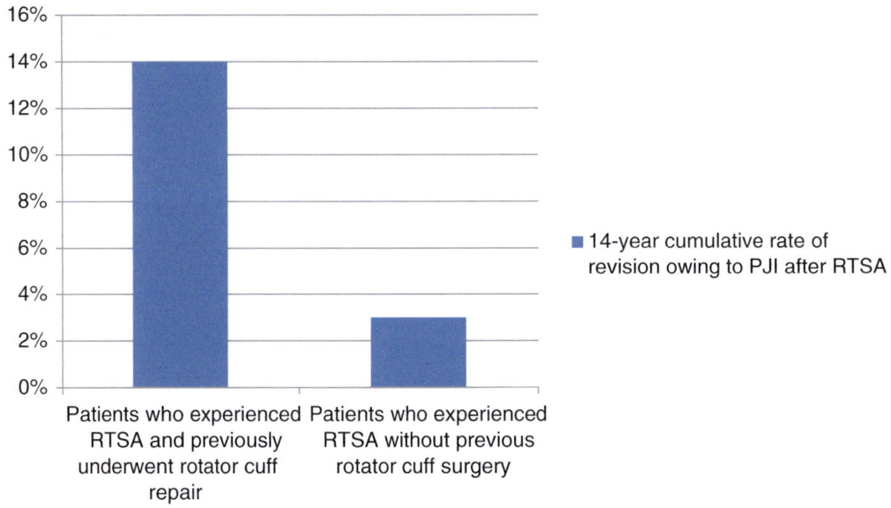

Fig. 4.5 Fourteen-year cumulative rate of revision owing to periprosthetic joint infection (PJI) after reverse total shoulder arthroplasty (RTSA): patients who experienced RTSA and previously underwent rotator cuff repair versus patients who experienced RTSA without previous rotator cuff surgery

4.6 Elevated Risk of PJI in Cannabis Users After TSA

There is emerging evidence that cannabis use may elevate the risk of PJI following shoulder arthroplasty, including total shoulder and reverse shoulder procedures. Studies indicate that cannabis use is associated with increased rates of complications after joint arthroplasty, including PJI. One study showed that cannabis users were significantly more likely to experience prosthetic infections post-surgery, with cannabis-only users exhibiting the highest odds of infection (OR: 5.79) compared with nonusers [11].

This finding is consistent with studies in other types of joint arthroplasty, such as knee and hip, where cannabis use has been linked to increased risk of infections and complications postoperatively [12–14]. The mechanisms are thought to involve the immunosuppressive effects of cannabis, which could impair wound healing and increase the vulnerability to infections after surgery. Given these findings, it is recommended that cannabis use be carefully considered as a potential risk factor for PJI in patients undergoing shoulder arthroplasty, especially when planning postoperative care and infection prevention strategies.

4.7 Conclusions

In conclusion, various modifiable and non-modifiable factors contribute to an increased risk of PJI after shoulder arthroplasty, highlighting the need for careful preoperative management. Modifiable factors include perioperative steroid injections, cannabis use, and poor glycemic control in diabetic patients, which have been linked to higher infection rates following TSA or RTSA. Previous rotator cuff repair and prior non-shoulder PJI are significant non-modifiable risk factors that further predispose patients to infectious complications and the need for revision surgery. Evidence suggests that prior rotator cuff surgeries compromise tissue integrity, impair healing, and increase vulnerability to infection. Furthermore, prior non-shoulder infections can alter the immune response, raising the risk of subsequent infections in shoulder arthroplasty patients. Minimizing these risks through preoperative screening and tailored management strategies is essential for reducing the incidence of PJI and improving surgical outcomes in high-risk patients.

References

1. Kunutsor SK, Barrett MC, Whitehouse MR, Craig RS, Lenguerrand E, Beswick AD, et al. Incidence, temporal trends and potential risk factors for prosthetic joint infection after primary total shoulder and elbow replacement: systematic review and meta-analysis. J Infect. 2020;80(4):426–36. https://doi.org/10.1016/j.jinf.2020.01.008.
2. Seok HG, Park JJ, Park SG. Risk factors for periprosthetic joint infection after shoulder arthroplasty: systematic review and meta-analysis. J Clin Med. 2022;11(14):4245. https://doi.org/10.3390/jcm11144245.
3. Walocha D, Bogdan P, Gordon AM, Magruder ML, Conway CA, Razi AE, et al. Risk factors for the development of a peri-prosthetic joint infection up to 2 years following primary reverse shoulder arthroplasty. J Orthop. 2022;35:69–73. https://doi.org/10.1016/j.jor.2022.11.007.
4. Agarwal AR, Wang KY, Mikula JD, Berger P, Kreulen RT, Nayar SK, et al. Prior non-shoulder periprosthetic joint infection increases the risk of surgical site infection, sepsis, and all-cause revision after primary total shoulder arthroplasty. J Am Acad Orthop Surg. 2022;30(3):133–9. https://doi.org/10.5435/JAAOS-D-21-00745.
5. Wickman JR, Goltz DE, Levin JM, Lassiter T, Anakwenze OA, Klifto CS. Early aseptic reoperation after shoulder arthroplasty increases risk of subsequent prosthetic joint infection. JSES Int. 2021;5(6):1067–71. https://doi.org/10.1016/j.jseint.2021.06.002.
6. Baksh N, Nadarajah V, Connors KM, Bains SS, Chen Z, Dubin JA, et al. Does preoperative corticosteroid injection increase the risk of periprosthetic joint infection after reverse shoulder arthroplasty? J Shoulder Elbow Surg. 2023;32(7):1459–64. https://doi.org/10.1016/j.jse.2023.01.008.
7. Baksh N, Etcheson JI, Liu S, Ikwuazom CP, Chen Z, Dubin JA, et al. Pre-operative corticosteroid injection within 1 month of total shoulder arthroplasty is associated with increased risk of periprosthetic joint infection. Arch Orthop Trauma Surg. 2023;143(9):5609–14. https://doi.org/10.1007/s00402-023-04866-2.
8. Morris BJ, Schairer WW, Kauffman JB. The impact of prior rotator cuff surgery on complications after reverse shoulder arthroplasty. J Shoulder Elbow Surg. 2015;24(6):867–73. https://doi.org/10.1016/j.jse.2015.01.036.
9. Jensen ML, Jensen SL, Bolder M, Hanisch KWJ, Sørensen AKB, Olsen BS, et al. Previous rotator cuff repair increases the risk of revision surgery for periprosthetic joint infection after reverse shoulder arthroplasty. J Shoulder Elbow Surg. 2023;32(1):111–20. https://doi.org/10.1016/j.jse.2022.07.001.
10. Boileau P, Watkinson DJ, Hovorka I, Lädermann A. Risk factors for infection following reverse shoulder arthroplasty. J Bone Joint Surg Am. 2016;98(24):2096–103. https://doi.org/10.2106/JBJS.16.00502.
11. Remily EA, Bains SS, Dubin J, Hameed D, Reich J, Livesey MG, et al. Elevated risk of prosthetic infections in cannabis users after shoulder arthroplasty. Eur J Orthop Surg Traumatol. 2024;34(3):1381–7. https://doi.org/10.1007/s00590-023-03802-9.
12. Law TY, Kurowicki J, Rosas S, Sabeh K, Summers S, Hubbard Z, et al. Cannabis use increases risk for revision after total knee arthroplasty. J Long Term Eff Med Implants. 2018;28(2):125–30. https://doi.org/10.1615/JLongTermEffMedImplants.2018027401.
13. Vakharia RM, Mannino A, Salem HS, Roche MW, Wong CHJ, Mont MA. The association between cannabis use disorder and the outcome following primary total hip arthroplasty. Bone Joint J. 2021;103(1):111–5. https://doi.org/10.1302/0301-620X.103B7.BJJ-2020-2424.R1.
14. Weisberg MD, Ng MK, Magruder ML, Vakharia RM, Roche MW, Erez O. The association of cannabis use disorder and perioperative complications after primary total knee arthroplasty. J Am Acad Orthop Surg. 2022;30(5):313–20. https://doi.org/10.5435/JAAOS-D-21-00703.

Open Debridement, Antibiotic, and Implant Retention (DAIR) for Periprosthetic Joint Infection in Total Shoulder Arthroplasty

5

E. Carlos Rodríguez-Merchán
and Alfonso Vaquero-Picado

5.1 Introduction

Periprosthetic joint infection (PJI) remains a devastating complication following total shoulder arthroplasty (TSA) [1, 2]. Although staged revision arthroplasty is the standard treatment in many cases, surgical intervention with open debridement, antibiotics, and implant retention (DAIR) can be an effective alternative for acute PJI [2].

According to Boyer and Cazorla (2021), PJI is an uncommon but serious complication of TSA requiring multidisciplinary care. Given the dual objective of eradicating the infection while preserving satisfactory function, it is crucial to determine when implant retention is feasible. Bacteria and fungi form biofilms that shield them from antibiotics and immune responses [3]. In shoulder PJI, a high prevalence of *Cutibacterium acnes* infections has been reported [4], a commensal skin bacterium responsible for joint infections, often presenting with mild symptoms or stiffness [5, 6].

In 2021, Bdeir et al. analyzed the 5-year outcomes of patients with shoulder PJI treated according to established treatment algorithms originally designed for hip and knee PJIs [1]. They categorized outcomes as treatment failure or infection resolution. *Staphylococcus epidermidis* and *Staphylococcus aureus* were the most common pathogens. Acute PJI was primarily treated with open DAIR, while chronic cases required two-stage or multiple-stage exchanges. The management failure rate was 10.5%. Preoperative C-reactive protein (CRP) levels were elevated in 68.4% of patients. The mean number of operative revisions was 3.6, and the mean duration of antibiotic therapy was 72.4 days, with clindamycin and fluoroquinolone being the most frequently used antibiotics. This study suggested that PJI treatment protocols for hip and knee could be effectively applied to shoulder PJI [1].

For reverse shoulder arthroplasty (RSA), Jacquot et al. (2015) reported healing rates of approximately 75% after open DAIR, similar to hip and knee PJI outcomes [7].

This chapter aims to analyze the latest data on open DAIR for several conditions of PJI, with special focus on TSA.

5.2 DAIR in Gram-Negative PJI

In 2014, Rodriguez-Pardo et al. investigated the epidemiology and outcomes of gram-negative PJIs treated with open DAIR [8]. They conducted a multicenter retrospective study analyzing 242 episodes of gram-negative PJI. The implants included 150 (62%) hip, 85 (35%) knee, 5 (2%) shoulder, and 2 (1%) elbow arthroplasties. Among

E. C. Rodríguez-Merchán (✉) · A. Vaquero-Picado
Department of Orthopedic Surgery, Hospital Universitario La Paz, Madrid, Madrid, Spain

E. C. Rodríguez-Merchán (ed.), *Advances in Periprosthetic Joint Infection*,
https://doi.org/10.1007/978-3-032-02945-4_5

these, 189 (78%) were acute infections. The primary pathogens were *Enterobacteriaceae* (78%), *Pseudomonas* spp. (20%), and other gram-negative bacilli (2%). Ciprofloxacin-resistant isolates constituted 19% of cases. Open DAIR in ciprofloxacin-susceptible gram-negative PJIs treated with ciprofloxacin was employed in 174 (72%) patients, achieving a 79% success rate after an average follow-up of 2 years. Ciprofloxacin treatment was independently protective, while chronic renal impairment predicted failure [8].

5.3 Open DAIR + Linezolid

Morata et al. (2014) identified open DAIR combined with a prolonged antibiotic regimen, including rifampicin, as a viable strategy when symptoms persist for less than four weeks and radiological signs of loosening are absent. Previous studies reported success rates ranging from 60% to 90% [9]. Morata et al. retrospectively reviewed 39 patients treated with open DAIR and linezolid, with or without rifampicin. The mean patient age was 70.5 years, and 23% had diabetes mellitus. The study cohort included 25 knee (64%), 13 hip (33%), and 1 shoulder (3%) prostheses. The mean time from arthroplasty to infection diagnosis was 17 days, and 85% were diagnosed within the first 60 days. Antibiotic therapy lasted an average of 70.5 days, with 44.5 days of linezolid treatment. Adverse events occurred in 38% of patients, primarily gastrointestinal complaints and anemia. After a mean follow-up of 2.5 years, the failure rate was 28%, higher in the rifampicin cohort (36% vs. 18%), mostly due to relapses. Linezolid was a promising alternative for fluoroquinolone- and rifampicin-resistant staphylococcal infections [9].

5.4 Open DAIR with Exchange of Mobile Parts

Hirsiger et al. (2019) evaluated the role of mobile prosthetic component exchange during open DAIR [10]. Some studies suggest that not exchanging mobile parts leads to failure, while others consider it optional. Hirsiger et al. retrospectively analyzed 112 PJIs treated with open DAIR, including 69 total hip, 9 medullary hip, 41 total knee, and 1 TSA. Among them, 48 cases (43%) involved mobile part exchange, while 64 did not. After a mean follow-up of 3.3 years, 84% of patients remained in remission. Remission was not associated with PJI localization, pathogen type, number of surgical debridements, antibiotic duration, immunosuppression, or age. However, exchanging mobile components nearly doubled the likelihood of long-term remission [10].

5.5 Factors Negatively Impacting DAIR Success

Boyer and Cazorla (2021) identified risk factors reducing DAIR success: fracture or revision arthroplasty, cement use, bacteremia, kidney/liver failure, immunosuppression, and elevated CRP. Hematogenous infections had worse prognoses than early postoperative infections (Fig. 5.1). Open DAIR resolved infections in approximately 75% of cases, with functional outcomes comparable to primary hip/knee arthroplasties. A second DAIR procedure was not recommended if the first failed. *Cutibacterium acnes* infections require special attention in RSA due to diagnostic challenges [3].

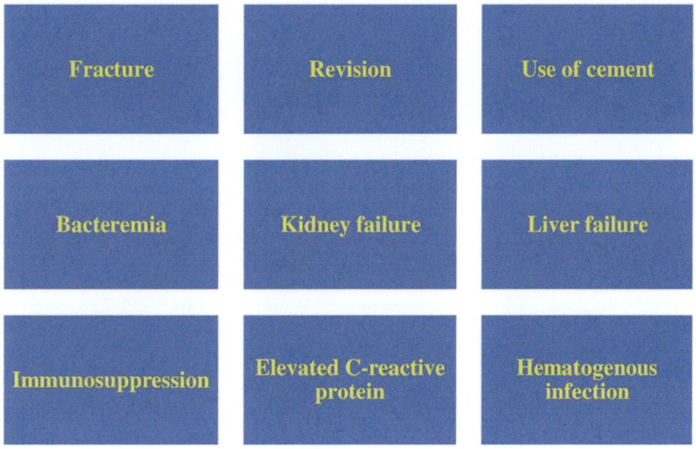

Fig. 5.1 Factors that negatively influence the likelihood of a successful open DAIR (debridement, antibiotic, and implant retention) procedure

5.6 Open DAIR for *Serratia marcescens* Infections

Lim et al. (2022) reported a case of infected RSA in a 73-year-old man previously treated for methicillin-resistant *Staphylococcus epidermidis* nonunion. The patient developed a sinus tract 16 days post-RSA implantation and was diagnosed with *Serratia marcescens* PJI. Successful treatment with open DAIR led to infection resolution after 4 years [2].

5.7 Effect of Rifampicin Resistance on Recovery Rates

Krizsán et al. (2023) analyzed rifampicin resistance in DAIR-treated PJIs, involving 67 patients (44 hip, 21 knee, 1 shoulder, 1 elbow) [11]. Rifampicin-sensitive infections were found in 47 cases, with 72.3% recovery in the sensitive and 76.9% in the resistant cohort. No significant difference was observed between groups, but age and diabetes negatively influenced recovery rates. *Staphylococcus aureus* and coagulase-negative *Staphylococci* were predominant in rifampicin-sensitive cases, while gram-negative rods prevailed in resistant cases. Rifampicin resistance had no significant clinical impact on recovery [11].

5.8 Open DAIR Versus Revision Strategies in Shoulder PJI

Lemmens et al. (2021) compared open DAIR, one-stage, and two-stage revision for shoulder PJI in 36 patients [12]. Recurrence was found in four patients (11%), all initially treated with open DAIR. Implant exchange did not compromise functional outcomes, supporting revision over DAIR for chronic infections. Kew et al. (2024) evaluated 65 patients treated with DAIR (26%), one-stage revision (9%), and two-stage revision (65%) [13]. No differences were observed in reinfection or complication rates across groups. Individuals experiencing open DAIR were diagnosed substantially earlier than those experiencing one- and two-stage revision procedures (Fig. 5.2).

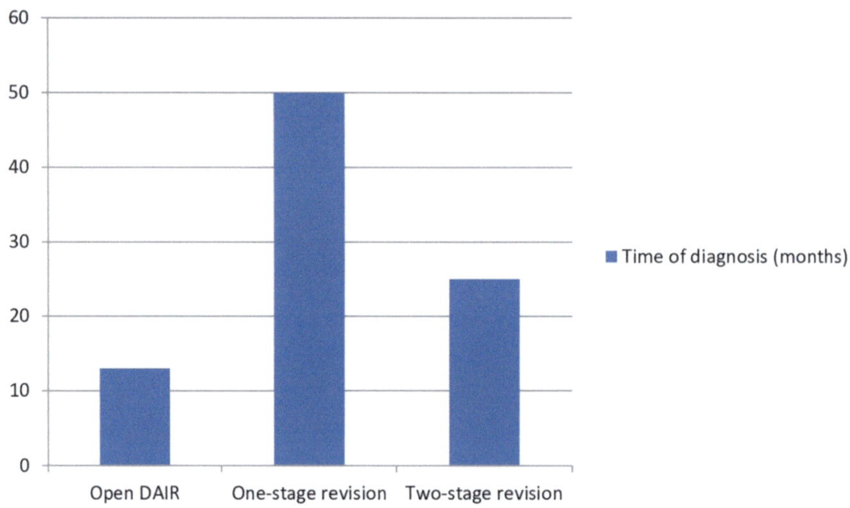

Fig. 5.2 Individuals experiencing open DAIR (debridement, antibiotic, and implant retention) were diagnosed substantially earlier than those experiencing one- and two-stage revision procedures

5.9 Conclusion

Open DAIR resolves the infection in about 75% of acute infections of shoulder arthroplasty. It is not advised to perform a second open DAIR if the first one fails. Changing mobile parts of PJI during the open DAIR procedure almost doubles the likelihood of long-run remission.

References

1. Bdeir M, Dally FJ, Assaf E, Gravius S, Mohs E, Hetjens S, et al. Periprosthetic infections of the shoulder joint: characteristics and 5-year outcome of a single-center series of 19 cases. Antibiotics (Basel). 2021;10(9):1125. https://doi.org/10.3390/antibiotics10091125.
2. Lim S, Lee JB, Shin MY, Jeon IH. Debridement, antibiotics, and implant retention in infected shoulder arthroplasty caused by Serratia marcescens: a case report. Clin Shoulder Elb. 2022;25(2):154–7. https://doi.org/10.5397/cise.2021.00479.
3. Boyer B, Cazorla C. Methods and probability of success after early revision of prosthetic joint infections with debridement, antibiotics and implant retention. Orthop Traumatol Surg Res. 2021;107(1S):102774. https://doi.org/10.1016/j.otsr.2020.102774.
4. Levy PY, Fenollar F, Stein A, Borrione F, Cohen E, Lebail B, et al. Propionibacterium acnes postoperative shoulder arthritis: an emerging clinical entity. Clin Infect Dis. 2008;46(12):1884–6. https://doi.org/10.1086/588477.
5. Boisrenoult P. Cutibacterium acnes prosthetic joint infection: diagnosis and treatment. Orthop Traumatol Surg Res. 2018;104(1S):S19–24. https://doi.org/10.1016/j.otsr.2017.05.030.
6. Lutz M-F, Berthelot P, Fresard A, Cazorla C, Carricajo A, Vautrin A-C, et al. Arthroplastic and osteosynthetic infections due to Propionibacterium acnes: a retrospective study of 52 cases, 1995–2002. Eur J Clin Microbiol Infect Dis. 2005;24(11):739–44. https://doi.org/10.1007/s10096-005-0040-8.
7. Jacquot A, Sirveaux F, Roche O, Favard L, Clavert P, Molé D. Surgical management of the infected reversed shoulder arthroplasty: a French multicenter study of reoperation in 32 patients. J Shoulder Elbow Surg. 2015;24(11):1713–22. https://doi.org/10.1016/j.jse.2015.03.007.
8. Rodríguez-Pardo D, Pigrau C, Lora-Tamayo J, Soriano A, del Toro MD, Cobo J, et al. REIPI Group for the Study of Prosthetic Infection. Gram-negative prosthetic joint infection: outcome of a debridement, antibiotics and implant retention approach. A large multicentre study. Clin

Microbiol Infect. 2014;20(11):O911–9. https://doi.org/10.1111/1469-0691.12649.
9. Morata L, Senneville E, Bernard L, Nguyen S, Buzelé R, Druon J, et al. A retrospective review of the clinical experience of linezolid with or without rifampicin in prosthetic joint infections treated with debridement and implant retention. Infect Dis Ther. 2014;3(2):235–43. https://doi.org/10.1007/s40121-014-0032-z.
10. Hirsiger S, Betz M, Stafylakis D, Götschi T, Lew D, Uçkay I. The benefice of mobile parts' exchange in the management of infected total joint arthroplasties with prosthesis retention (DAIR procedure). J Clin Med. 2019;8(2):226. https://doi.org/10.3390/jcm8020226.
11. Krizsán G, Sallai I, Veres DS, Prinz G, Kovács M, Skaliczki G. Investigation of the effect of rifampicin resistance and risk factors on recovery rates after DAIR procedure in patients with prosthetic joint infection. J Orthop Surg Res. 2023;18(1):611. https://doi.org/10.1186/s13018-023-04091-y.
12. Lemmens L, Geelen H, Depypere M, De Munter P, Verhaegen F, Zimmerli W, et al. Management of periprosthetic infection after reverse shoulder arthroplasty. J Shoulder Elbow Surg. 2021;30(11):2514–22. https://doi.org/10.1016/j.jse.2021.04.014.
13. Kew ME, Mathew JI, Wimberly AC, Fu MC, Taylor SA, Blaine TA, et al. Outcomes after débridement, antibiotics, and implant retention for prosthetic joint infection in shoulder arthroplasty. J Shoulder Elbow Surg. 2024;33(2):e68–78. https://doi.org/10.1016/j.jse.2023.06.012.

6 Revision Total Shoulder Arthroplasty for Periprosthetic Joint Infection

E. Carlos Rodríguez-Merchán
and Alfonso Vaquero-Picado

6.1 Introduction

Periprosthetic joint infection (PJI) can be a devastating complication following total shoulder arthroplasty (TSA) [1]. The global incidence of prosthetic joint infection ranges from 0.7% to 7% [2]. The most frequent organisms related to shoulder PJI are *Propionibacterium acnes*, *Staphylococcus aureus*, *Staphylococcus epidermidis*, and coagulase-negative *Staphylococcus* [2]. In a level 3 of evidence study published in 2022 by Austin et al., 1160 revision shoulder prosthesis procedures were classified as either septic (21.8%) or aseptic (78.2%). The most frequent bacterium isolated was *Cutibacterium acnes* (64.4%) [1]. The purpose of this chapter is to analyze the most recent data on open revision arthroplasty for PJI in TSA.

6.2 Outcomes of Revision Before 2020

According to Egglestone et al. (2019), eradication rates of shoulder PJI varied from 54% to 100% for DAIR (debridement, antibiotics, and implant retention) procedures; 66–100% for permanent spacers; 50–100% following one-stage revision; 60–100% following two-stage revision; and 66–100% following resection arthroplasty [2]. This data reflect that there is a wide variability in eradication rate of PJI depending on the author and treatment.

In a scoping review published in 2019 by Mercurio et al., it was found that *Cutibacterium acnes* was the most frequent microorganism causing shoulder PJI (33%). It is also the main cause of persistent infections (40%) [3]. These data have also been reported in other studies [1, 2]. In the study by Mercurio et al., eradication rate was 96% with one-stage revision, 93% with permanent spacers, 86% with two-stage revision, 85% with resection arthroplasty, and 65% with DAIR. One-stage revision was also the best option when considering postoperative function (especially in postoperative flexion and abduction), compared with resection arthroplasty, permanent spacers, and two-stage revision. One-stage revision also exhibited fewer postoperative complications than DAIR, resection arthroplasty, and two-stage revision. Mercurio et al. suggested that a one-stage revision could be the best option to treat shoulder PJI. The authors recommend reserving two-stage revision for selected individuals in whom the implicated bacterium is unknown [3].

E. C. Rodríguez-Merchán (✉) · A. Vaquero-Picado
Department of Orthopedic Surgery, Hospital Universitario La Paz, Madrid, Madrid, Spain

E. C. Rodríguez-Merchán (ed.), *Advances in Periprosthetic Joint Infection*,
https://doi.org/10.1007/978-3-032-02945-4_6

6.3 Outcomes of Revision After 2000

6.3.1 One-Stage Revision

In 2023, Bastard et al. analyzed 37 individuals with chronic shoulder PJI who underwent single-stage revision. The most frequently isolated pathogen was *Cutibacterium acnes* (68%), isolated alone (15 individuals, 41%) or as a part of polymicrobial infections (10 individuals, 27%). The primary outcome was the 2-year reinfection-free rate. The reinfection-free rate was 94.6% (35/37 cases). Outcomes from this study suggested that one-stage revision could be a good treatment option with a low infection recurrence rate [4].

In 2023, El Amiri et al. reported the results (infection eradication, functional, and radiographic outcomes) after systematic one-stage revision, without preoperative selection of individuals, in chronic (more than 3 weeks) shoulder PJI [5]. They analyzed 40 individuals (14 women and 26 men). The primary endpoint was the lack of signs of persistent infection at a minimum 2-year follow-up. Secondary endpoints were clinical and radiological results. At final follow-up, 36/40 (90%) individuals had no recurrence of infection. In 45% (18/40) of the individuals, the microbial organism was unknown at the time of surgery. *Cutibacterium acnes* was the most common pathogen, encountered in 67.5% (27/40) of the individuals. The infection was polymicrobial in 40% (16/40) of the individuals. At final follow-up, mean absolute constant score was 48.4 and weighted score was 65.5%, and satisfaction was assessed by the individuals as excellent or good in 75% (30/40). Approximately 20% (8/40) of the individuals had a postoperative complication. The authors concluded that one-stage revision procedure, combined with appropriate antibiotic therapy, made it possible to eradicate the PJI in 90% of the shoulders, with satisfactory functional results.

6.3.2 Two-Stage Revision

In 2020, Brown et al. reported the outcomes of two-stage revision arthroplasty, including eradication of infection and reoperation rates [6]. They retrospectively reviewed individuals who experienced revision arthroplasty for shoulder PJI between 2006 and 2015. Cases were confirmed using Musculoskeletal Infection Society (MSIS) and American Academy of Orthopedic Surgeons (AAOS) guidelines. Their protocol included total shoulder arthroplasty removal, debridement and irrigation, insertion of an antibiotic-loaded cement spacer, and a minimum of 6 weeks of intravenous antibiotics. Reimplantation was performed as a second stage following a negative aspirate. Twenty-eight individuals underwent a first-stage procedure (mean age 69 years; 16 male, 12 female). *Cutibacterium acnes,* methicillin-sensitive *Staphylococcus aureus,* coagulase-negative *Staphylococcus* spp., and *Staphylococcus epidermidis* were the most frequent microorganisms cultured. Five individuals had mixed growths and six individuals had no growth. Three individuals did not proceed to a second stage. Twenty-five individuals experienced reimplantation (mean interval 6.7 months), with 80% remaining infection-free (mean follow-up 38.3 months). Thus, in this study, the authors concluded that managing complex and late presentation shoulder PJI with two-stage revision was associated with high rates of infection eradication (80%) [6].

In 2021, Klingebiel et al. analyzed 16 individuals experiencing two-stage revision after shoulder PJI [7]. Postoperative scores and range of motion (ROM) were compared in a subgroup analysis according to different reimplanted prosthesis types. The reinfection-free implant survival was 81% after 1 year and at final follow-up (mean 33.2 months). The overall revision-free survival was 56% after 1 year and at final follow-up. So, even if the infection was well addressed in almost four out of five cases, almost 25% of the successful cases needed additional surgery.

Individuals who underwent reverse shoulder arthroplasty (RSA) as part of reimplantation had less disability and long-term complications. This cohort showed better subjective stability and function compared with individuals revised to megaprostheses or large-head hemiarthroplasties. Two-stage revision following PJI of the shoulder allowed adequate infection control in the majority of individuals. However, the overall complications and revision rates due to mechanical failure or reinfection were high. Reimplantation of RSA appeared superior to alternative prosthesis models in terms of function and patient satisfaction [7]. Thus, in comparison with the classical approach to infected arthroplasties, reconstruction with RSA provides a similar rate of infection control while improving mechanical function after surgery.

In 2023, Lo et al. analyzed 38 individuals who underwent a staged RSA for the treatment of PJI [8]. All individuals underwent the first stage with implant removal, irrigation, debridement, and antibiotic spacer placement. Next, intravenous antibiotics were administered for a minimum of 6 weeks. Infection workup was then repeated and, if normalized, final-stage revision started with antibiotic spacer removal and revision to RSA. If indices were persistently abnormal, an additional stage of debridement and spacer placement procedure was carried out. Treatment failure was defined as recurrent PJI after final prosthesis implantation or persistently elevated indices despite appropriate debridement and spacer placement. Mean age of the cohort was 68 years and mean follow-up was 33 months, with 34 Cierny-Mader C hosts and 4 B hosts. Individuals underwent a mean of two previous surgeries. The staged revision protocol was successful in 34 (89.5%) individuals for management of PJI. Four individuals (10.5%) were considered failures with recurrent infections at a mean of 13 months after the final RSA implantation and experienced repeat staged revisions. Of the 34 individuals who had successful infection eradication, 31 had two-stage treatment and 3 had to undergo three stages (7.9% of initial PJI). There were no treatment-associated mortalities and 10 major complications (26%), including permanent neuropathy, instability, and periprosthetic fractures. The most frequently cultured microorganism was *Cutibacterium acnes* (18%), with no polymicrobial infections observed. It seemed that staged revision provides an efficacious therapeutic alternative. Although there were several individuals who needed an additional stage of treatment, and a substantial complication rate, staged revision RSA proved successful in the eradication of shoulder PJI [8].

6.4 Single-Stage Versus Two-Stage Revision

In a systematic review and meta-analysis published in 2020, Belay et al. compared the role of single- and two-stage shoulder arthroplasty revision for PJI [9]. Inclusion criteria for this systematic review were studies that reported on one-stage or two-stage revision, with infection eradication and a minimum follow-up of 12 months and a minimum of five individuals for analysis. The majority of positive cultures from one-stage revision for PJI identified *Cutibacterium acnes* in 113 of 232 (48.7%) reported cases compared with 190 of 566 (33.7%) reported cases for two-stage revision. There was a lower percentage of methicillin-resistant *Staphylococcus aureus* positive cultures, with 2.5% for one-stage compared with 9.7% for two-stage revision. Reinfection rate was 6.3% for one-stage and 10.1% for two-stage revision, but there was no statistical significance. Based on this systematic review and meta-analysis, one-stage revision for shoulder PJI was an effective treatment, with a better eradication rate. However, this was likely confounded by a treatment bias given the higher propensity of virulent and drug-resistant bacteria treated with two-stage in the published literature [9].

In another systematic review published in 2023, Fiore et al. compared the outcomes in the literature in one-stage and two-stage protocols in the treatment of shoulder PJI [10]. A total of 486 shoulder PJIs were included: 137 treated with one-stage and 349 with two-stage procedure. A similar distribution between early and not-early infections (19.1% vs. 80.9%) was encountered between the two cohorts. The overall rate of success in terms of PJI eradication was significantly higher in the one-stage cohort (95.6% vs. 85.7%). The noninfection-related complications rate was 13.8% in the one-stage cohort and 37.6% in the two-stage cohort, while the noninfection-related

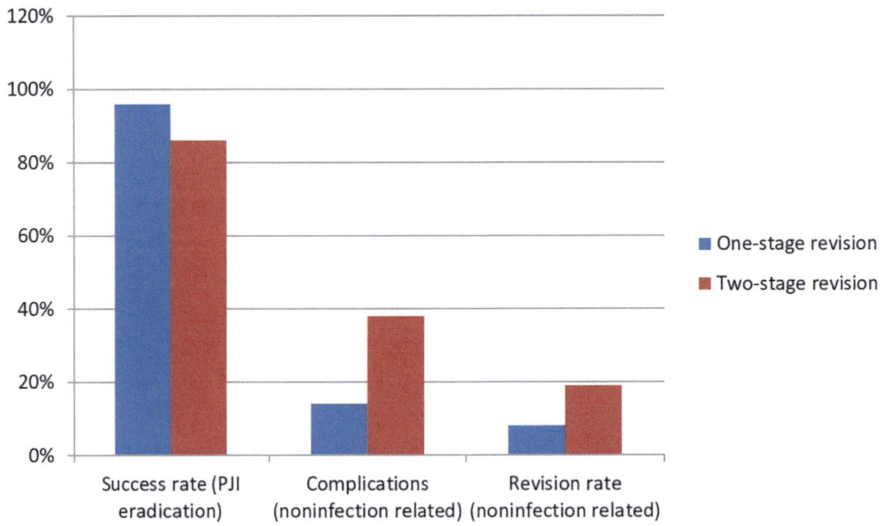

Fig. 6.1 One-stage revision shoulder arthroplasty versus two-stage revision shoulder arthroplasty in periprosthetic joint infection (PJI): rates of success (in terms of PJI eradication), noninfected-related complications, and noninfection-related revision

revision rate was 8% and 18.9%, respectively (Fig. 6.1). The single-phase protocol showed a higher success rate in eradicating the infection and a lower complication rate. However, the low number of individuals, the low quality of the articles, and the lack of data on clinical severity and bacteriological virulence suggested caution in conclusions [10].

In 2023, Rodrigues-Lopes et al. performed another systematic review of the literature and meta-analysis [11]. A total of 185 shoulders were reported in one-stage revision studies, whereas 526 shoulders were reported in two-stage revision studies. The overall pooled random-effects reinfection rate was 6.68%. One-stage revision exhibited a reinfection rate of 1.14%, whereas two-stage revision analysis showed a reinfection rate of 8.81%. This difference was statistically significant. The overall pooled rate for other clinical complications was 16.76%. One-stage revision had a complication rate of 6.11%, whereas the two-stage revision complication rate was 21.26% (Fig. 6.2). According to Rodrigues-Lopes et al., this was the first systematic review and meta-analysis demonstrating significant statistical differences between one-stage and two-stage revision in infected shoulder arthroplasties [11].

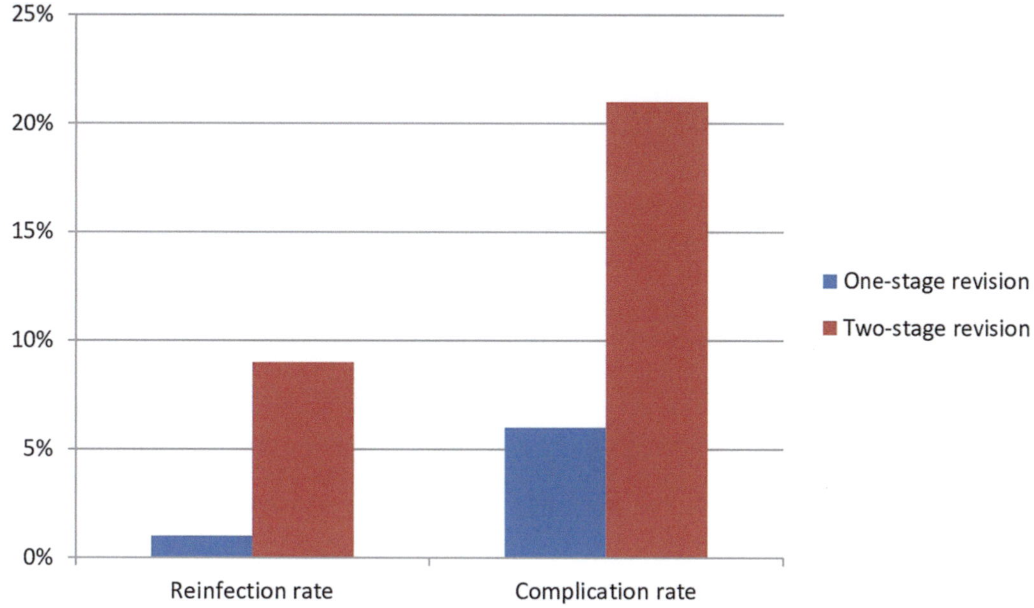

Fig. 6.2 One-stage revision shoulder arthroplasty versus two-stage revision shoulder arthroplasty in periprosthetic joint infection (PJI): rates of reinfection and complication

6.5 A Three-Stage Protocol

In 2019, Tseng et al. assessed results after treatment of shoulder PJI with a three-stage revision protocol consisting of (1) debridement, explantation, and cement spacer placement, followed by parenteral antibiotics; (2) open biopsy and debridement; and (3) reimplantation if cultures were negative [12]. They retrospectively analyzed a prospectively collected revision shoulder arthroplasty group to identify individuals with shoulder PJI treated with a three-stage protocol. Outcomes for individuals with shoulder PJI and revision to RSA were compared with individuals revised to RSA for noninfectious indications. There were 28 cases of shoulder PJI in 27 individuals (mean age, 66.4 years); of these, 21 shoulders were revised to RSA, and 7 shoulders were revised to hemiarthroplasty. There was no recurrent infection in this cohort at a mean 32-month follow-up. The 21 shoulders with PJI revised to RSA had no differences in functional and subjective outcomes compared with revision RSA without shoulder PJI. A three-stage revision protocol for shoulder PJI dependably eradicated infection. Individuals with PJI revised to RSA can have similar results as individuals with noninfectious revision to RSA [12].

6.6 Pyrocarbon as a Functional Spacer for the Treatment of Recalcitrant Shoulder Infections

According to Barret and Boileau (2024), the most frequent treatment approach in chronic shoulder PJI is a two-stage revision involving interval placement of an antibiotic cement spacer or resection arthroplasty [13]. In their study, they assessed whether Pyrocarbon spacers could be used as a temporary or permanent functional spacer.

The primary objective was to evaluate the rate of infection eradication after temporary or definitive implantation of Pyrocarbon Interposition Shoulder Arthroplasty (PISA) in individuals with recalcitrant chronic PJI. The secondary objective was to evaluate mid-run clinical and radiographic results. Fifteen individuals (mean age: 52 years) with chronic shoulder infection experienced, after joint debridement, implantation of PISA (InSpyre; Tornier-Stryker, Kalamazoo, MI, USA) with tailored perioperative antibiotics. In 7 cases, PJI occurred after hemiarthroplasty (N = 2), reverse shoulder arthroplasty (N = 2), hemireverse (N = 2), and resurfacing arthroplasty (N = 1). In the remaining 8 cases, PJI occurred in the context of failed surgery after fracture sequelae (N = 4), instability (N = 2), and cuff arthropathy (N = 2). Preoperatively, individuals had a mean of 3 previous failed surgeries prior to PISA implantation. Individuals were assessed with clinical, laboratory, and radiographic evaluation at a minimum of 2 years after surgery. At a mean follow-up of 55 months, no individual experienced reinfection after temporary (3 cases) or definitive (12 cases) PISA implantation. On final radiographs of definitive PISA, complete humeral densification, or a neocortex, formed around the implant in 64% (7/11). This study suggested that, after washout, debridement and tailored antibiotics, PISA can be utilized as a temporary or definitive functional spacer for the management of recalcitrant shoulder PJI and presents the following advantages: (1) PISA does not appear to be a risk for recurrent infection thanks to the antibacterial property of Pyrocarbon; (2) PISA can be utilized as a temporary or a definitive spacer without causing bone erosion, thanks to the low modulus of elasticity of Pyrocarbon; (3) PISA can be utilized as a salvage procedure in case of complete glenoid or humeral destruction, thanks to the sphericity of the implant requiring no implant anchorage [13].

6.7 Conclusions

Sometimes, septic loosening is not well observed in short term, especially in low-grade infections. In Fig. 6.3, the patient complained of pain for two years. The initial X-ray did not show any change [image (a)]. In image (b), resorption of bone around the humeral without stem loosening was observed. In this case, the surgeon's preference was to perform revision in a two-stage fashion because of the bone defect, long-term infection, and the high charge of microorganisms.

As we have seen above, recent literature analysis on revision shoulder arthroplasty after PJI reveals that one-stage procedures showed better results in eradication of infection, reinfection, and a lower rate of complications in comparison with two-stage procedures. Although many of the reports that exist in literature are lacking of enough number of cases for analysis, aggregated data on systematic reviews and meta-analyses confirmed this trend. However, these are very complex problems that depend on the patient characteristics, shoulder conditions, implants, and microorganisms, so more prospective, randomized, and multicenter studies are needed to elucidate what is the best treatment for each patient.

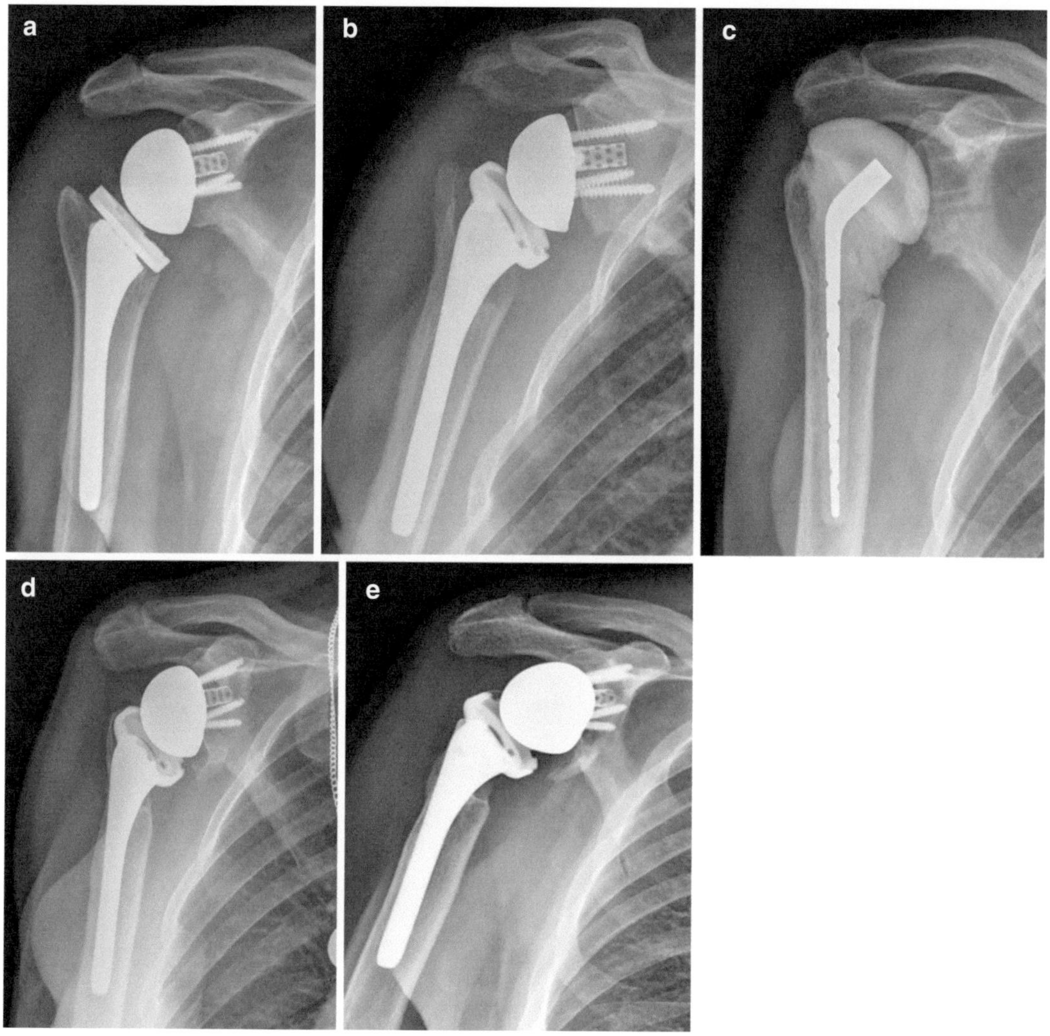

Fig. 6.3 (**a**–**e**). Sometimes, septic loosening is not well observed in short term, especially in low-grade infections. In this case, the patient complained of pain for two years. Initial X-ray did not show any change (**a**). In image (**b**), resorption of bone around the humeral component without stem loosening was observed. In this case, the surgeon's preference was to perform revision in a two-stage fashion because of the bone defect, long-term infection, and the high charge of microorganisms (**c**–**e**)

References

1. Austin DC, Townsley SH, Rogers TH, Barlow JD, Morrey ME, Sperling JW, et al. Shoulder periprosthetic joint infection and all-cause mortality: a worrisome association. JB JS Open Access. 2022;7(1):e21.00118. https://doi.org/10.2106/JBJS.OA.21.00118.
2. Egglestone A, Ingoe H, Rees J, Thomas M, Jeavons R, Rangan A. Scoping review: diagnosis and management of periprosthetic joint infection in shoulder arthroplasty. Shoulder Elbow. 2019;11(3):167–81. https://doi.org/10.1177/1758573218779076.
3. Mercurio M, Castioni D, Iannò B, Gasparini G, Galasso O. Outcomes of revision surgery after periprosthetic shoulder infection: a systematic review. J Shoulder Elbow Surg. 2019;28(6):1193–203. https://doi.org/10.1016/j.jse.2019.02.014.
4. Bastard C, Aïm F, Meyssonnier V, Kerroumi Y, Marion B, Zeller V, et al. One-stage revision for infected shoulder arthroplasty: prospective, observational study of 37 patients. JSES Int. 2023;7(6):2433–9. https://doi.org/10.1016/j.jseint.2023.06.021.

5. El Amiri L, Clavert P, Gaudias J, Klein S, Rondé Oustau C, Antoni M. High infection control rate after systematic one-stage procedure for shoulder arthroplasty chronic infection. Int Orthop. 2023;47(11):2809–26. https://doi.org/10.1007/s00264-023-05927-2.
6. Brown M, Eseonu K, Rudge W, Warren S, Majed A, Bayley I, et al. The management of infected shoulder arthroplasty by two-stage revision. Shoulder Elbow. 2020;12(1 Suppl):70–80. https://doi.org/10.1177/1758573219841057.
7. Klingebiel S, Theil C, Gosheger G, Schneider KN, Ackmann T, Timme M, et al. Clinical outcome of two-stage revision after periprosthetic shoulder infection. J Clin Med. 2021;10(2):218. https://doi.org/10.3390/jcm10020218.
8. Lo EY, Ouseph A, Badejo M, Lund J, Bettacchi C, Garofalo R, et al. Success of staged revision reverse total shoulder arthroplasty in eradication of periprosthetic joint infection. J Shoulder Elbow Surg. 2023;32(3):625–35. https://doi.org/10.1016/j.jse.2022.09.006.
9. Belay ES, Danilkowicz R, Bullock G, Wall K, Garrigues GE. Single-stage versus two-stage revision for shoulder periprosthetic joint infection: a systematic review and meta-analysis. J Shoulder Elbow Surg. 2020;29(12):2476–86. https://doi.org/10.1016/j.jse.2020.05.034.
10. Fiore M, Ferra L, Giannini C, Sambri A, Filippini M, Tedeschi S, et al. Management of periprosthetic joint infection of shoulder arthroplasty: single-stage versus two-stage protocols. A systematic review and meta-analysis of the literature. Shoulder Elbow. 2023;15(1 Suppl):25–40. https://doi.org/10.1177/17585732221116839.
11. Rodrigues-Lopes R, Silva F, Torres J. Periprosthetic shoulder infection management: one-stage should be the way: a systematic review and meta-analysis. J Shoulder Elbow Surg. 2024;33(3):722–37. https://doi.org/10.1016/j.jse.2023.09.007.
12. Tseng WJ, Lansdown DA, Grace T, Zhang AL, Feeley BT, Hung LW, et al. Outcomes of revision arthroplasty for shoulder periprosthetic joint infection: a three-stage revision protocol. J Shoulder Elbow Surg. 2019;28(2):268–75. https://doi.org/10.1016/j.jse.2018.07.014.
13. Barret H, Boileau P. Can Pyrocarbon be used as a functional spacer for the treatment of recalcitrant shoulder infections? JSES Int. 2024;8(1):167–75. https://doi.org/10.1016/j.jseint.2023.09.005.

Periprosthetic Joint Infection in Total Elbow Arthroplasty

7

E. Carlos Rodríguez-Merchán
and Amir R. Kachooei

7.1 Introduction

Periprosthetic joint infection (PJI) is a relatively frequent and oftentimes devastating complication after total elbow arthroplasty (TEA) [1]. In the study of Somerson et al. (2019) of 1452 individuals, the rate of PJI after TEA was 3.7% (54/1452). There were 30 (56%) early infections, 17 (31%) delayed infections, and 7 (13%) late infections [2] (Fig. 7.1). According to Gutman et al. (2020), *Staphylococcus aureus* was the most frequently isolated organism (42.4%), followed by coagulase-negative staphylococci (32.6%) [3]. This chapter aims to analyze the most recent data on open revision arthroplasty for PJI in TEA.

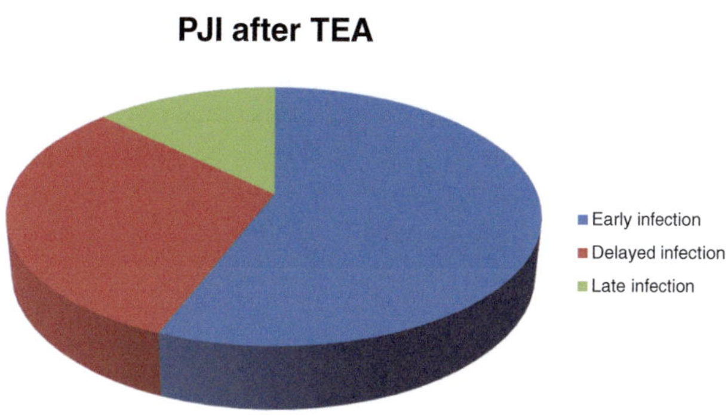

Fig. 7.1 Types of periprosthetic joint infection (PJI) after total elbow arthroplasty (TEA)

E. C. Rodríguez-Merchán (✉)
Department of Orthopedic Surgery, Hospital Universitario La Paz, Madrid, Madrid, Spain

A. R. Kachooei
Department of Orthopedic Surgery, Rothman Orthopedics Florida at AdventHealth, Orlando, FL, USA

E. C. Rodríguez-Merchán (ed.), *Advances in Periprosthetic Joint Infection*,
https://doi.org/10.1007/978-3-032-02945-4_7

7.2 Diagnosis

Flurin et al. (2021) found that the combination of sonicate fluid and periprosthetic tissue culture had a greater sensitivity than that for microbiologic diagnosis of PJI after TEA [1]. They retrospectively analyzed 112 sonicate fluid cultures from individuals who experienced revision of a TEA, comparing results with those of periprosthetic tissue cultures. They excluded individuals who had fewer than two tissues submitted for culture. Utilizing the Infectious Diseases Society of America guidelines to define PJI, 49 infected and 63 noninfected cases were found. The median ages in the PJI and noninfected cohorts were 66 and 61, respectively. In the noninfected cohort, 65% were women versus 63% in the PJI cohort. Flurin et al. calculated the sensitivity and specificity of periprosthetic tissue culture compared with sonicate fluid culture. Besides, they compared the sensitivity of periprosthetic tissue culture to the combination of periprosthetic tissue culture and sonicate fluid culture. The most frequent pathogens were coagulase-negative *Staphylococcus saprophyticus* (49%), followed by *Staphylococcus aureus* (12%). The sensitivity of periprosthetic tissue culture was 63%, and sonicate fluid culture was 76%. The specificity of periprosthetic tissue culture was 94%, and the specificity of sonicate fluid culture was 100%. The sensitivity of sonicate fluid culture in combination with periprosthetic tissue culture was 84% [1].

In 2021, Flurin et al. compared 16S ribosomal RNA (rRNA) gene PCR (*polymerase chain reaction*) followed by next-generation sequencing (NGS) to a culture of sonicate fluid derived from TEA for PJI diagnosis [4]. They found that 16S rRNA gene-based targeted metagenomic analysis of sonicate fluid was more sensitive than culture. Sonicate fluids collected from individuals who experienced TEA revision were analyzed retrospectively. PCR amplification of the V1–V3 region of the 16S rRNA gene was carried out, followed by NGS utilizing an Illumina MiSeq. Results were compared with those of a sonicate fluid culture using McNemar's test of paired proportions. Forty-seven periprosthetic joint infections and 58 noninfectious arthroplasty failures were studied. The sensitivity of targeted NGS was 85%, compared with 77% for culture. Specificity and positive and negative predictive values of targeted NGS were 98%, 98%, and 89%, respectively, compared with 100%, 100%, and 84%, respectively, for culture. 16S rRNA gene-based targeted metagenomic analysis of sonicate fluid was more sensitive than culture [4].

7.3 Risk Factors for Elbow PJI

In a study with level 3 of evidence, Somerson et al. (2019) demonstrated that significant risk factors for PJI were hypothyroidism, tobacco use disorder, and rheumatoid arthritis. Preoperative optimization of thyroid function, smoking cessation, and treatment of rheumatoid arthritis might be considered in surgical candidates for TEA [2]. According to Gutman et al. (2020), risk factors for developing elbow PJI include rheumatoid arthritis, steroid use, an immunocompromised state, and previous elbow surgery [3]. Figure 7.2 summarizes the main risk factors for elbow PJI.

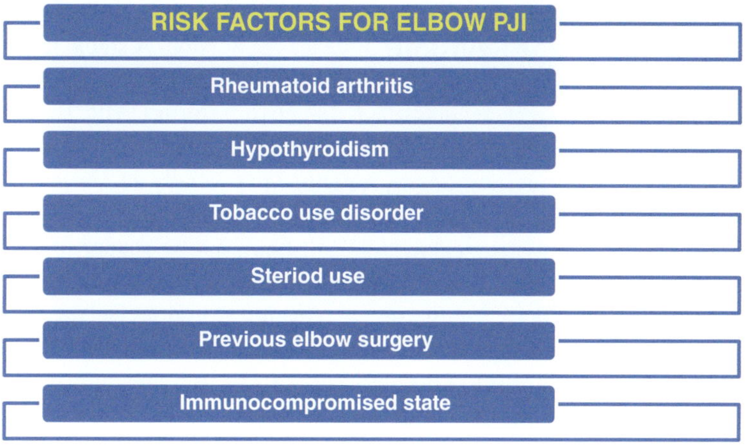

Fig. 7.2 Risk factors for periprosthetic joint infection (PJI) after total elbow arthroplasty (TEA)

7.4 Perioperative Antibiotic Choice Affects Rates of PJI in TEA

In 2023, Nieboer et al. reported that in primary TEA, cefazolin administration was associated with substantially lower PJI rates than non-cefazolin antibiotics, even in individuals with more prior surgeries. For individuals with penicillin or cephalosporin allergies, preoperative allergy testing or a cefazolin test dose should be considered prior to administering non-cefazolin alternatives [5].

7.5 Treatment of Elbow PJI

7.5.1 Open Debridement, Antibiotics, and Implant Retention (DAIR)

In 2023, Tai et al. analyzed the outcomes of 26 DAIR procedures [6]. DAIR failed in 17 cases of elbow PJI with a failure rate of 65% at 2 years. The median time to failure from DAIR was 43 days. It was found that DAIR failed in all cases with sinus tracts or negative cultures. The group with favorable results had a shorter median duration of symptoms (5 vs. 18 days) and a higher proportion of monomicrobial infections (58.8% vs. 88.9%) than those with unfavorable results. DAIR for elbow PJI was associated with high rates of failure. Possible risk factors for failure may include the presence of sinus tract, longer duration of symptoms, and culture-negative infection. Although the relatively low morbidity of DAIR compared with TEA implant resection for a one-stage or two-stage revision is attractive, individuals considered for DAIR must know that the chance of success is limited to about 35% [6].

7.5.2 Two-Stage Revision

In 2022, Martinez-Catalan studied the infection eradication rates, complications, and results in a group of individuals treated with two-stage revision for deep PJI following TEA [7]. They analyzed 52 elbows that underwent a two-stage revision for PJI after TEA. There were 22 men and 30 women, with a mean age of 61. The most common bacterium was *Staphylococcus epidermidis* (28 elbows). The mean follow-up time was 6 years. PJI was eradicated in 36 elbows (69%). The remaining 16 elbows were considered treatment failures secondary to recurrent infection. The risk of persistent infection was 3.3 times higher in elbows with retained cement and 3.5 times higher when the infecting organism was *Staphylococcus epidermidis* [7].

7.6 One-Stage Revision or Two-Stage Revision?

In a systematic review published in 2019, Kunutsor et al. compared the clinical efficacy of one- and two-stage revision surgery for elbow PJI utilizing reinfection (recurrent and new infections) rates; mortality; clinical measures of function, pain, and satisfaction; and noninfection-related adverse events. *Staphylococcus aureus* was the most frequent causative organism for PJI of the elbow (24 of 71 elbow PJIs). The reinfection rate for one-stage ranged from 0% to 16.7%, and that for two-stage revision ranged from 0% to 20%. Noninfection-related adverse event rate for one-stage was 16.7%, and that for two-stage ranged from 11.8% to 20%. No strong conclusions could be drawn because of limited data [8].

7.7 Results of Different Treatments for Elbow PJI

According to Goyal et al. (2020), evidence regarding an optimal treatment algorithm for PJI after TEA is limited. Initial management typically consists of either DAIR or a two-stage revision. A stable implant, a functioning triceps, and an intact soft tissue envelope are required to perform DAIR. Besides, DAIR is associated with a relatively high risk of infection recurrence, especially in chronic infections. Two-stage revision offers a lower recurrence risk, although there is a 25% chance of not completing the second stage. Resection arthroplasty, arthrodesis, and amputation are salvage options, whereas medical treatment, in the form of antibiotics alone, is reserved for poor surgical candidates [9].

In the systematic review reported by Gutman et al. (2020), the rate of successful infection eradication was highest with two-stage revision (81.2%) and lowest with DAIR (55.8%) [3] (Fig. 7.3). According to Rodriguez-Merchan et al. (2022), the rate of eradication of PJI is 73% with two-stage, 71% with resection arthroplasty, 67% with one-stage, 58% with DAIR, and 40% with elbow arthrodesis [10] (Fig. 7.4).

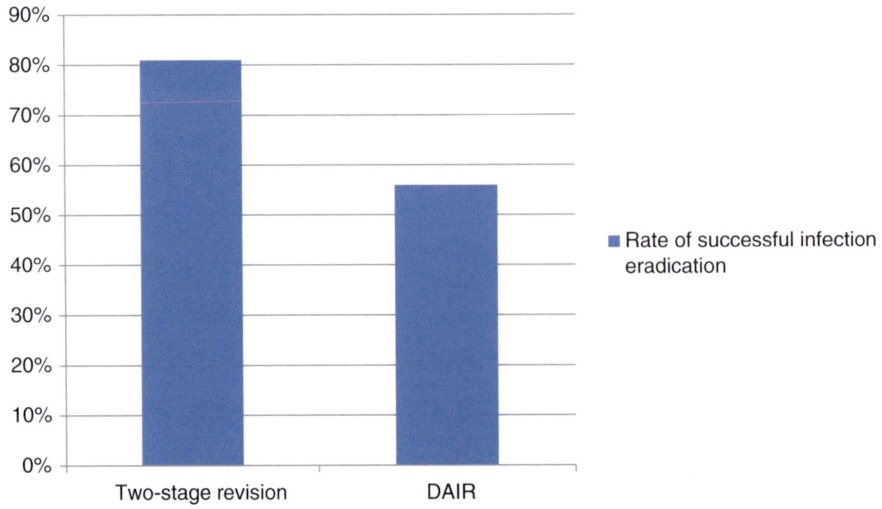

Fig. 7.3 Periprosthetic joint infection (PJI) after total elbow arthroplasty (TEA): Rates of successful infection eradication: Two-stage revision versus DAIR (debridement, antibiotics, and implant retention)

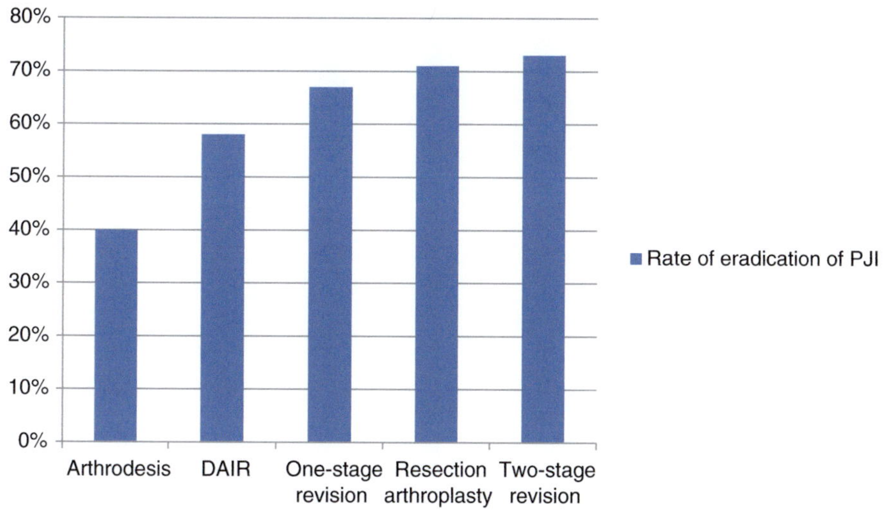

Fig. 7.4 Periprosthetic joint infection (PJI) after total elbow arthroplasty (TEA): Rates of successful infection eradication of different surgical procedures. DAIR = debridement, antibiotics, and implant retention

7.8 Impact of the Etiology of Primary TEA Failure on the Failure Rate of Revision Surgery

In 2020, DeBernardis et al. studied the impact of primary TEA failure etiology on the revision surgery failure rate [11]. A total of 46 individuals with a mean age of 62.7 years and a minimum 2-year follow-up were included. The etiologies of failure identified were infection (N = 20), aseptic loosening (N = 17), periprosthetic fracture (N = 6), and bushing wear (N = 3). All noninfectious etiologies were grouped into an additional cohort. Individuals who experienced revision for infection showed a substantially greater failure rate and a greater number of further revisions per patient than those with aseptic loosening, those with periprosthetic fracture, and the noninfectious cohort, as well as a shorter time to failure than the noninfectious cohort. Individuals whose primary TEA failed because of infection were more likely to experience revision failure and need a greater number of subsequent operations than individuals with other etiologies of primary TEA failure [11] (Fig. 7.5).

7.9 Conclusions

Periprosthetic joint infection (PJI) is a relatively frequent and oftentimes devastating complication after total elbow arthroplasty (TEA). The reported rate of PJI after TEA is around 4%. Risk factors for the development of elbow PJI include rheumatoid arthritis, hypothyroidism, tobacco use disorder, steroid use, previous elbow surgery, and immunocompromised state. Possible treatments of PJI after TEA are arthrodesis, DAIR (debridement, antibiotics, and implant retention), one-stage revision, two-stage revision and resection arthroplasty. The reported rates of eradication of PJI are 73% with two-stage, 71% with resection arthroplasty, 67% with one-stage, 58% with DAIR (open debridement, antibiotics, and implant retention), and 40% with elbow arthrodesis. Individuals in whom primary TEA failed because of infection were more likely to experience revision failure and need a greater number of subsequent operations than individuals with other etiologies of primary TEA failure.

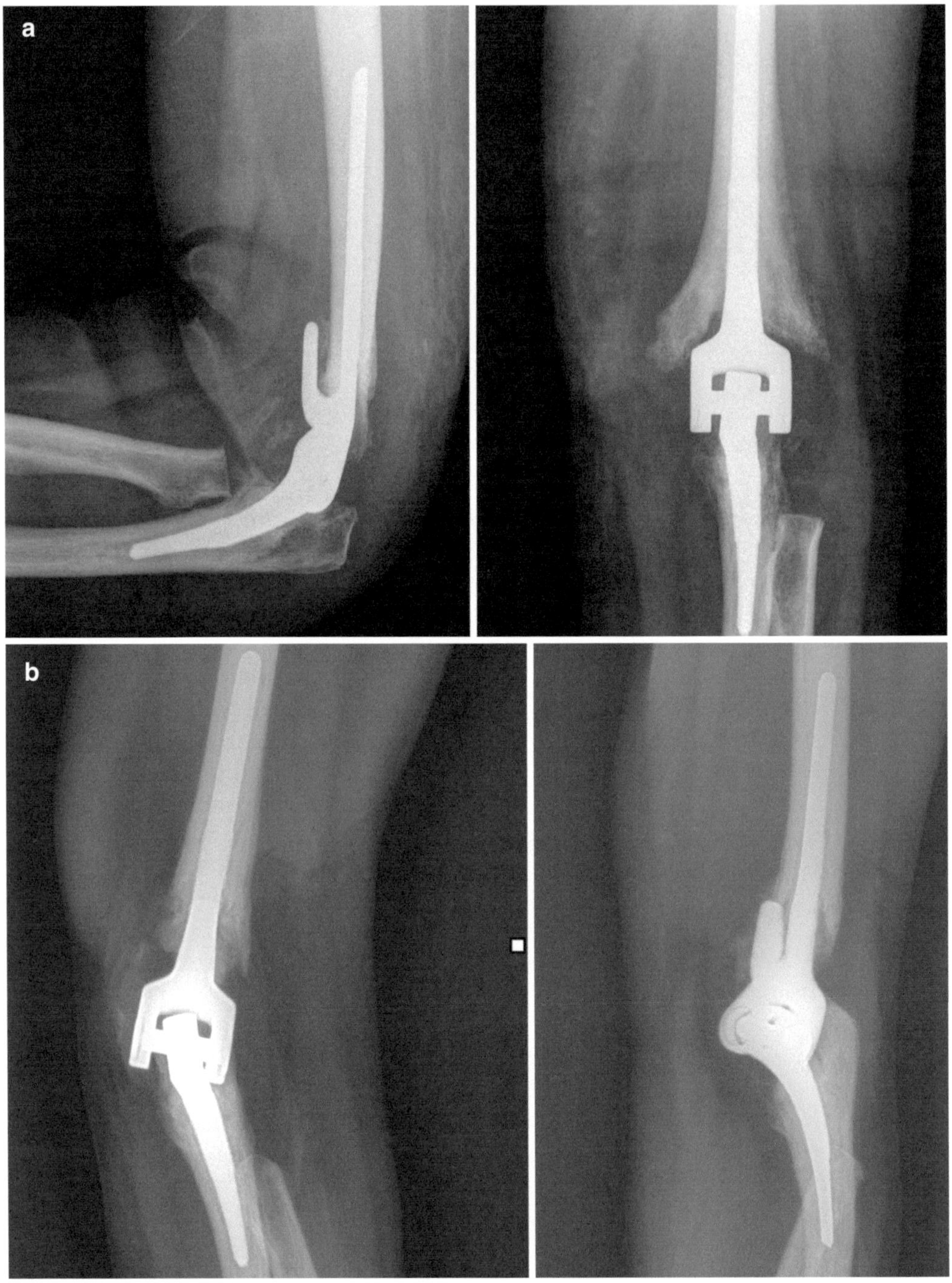

Fig. 7.5 (**a**–**f**). The image depicts the medical history of a 69-year-old female who underwent a total elbow arthroplasty (TEA) in 2007 due to posttraumatic arthritis (**a**). Over the years, she experienced complications, including squeaking, which led to bushing exchanges in 2014 and 2018 (**b**). In 2019, she required revision surgery with a cortical bone graft following a periprosthetic fracture (**c**). Unfortunately, a fall 1-month post-revision necessitated irrigation, debridement due to wound dehiscence, and another bushing exchange. Persistent drainage led to resection arthroplasty with removal of the humeral component and placement of an antibiotic-impregnated bone cement spacer two months later (**d**). Despite long-term antibiotics, the distal humerus fracture displaced further, causing increased disability and elevated C-reactive protein (CRP) levels (**e**). Recurrent drainage two months later prompted complete resection arthroplasty of the ulnar component with spacer placement, which ultimately resolved the infection (**f**). This case highlights the complexities and challenges of managing complications following TEA, including infections, implant failures, and the need for multiple revision surgeries

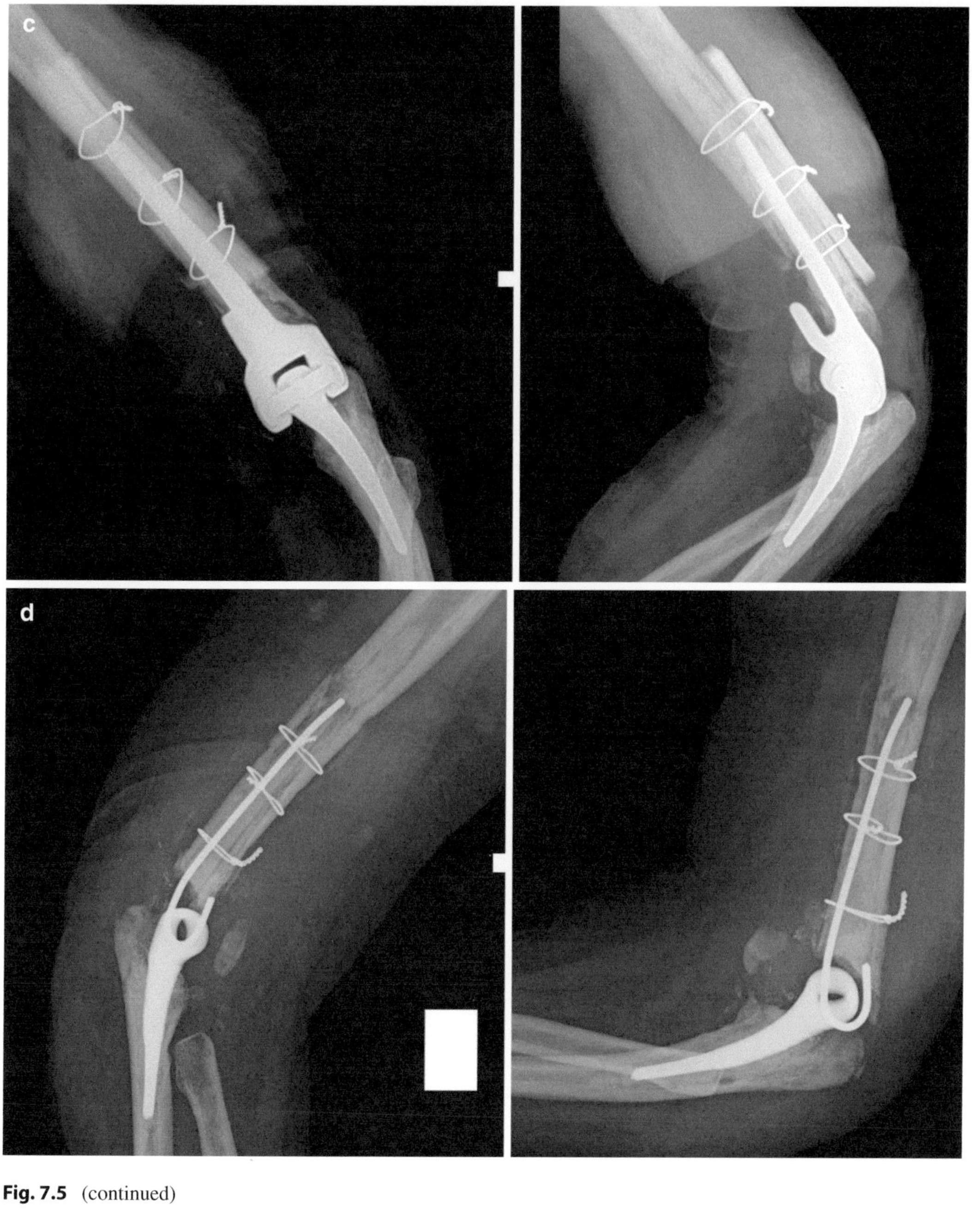

Fig. 7.5 (continued)

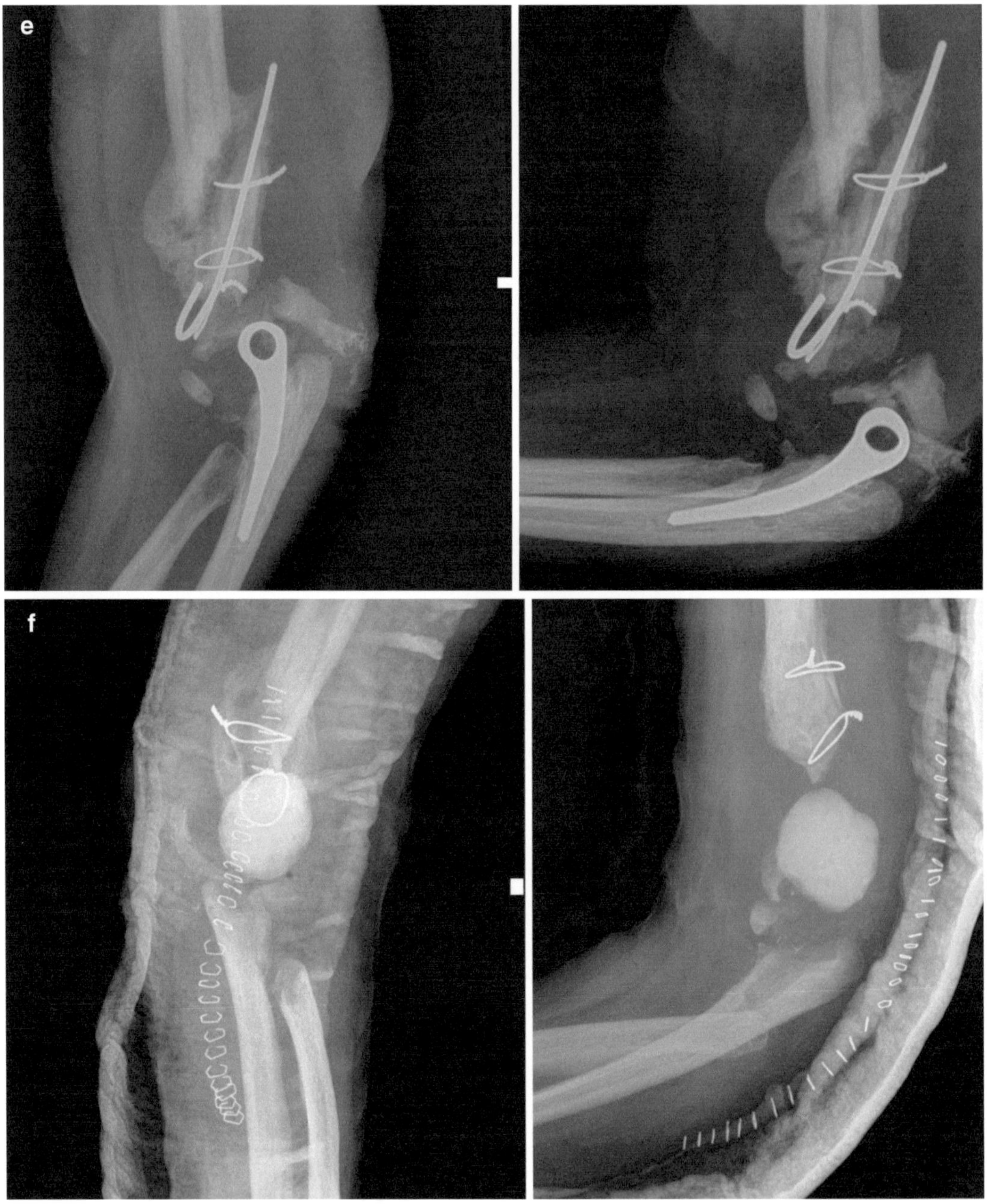

Fig. 7.5 (continued)

References

1. Flurin L, Greenwood-Quaintance KE, Esper RN, Sanchez-Sotelo J, Patel R. Sonication improves microbiologic diagnosis of periprosthetic elbow infection. J Shoulder Elbow Surg. 2021;30(8):1741–9. https://doi.org/10.1016/j.jse.2021.01.023.
2. Somerson JS, Boylan MR, Hug KT, Naziri Q, Paulino CB, Huang JI, JI. Risk factors associated with periprosthetic joint infection after total elbow arthroplasty. Shoulder Elbow. 2019;11(2):116–20. https://doi.org/10.1177/1758573217741318.
3. Gutman MJ, Stone MA, Namdari S, Abboud JA. Treatment of elbow periprosthetic joint infection: a systematic review of clinical outcomes. J Shoulder Elbow Surg. 2020;29(2):411–9. https://doi.org/10.1016/j.jse.2019.10.002.
4. Flurin L, Wolf MJ, Greenwood-Quaintance KE, Sanchez-Sotelo J, Patel R. Targeted next generation sequencing for elbow periprosthetic joint infection diagnosis. Diagn Microbiol Infect Dis. 2021;101(2):115448. https://doi.org/10.1016/j.diagmicrobio.2021.115448.
5. Nieboer M, Braig Z, Rosenow C, Marigi E, Tande A, Barlow J, et al. Non-cefazolin antibiotic prophylaxis is associated with higher rates of elbow periprosthetic joint infection. J Shoulder Elbow Surg. 2024;33(4):940–7. https://doi.org/10.1016/j.jse.2023.10.029.
6. Tai DBG, Hanson S, Brennan P, Suh GA, Esper RN, Sanchez-Sotelo J. Outcomes and risk factors for failure after débridement, antibiotics, and implant retention for elbow periprosthetic joint infection. J Shoulder Elbow Surg. 2023;32(3):475–9. https://doi.org/10.1016/j.jse.2022.11.009.
7. Martinez-Catalan N, Nguyen NTV, Morrey ME, O'Driscoll SW, Sanchez-Sotelo J. Two-stage reimplantation for deep infection after total elbow arthroplasty. Shoulder Elbow. 2022;14(6):668–76. https://doi.org/10.1177/17585732211043524.
8. Kunutsor SK, Beswick AD, Whitehouse MR, Blom AW. One- and two-stage surgical revision of infected elbow prostheses following total joint replacement: a systematic review. BMC Musculoskelet Disord. 2019;20(1):467. https://doi.org/10.1186/s12891-019-2848-x.
9. Goyal N, Luchetti TJ, Wysocki RW, Cohen MS. Management of periprosthetic joint infection in total elbow arthroplasty. J Hand Surg Am. 2020;45(10):957–70. https://doi.org/10.1016/j.jhsa.2020.05.020.
10. Rodriguez-Merchan EC, Kachooei AR, Tabeayo E. Elbow arthroplasty: a concise literature update. Arch Bone Jt Surg. 2023;11(7):465–72. https://doi.org/10.22038/ABJS.2023.71082.3323.
11. DeBernardis DA, Horneff JG, Davis DE, Ramsey ML, Pontes MC, Austin LS. Revision total elbow arthroplasty failure rates: the impact of primary arthroplasty failure etiology on subsequent revisions. J Shoulder Elbow Surg. 2020;29(2):321–8. https://doi.org/10.1016/j.jse.2019.10.010.

Periprosthetic Joint Infection in Total Hip Arthroplasty: Diagnosis

8

E. Carlos Rodríguez-Merchán
and Alberto D. Delgado-Martínez

8.1 Introduction

Periprosthetic joint infection (PJI) is a dangerous complication following total hip arthroplasty (THA), which is associated with substantial health costs, morbidity, and mortality (Figs. 8.1 and 8.2). There is currently no agreement on the optimal definition of PJI, and diagnosing PJI is challenging because of conflicting guidelines, many tests, and insufficient evidence, with no single test rendering a sensitivity and specificity of 100%. Furthermore, culture-negative PJI happens in 5% to 12% of cases and is caused by low-grade infection as well as by previous or concomitant antibiotic therapy. Unfortunately, delayed diagnosis of PJI is associated with poorer results [1].

In a recent article, Lutro et al. (2024) investigated how effectively surgeons diagnosed PJI at the time of revision THA, based on preoperative and intraoperative assessments. They investigated the causes for revision potentially related to PJI following primary THA: infection, aseptic loosening, prolonged wound drainage, and pain only, reported to the Norwegian Arthroplasty Register (NAR) from surgeons in the region of Western Norway from 2010 to 2020. The accuracy of surgeon-reported revisions due to infection as representing PJI was 87% in the NAR [2].

The purpose of this chapter is to analyze the most recent data on the diagnosis of PJI in THA.

E. C. Rodríguez-Merchán (✉)
Department of Orthopedic Surgery, Hospital Universitario La Paz, Madrid, Madrid, Spain

A. D. Delgado-Martínez
Department of Orthopedic Surgery, Hospital Universitario de Jaén, Jaén, Spain

E. C. Rodríguez-Merchán (ed.), *Advances in Periprosthetic Joint Infection*,
https://doi.org/10.1007/978-3-032-02945-4_8

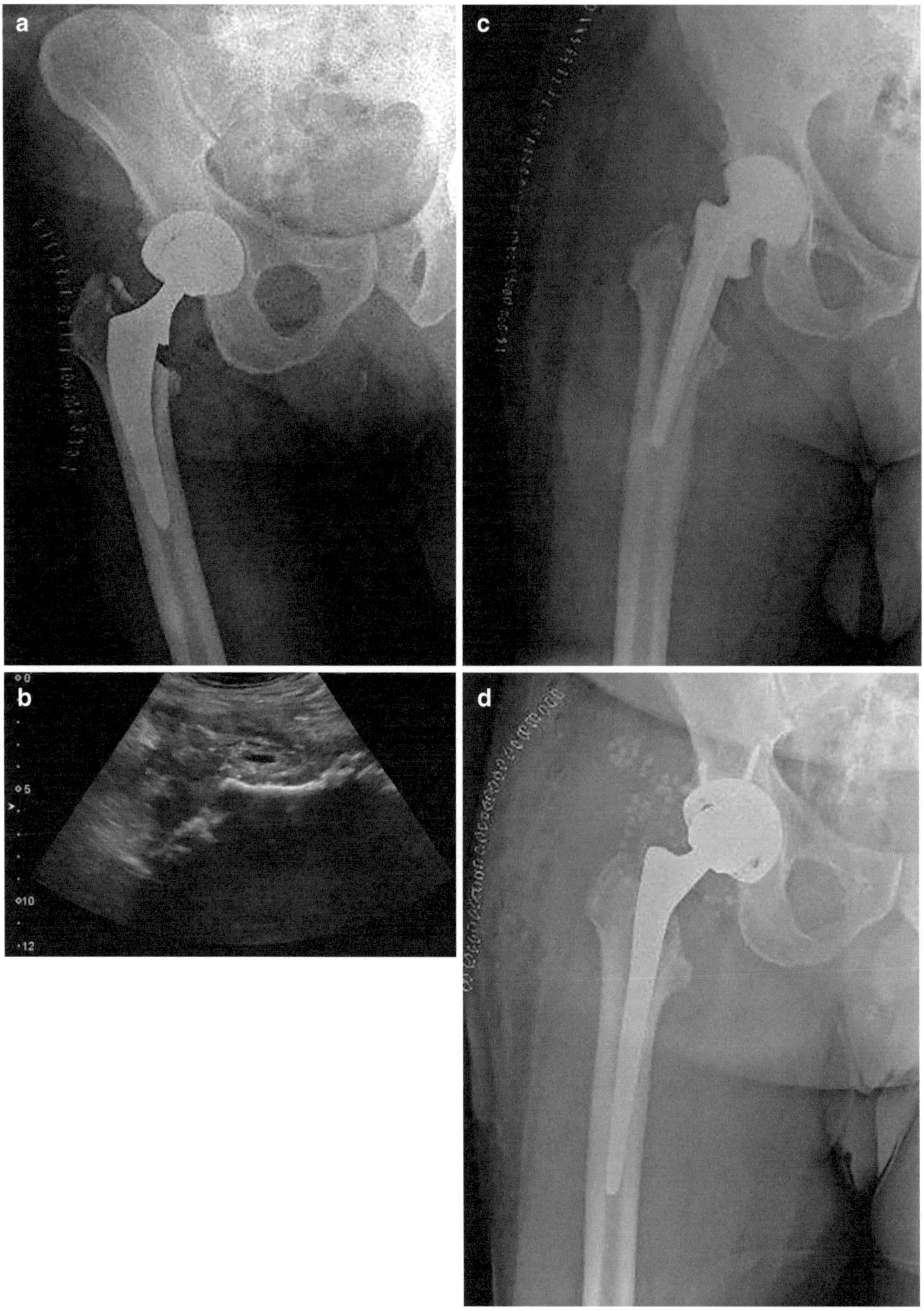

Fig. 8.1 (**a**–**d**). Two-stage revision hip arthroplasty due to periprosthetic joint infection (PJI): A 61-year-old patient with coxarthrosis underwent total hip arthroplasty by anterior approach with short femoral stem (**a**); after 2 months he started with fever and poor wound condition; ultrasonography was performed which detected a periprosthetic cyst that was punctured and cultured with a positive result for *Staphylococcus epidermidis* (**b**); the following month, the first-stage of revision arthroplasty was carried out via posterior approach with placement of cement spacer (**c**); antibiotic treatment with linezolid was started; at 3 months the second stage of revision arthroplasty was performed, with placement of antibiotic beads (calcium sulfate beads with gentamicin) (Stimulan®) (**d**); antibiotic treatment continued with oritavancin

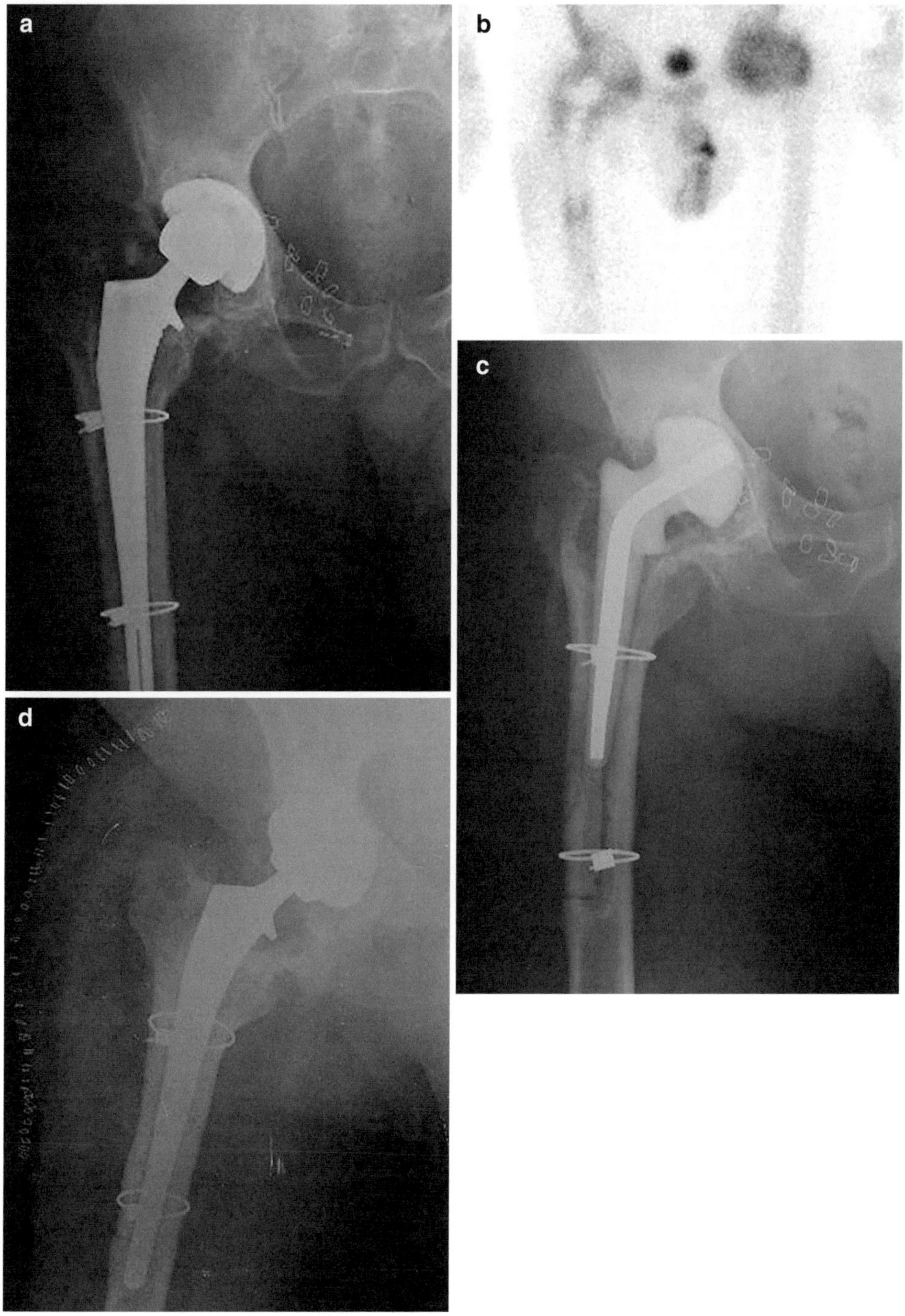

Fig. 8.2 (**a**–**d**). Two-stage revision hip arthroplasty due to periprosthetic joint infection (PJI): Radiographs of a 55-year-old patient, with a total hip prosthesis implanted 15 years earlier, who suddenly presented pain and fever (**a**); bone scintigraphy showed loosening of the implant, without determining whether it was septic or aseptic; C-reactive protein (CRP) and erythrocyte sedimentation rate (ESR) values were elevated (**b**); the first stage of revision arthroplasty was performed through an extended trochanteric approach and placement of a spacer (**c**); cultures were positive for *Staphylococcus epidermidis*; antibiotic treatment was carried out with ciprofloxacin and rifampicin; three months later, the second stage of revision arthroplasty was performed (**d**); cultures were negative; antibiotics were maintained for another month and then discontinued; at 7 months, CRP was normalized and ESR was 28; the patient was clinically well

8.2 Methylene Blue (MB) Infiltration as a Method for Differentiating Superficial and Deep Infections

In 2024, Fraval et al. reported a technique of differentiating superficial and deep infections by infiltrating MB into a prosthetic hip [3]. An analysis was performed on 35 individuals who preoperatively received an injection of MB under radiological guidance to their THA. When established PJI criteria were not met, without signs of MB beyond the deep fascia, the infection was deemed superficial, and debridement remained superficial to the deep fascia. When the diagnosis of PJI was confirmed preoperatively or the presence of MB in the wound cavity confirmed deep contamination, the prosthesis was addressed, with MB staining defining the joint cavity as a guide for debridement. There were 11 individuals who had no MB extrusion into the superficial compartment and did not meet PJI criteria. Eight individuals failed to meet PJI criteria preoperatively, but had extrusion of MB, confirming a deep infection intra-operatively. There were 16 individuals who met PJI criteria before surgery, with MB acting as a visual guide to the joint space. Therefore, infiltrating MB in a prosthetic hip seemed useful in distinguishing between superficial or deep infections when PJI workup was indeterminate [3].

8.3 Platelet-to-Lymphocyte Ratio (PLR) and Platelet-to-Volume Ratio (PVR) Calculated from Complete Blood Counts When Combined with Serum [Erythrocyte Sedimentation Rate (ESR), C-Reactive Protein (CRP)] and Synovial Fluid Markers [Synovial White Blood Cell (Syn. WBC), Synovial Polymorphonuclear Neutrophil Percentage (Syn. PMN%)]

In a study with level 3 of evidence, Klemt et al. (2023) analyzed 464 individuals that experienced revision THA with calculable PLR and PVR [4]. They evaluated two cohorts: individuals with a preoperative diagnosis of PJI (N = 191), and matched individuals treated for revision THA for aseptic complications (N = 273). The sensitivity and specificity of PLR combined with ESR, CRP, Syn. WBC, and Syn. PMN% (97.9%; 98.5%) were substantially higher than only ESR combined with CRP, Syn. WBC and Syn. PMN% (94.2%; 94.5%). The sensitivity and specificity of PVR combined with ESR, CRP, Syn. WBC, and Syn. PMN (98%; 98%) were higher than only ESR combined with CRP, Syn. WBC, and Syn. PMN% (94%; 94%) (Fig. 8.3). This study showed that both PLR and PVR calculated from

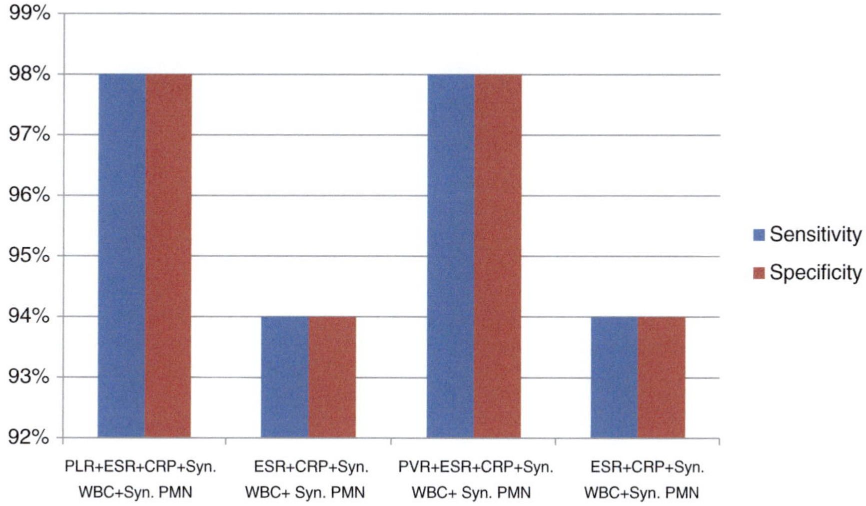

Fig. 8.3 Diagnosing periprosthetic joint infection (PJI) in total hip arthroplasty (THA) individuals: The sensitivity and specificity of platelet-to-lymphocyte ratio (PLR) combined with erythrocyte sedimentation rate (ESR), C-reactive protein (CRP), synovial white blood cell count (Syn. WBC), and synovial polymorphonuclear leukocytes (Syn. PMN) (98%; 98%) were substantially higher than only ESR combined with CRP, synovial WBC and synovial PMN (94%; 94%). The sensitivity and specificity of platelet-to-volume ratio (PVR) combined with ESR, CRP, and synovial WBC, and synovial PMN (98%; 98%) were higher than only ESR combined with CRP, Syn. WBC and Syn. PMN (94%; 94%)

complete blood counts when combined with serum and synovial fluid markers had increased diagnostic sensitivity and specificity in diagnosing PJI in individuals with THA [4].

In 2023, Denyer et al. aimed to validate the effectiveness of PVR and PLR in diagnosing PJI [5]. A retrospective review was performed to evaluate the accuracy of different marker combinations for diagnosing chronic PJI. A total of 573 individuals were included in the study, 124 of whom had TKAs and 122 had THAs with a diagnosis of chronic PJI. Complete blood count and synovial fluid analyses were collected. Recently published blood cell ratio cut-off points were applied to receiver operating characteristic curves for all markers and combinations. The area under the curve (AUC), sensitivity, specificity, and positive and negative predictive values were calculated. The results of the analysis showed that the combination of ESR, CRP, Syn. WBC, and Syn. PMN% with PVR had the highest AUC of 0.99 for knees, with sensitivity of 97.73% and specificity of 100%. Similarly, for hips, this combination had an AUC of 0.98, sensitivity of 96.15%, and specificity of 100% (Fig. 8.4). Therefore,

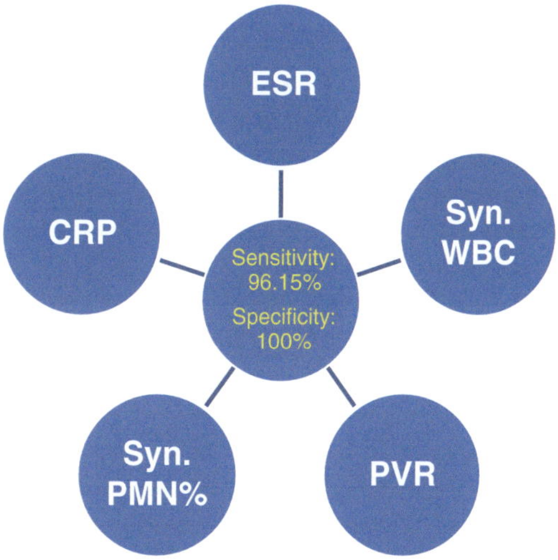

Fig. 8.4 Diagnosis of periprosthetic joint infection (PJI) in total hip arthroplasty (THA): the combination of erythrocyte sedimentation rate (ESR), C-reactive protein (CRP), synovial white blood cell count (Syn. WBC), and synovial polymorphonuclear neutrophil percentage (Syn. PMN%) with platelet-to-volume ratio (PVR) had a sensitivity of 96%, and a specificity of 100%

PVR calculated from readily available complete blood counts, when combined with established markers improved the accuracy in diagnosing chronic PJI in THA [5].

8.4 Synovial Long Pentraxin 3 (PTX3)

Loppini et al. (2023) assessed the potential of synovial and plasmatic PTX3 in the diagnosis of PJI after THA and TKA [6]. Consecutive THA/TKA revisions were prospectively included and classified as septic or aseptic according to the European Bone and Joint Infection Society (EBJIS) [7] and Musculoskeletal Infection Society (MSIS) criteria [8]. The concentration of PTX3 in plasma and synovial fluid samples was measured using ELISA (Enzyme-Linked ImmunoSorbent Assay). The AUC, threshold value, sensitivity, specificity, and positive and negative likelihood ratios were calculated using the receiver operating characteristic (ROC) curve method. The study population included 128 patients (94 THAs; 34 TKAs). The AUC of the synovial PTX3 based on EBJIS criteria was 0.85, with a sensitivity of 81.13% and a specificity of 93.33%. The AUC based on MSIS criteria was 0.95, with a sensitivity of 91.43% and a specificity of 89.25%. Plasmatic PTX3 failed to discriminate infected from noninfected patients. Synovial PTX3 demonstrated an excellent diagnostic potential in hip and knee PJIs, with a very high specificity irrespective of the diagnostic criteria for PJI [6] (Fig. 8.5).

In a prospective and multicenter study, Logroscino et al. (2023) aimed to establish the efficacy of plasma PTX3 trends in individuals undergoing primary THA, and to assess the diagnostic accuracy of blood and synovial PTX3 in individuals undergoing prosthetic revision of infected THA. Human PTX3 was measured using ELISA in two cohorts of individuals: ten individuals undergoing primary THA for osteoarthritis and nine individuals with infected THA. The study showed that PTX3 was a viable biomarker for acute-phase inflammation. An increase in PTX3 protein concentration in the synovial fluid of individuals undergoing implant revision had a strong diagnostic capacity for PJI, showing 97% specificity [7].

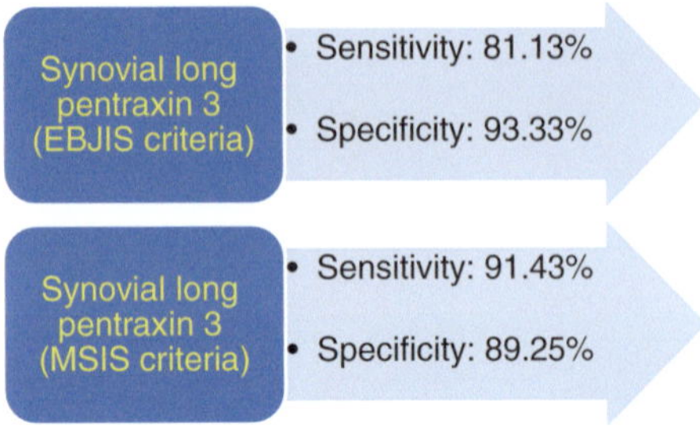

Fig. 8.5 Synovial long pentraxin 3 (PTX3) demonstrated an excellent diagnostic potential in hip periprosthetic joint infection (PJI), with a very high specificity irrespective of the diagnostic criteria for PJI. *EBJIS* European Bone and Joint Infection Society, *MSIS* Musculoskeletal Infection Society

8.5 C-Reactive Protein/Albumin and C-Reactive Protein/Fibrinogen Ratios

Wu et al. (2023) assessed the application of CRP/albumin ratio (CRP/Alb) and CRP/fibrinogen ratio (CRP/Fib) as new inflammation-based markers for the diagnosis of PJI [8]. They retrospectively assessed 445 individuals who experienced revision THA and revision TKA. Of these, 129 individuals with coagulation-related comorbidities were also independently assessed for PJI. The individuals were divided into two cohorts: the aseptic revision ($N = 268$) and PJI revision cohorts ($N = 187$). Then, they assessed the diagnostic value of the CRP/Alb and CRP/Fib ratios compared with other inflammation-based diagnoses utilizing the AUC values. The AUC values of the CRP/Alb and CRP/Fib ratios were 0.880 and 0.872, respectively, suggesting similar diagnostic potentials for PJI. The CRP/Alb and CRP/Fib ratios were better than the ESR, Alb, and Fib, whose AUC values were 0.765, 0.352, and 0.730, respectively, for the diagnosis of PJI. The optimal cut-off for the CRP/Alb ratio was 0.13, with good sensitivity (85%) and specificity (78.4%). The optimal cut-off CRP/Fib ratio was 2.04, with good sensitivity (81%) and speci-

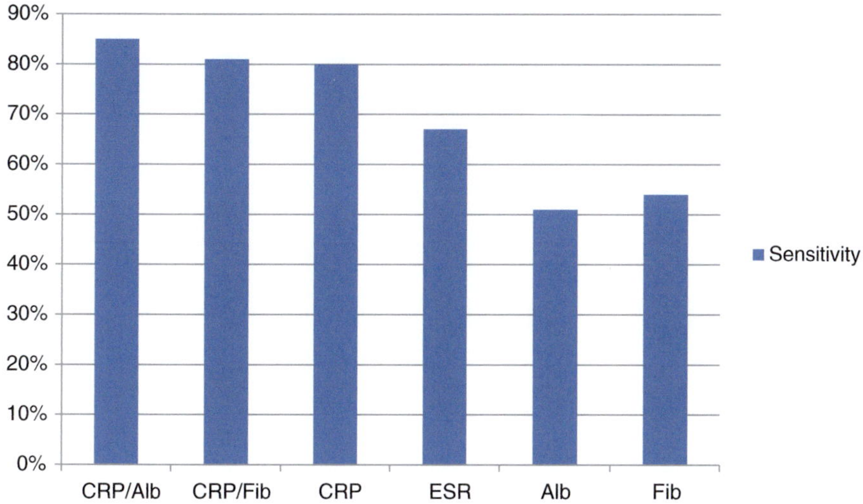

Fig. 8.6 Sensitivities of different tests in the diagnosis of hip periprosthetic joint infection (PJI). CRP/Alb = C-reactive protein/albumin ratio; CRP/Fib = C-reactive protein/fibrinogen ratio (CRP/Fib) ratio; CRP = C-reactive protein; ESR = erythrocyte sedimentation rate; Alb = albumin; Fib = fibrinogen

ficity (81%). Notably, the CRP/Alb and CRP/Fib ratios had the highest sensitivity, followed by CRP, ESR, Alb, and Fib, which had sensitivities of 80%, 67%, 51%, and 54%, respectively (Fig. 8.6). Similar findings were noted in individuals with coagulation-related comorbidities. Both the CRP/Alb and CRP/Fib ratios were substantially higher in individuals with PJI than in those with aseptic failure and demonstrated better sensitivity and specificity for diagnosing PJI than classical inflammatory markers [8].

8.6 Biopsy

Considering that, low-grade chronic PJI is frequently difficult to diagnose prior to revision THA, Simon et al. (2023) aimed to establish the diagnostic accuracy of open incisional tissue biopsy (OITB) for the prediction of PJI before THA revision in cases of culture-negative or dry tap joint aspirates [9]. This retrospective single-center study included 32 consecutive THA revision cases that presented with high clinical suspicion of low-grade chronic PJI of the hip, along with culture-negative or dry tap joint aspirates and without systemic signs of infection. OITB was performed prior to revision surgery. Periprosthetic tissue samples were analyzed by microbiology and histopathology for PJI. During definitive revision THA, identical diagnostic procedures were repeated. Results from both procedures were compared, and the sensitivity, specificity, and positive and negative predictive values of OITB for the final diagnosis were calculated. The average age at revision was 69.3 years. The sensitivity of the OITB procedure was 80% (microbiology), 69% (histology), and 82% for combined analyses (microbiology and histology). The specificity of OITB was 80% (microbiology), 94% (histology), and 60% for combined analyses (Fig. 8.7). Therefore, OITB performed in cases with culture-negative or inconclusive synovial fluid aspirates prior to THA revision had limited diagnostic accuracy for the prediction of PJI [9].

In 2023, Li et al. published a meta-analysis on the role of biopsy in diagnosing infection after THA and TKA [10]. Three biopsy-related tests were identified in 14 articles and further analyzed. The combined method had the highest value for the AUC (0.9805), followed by histology (0.9425) and microbiological tests (0.9292). In the subgroup, statistical differences were identified in sensitivity and specificity for PJI diagnosis between the synovial fluid culture and biopsy

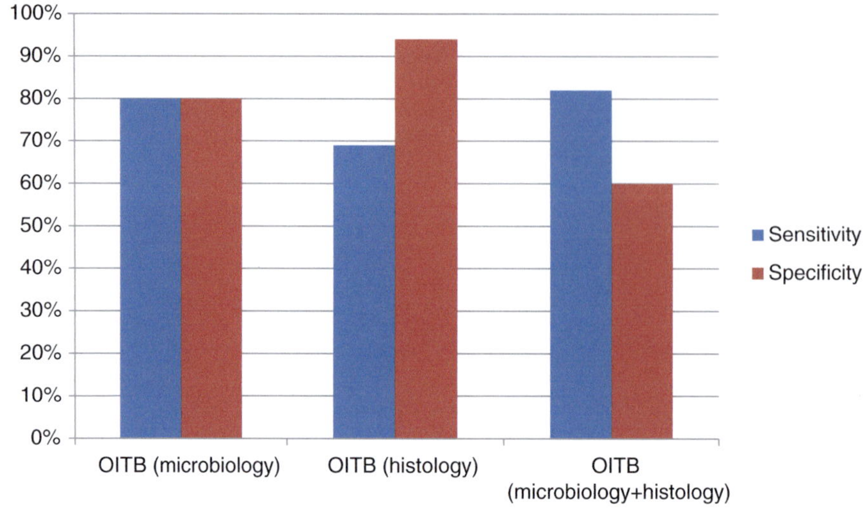

Fig. 8.7 The sensitivity of the open incisional tissue biopsy (OITB) was 80% (microbiology), 69% (histology), and 82% for combined analyses (microbiology and histology). Specificity of OITB was 80% (microbiology), 94% (histology), and 60% for combined analyses. Therefore, OITB carried out in cases with culture-negative or inconclusive synovial fluid aspirates before revision of THA had limited diagnostic accuracy for the prediction of periprosthetic joint infection (PJI) in total hip arthroplasty (THA)

culture group and between the biopsy-related combined method and serum CRP. Biopsy culture did not seem to be advantageous compared with synovial fluid culture in the preoperative diagnosis of PJI after THA and TKA. In contrast, the combined biopsy microbial culture with histology analysis showed great potential in improving the preoperative diagnosis of PJI [10].

8.7 Next-Generation Sequencing (NGS) of Blood Samples

In 2023, Zhang et al. analyzed the diagnostic value of blood sample NGS in individuals with early PJI after THA. The diagnostic value of NGS of blood samples from individuals with PJI after THA was assessed by comparing with drainage fluid NGS and bacterial culture [11]. Thirty-six infected individuals were diagnosed with PJI according to the MSIS criteria and fifty-seven volunteers were included in the study. NGS and bacterial culture were chosen to detect PJI after THA. Blood samples and drainage fluid were collected for NGS, and the drainage fluid, collected simultaneously with the NGS drainage fluid sample, was utilized for bacterial culture. In the infection cohort, 31 individuals showed positive results by blood sample NGS, 33 individuals showed positive results by drainage fluid NGS, and 17 individuals showed positive bacterial culture results. In the control cohort, the results of 2 blood sample NGS, 16 drainage fluid NGS, and 3 bacterial cultures were positive. The sensitivity, specificity, and accuracy of the blood sample were 0.86, 0.96, and 0.92, respectively. The sensitivity, specificity, and accuracy of the drainage fluid samples were 0.92, 0.72, and 0.80, respectively. The sensitivity, specificity, and accuracy of bacterial culture were 0.47, 0.95, and 0.79, respectively (Table 8.1). The study showed that both the sensitivity and specificity of NGS were higher than

Table 8.1 Periprosthetic joint infection (PJI) after total hip arthroplasty (THA): The diagnostic value of blood sample NGS was superior to that of drainage fluid NGS and bacterial culture

	Sensitivity	Specificity	Accuracy
NGS blood sample	0.86	0.96	0.92
NGS drainage fluid sample	0.92	0.72	0.80
Bacterial culture drainage fluid	0.47	0.95	0.79

NGS next-generation sequencing

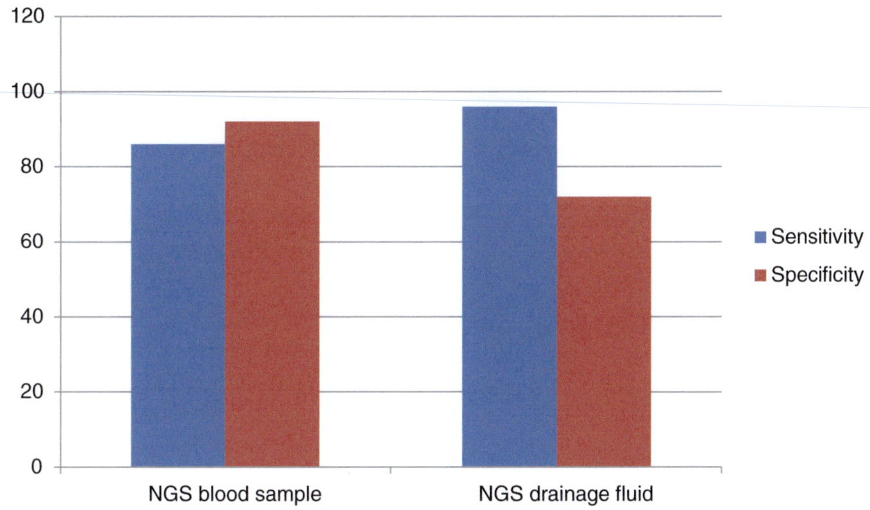

Fig. 8.8 Diagnosing periprosthetic joint infection (PJI) in total hip arthroplasty (THA) individuals: The diagnostic value of blood sample next-generation sequencing (NGS) was superior to that of drainage fluid NGS and bacterial culture. Compared with drainage fluid NGS, the sensitivity of blood sample NGS was slightly lower (0.86 vs. 0.92), but blood sample NGS showed higher specificity (0.96 vs. 0.72)

those of bacterial culture, regardless of the sample type. Compared with drainage fluid NGS, the sensitivity of blood sample NGS was slightly lower (0.86 vs. 0.92), but blood sample NGS showed higher specificity (0.96 vs. 0.72) (Fig. 8.8). The diagnostic value of blood sample NGS was superior to that of drainage fluid NGS and bacterial culture. Most infected individuals could be identified by blood sample NGS. Furthermore, because of its high specificity, blood sample NGS can not only detect infectious bacteria but also differentiate infectious from noninfectious bacteria, which is dramatically different from utilizing drainage fluid NGS [11].

8.8 The Synovial Fluid Calprotectin Lateral Flow Test (LFT)

According to Suren et al. (2023), calprotectin has been demonstrated to be an excellent diagnostic marker for PJI [12]. In their study, they aimed to assess an LFT in challenging individuals. They prospectively included individuals scheduled for arthroplasty exchange of THA or TKA. Synovial fluid samples were collected intra-operatively. They utilized the International Consensus Meeting of 2018 (ICM) score as the gold standard. They then compared the preoperative ICM score with the LFT result to calculate its diagnostic accuracy as a standalone preoperative marker and in combination with the ICM score as part of an expanded diagnostic workup. A total of 137 individuals with a mean age of 67 years with 53 THA and 84 TKA were included. Ninety-nine individuals (72.8%) were not infected, thirty-four (25%) were infected, and four (2.9%) had an inconclusive final score and could not be classified after surgery. The calprotectin LFT had a sensitivity of 0.94 and a specificity of 0.87. The AUC for the calprotectin LFT was 0.94. In nine cases with an inconclusive preoperative ICM score, the calprotectin LFT would have led to the correct diagnosis of PJI. The synovial fluid calprotectin LFT demonstrated excellent diagnostic metrics both as a rule-in and a rule-out test, even in a challenging group of individuals with cases of severe osteolysis, wear disease, many previous surgeries, and poor soft tissue conditions, which can impair the common diagnostic criteria. As it is accessible before surgery, this test may prove to be a very valuable supplement to the diagnostic algorithm [12].

8.9 Diagnostic Efficiency of [^{68}Ga]Ga-DOTA-FAPI-04 in Differentiating Periprosthetic Hip Joint Infection and Aseptic Failure

In 2023, Wang et al. evaluated the efficiency of [^{68}Ga]Ga-DOTA-FAPI-04 in diagnosing PJI after THA. [^{68}Ga]Ga-DOTA-FAPI-04 PET/CT was performed in individuals with symptomatic THA [13]. The reference standard was based on the 2018 Evidence-Based and Validation Criteria. Two diagnostic criteria, maximum standardized uptake value (SUVmax) and uptake pattern, were used to diagnose PJI. A total of 103 individuals were included, 28 of whom had PJI. The AUC of SUVmax was 0.898, which was better than that of all serological tests. The cutoff value of SUVmax was 7.53, and the sensitivity and specificity were 100% and 72%, respectively. The sensitivity, specificity, and accuracy of the uptake pattern were 100%, 93%, and 95%, respectively (Fig. 8.9). The efficiency of [^{68}Ga]Ga-DOTA-FAPI-04 PET/CT in diagnosing PJI exhibited encouraging results, and the diagnostic criteria of the uptake pattern were more clinically instructive. Radiomics (extraction of information from medical images using advanced feature analysis) also demonstrated some application prospects in the field of PJI [13].

8.10 Serum Procalcitonin (PCT)

In 2023, Sun et al. analyzed the value of procalcitonin (PCT) in the diagnosis of PJI. A retrospective review of 77 individuals with revision arthroplasties was performed. PJI was defined utilizing the modified MSIS criteria combined with follow-up results [14]. Forty-one individuals were identified as the PJI cohort (27 hips and 14 knees), while thirty-six individuals were identified as the aseptic loosening (AL) cohort (33 hips and 3 knees). The AUCs for CRP, ESR, platelets (PLT), fibrinogen (Fib), and PCT were 0.845, 0.817, 0.728, 0.810, and 0.504, respectively. Higher AUC values were obtained for the combinations of PCT and CRP (AUC = 0.870), PCT and ESR (AUC = 0.817), PCT and PLT (AUC = 0.731), and PCT and Fib (AUC = 0.815). The serum PCT indicated a sensitivity of 19.5% and a specificity of 83.3% for diagnosing PJI. When the optimal cut-off value for PCT was set as 0.05 ng/mL, its positive and negative likelihood ratios were 57.1% and 47.6%, respectively. In conclusion, serum PCT seemed not a depend-

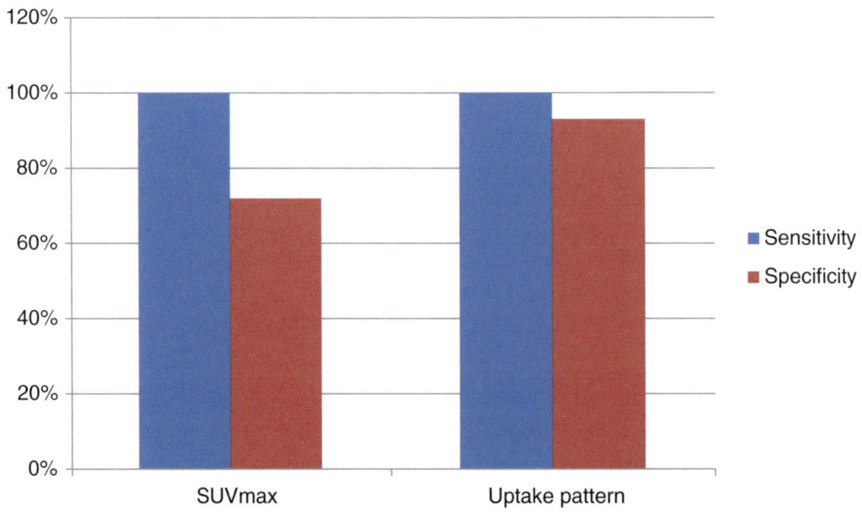

Fig. 8.9 Diagnostic efficiency of [68 Ga]Ga-DOTA-FAPI-04 in differentiating periprosthetic hip joint infection and aseptic failure: The sensitivity, specificity of the uptake pattern were 100% and 93%, respectively. The Maximum standardized uptake value (SUVmax) sensitivity and specificity were 100% and 72%, respectively

able biomarker in differentiating PJI from aseptic loosening prior to revision arthroplasties. Nonetheless, PCT combined with other biomarkers further increased the diagnostic accuracy [14].

8.11 Glycemic Control Markers

In a study with level 2 of evidence, Cetik et al. (2023) assessed the predictive value of hemoglobin A1c (HbA1c) and fructosamine for predicting PJI after THA and TKA. This cohort study included 304 individuals (mean age: 65 years, mean follow-up: 32 months) who underwent primary THA or TKA. Of these, 156 individuals had diabetes. Mean HbA1c was 6.5%, and fructosamine was 244 μmol/L. Individuals with and without diabetes were matched 1:1. HbA1c 7% and fructosamine 292 μmol/L were used as the cutoff. HbA1c was strongly associated with total complications, while fructosamine was associated with PJI [15].

8.12 Acidity (pH Value of Synovial Fluid)

In 2024, Judl et al. hypothesized that the pH value of synovial fluid could be an important indicator of the inflammatory status of the joint [16]. They investigated the potential of pH measurement as a diagnostic tool for PJI after THA and TKA. They recorded the pH values to be 7.55 and 7.46 in individuals in whom *Pseudomonas aeruginosa* was identified as the cause of the PJI. In other cases where the pH was higher, chronic mitigated infections were diagnosed, caused by strains of *Staphylococcus aureus*, *Streptococcus agalactiae*, and coagulase-negative *Staphylococcus*. In this group of 155 individuals with THA ($N = 85$) or TKA ($N = 70$) joint replacements, Judl et al. performed a prospective study with a pH measurement. Out of the whole group, 44 individuals had confirmed PJI (28.4%) (44/155). In 111 individuals, infection was ruled out (71.6%) (111/155). PJI was classified according to the criteria of the MSIS from 2018. The cohort of individuals with infection ($N = 44$) had a substantially lower synovial fluid pH (pH = 6.98) than the cohort of individuals with no infection ($N = 111$, pH = 7.82). The corresponding median pH values were 7.08 for the individuals with infection and 7.83 for the individuals with no infection. When Judl et al. determined the cut-off level of pH 7.4, the sensitivity level of infected replacements was 88.6%, and the specificity level of the measurement was 95.5%. The predictive value of a positive test was 88.6%, and the predictive value of a negative test was 95.5%. This study confirmed that it is appropriate to include a pH measurement in the diagnostic spectrum of total hip and knee arthroplasties [16].

8.13 Metal-Artifact-Reduction (MAR) MRI

Nakagawa et al. (2024) assessed the significant findings of PJI utilizing metal-artifact-reduction (MAR) magnetic resonance imaging (MRI) and compared the MRI results to other clinical markers [17]. Thirty-seven hip joints in 24 individuals (age = 73.9 years; 18 females) were included. Twelve hip joints (32%) had PJI; seven experienced a surgical intervention. The significant findings for hip PJI included periosteal edema of the acetabulum, intermuscular edema, intramuscular fluid collection, and lymphadenopathy. In the cases with surgical intervention, the significant findings included capsular distension, capsular thickening, an osteolysis-like pattern of the femur, subcutaneous fluid collection, and lymphadenopathy. The MRI impressions had high diagnostic significance for both hip PJI cases and those with surgical intervention. The MRI impression was more significant for hip PJI than the other clinical markers, while the other clinical markers were more significant in the cases with surgical intervention. Therefore, the utilization of MAR MRI demonstrated great diagnostic significance for hip PJI [17].

8.14 Conclusions

The diagnosis of PJI following THA is based on a mixture of clinical information, laboratory results from peripheral blood and synovial fluid, microbiological culture, histological assessment of periprosthetic tissue, radiological investigations, and intraoperative findings. Usually, a sinus tract communicating with the prosthesis and two positive cultures for the same pathogen are considered major criteria for the diagnosis. However, the availability of new serum and synovial biomarkers and molecular methods has demonstrated promising results.

PVR calculated from readily available complete blood counts (ESR, CRP, and PMN%), combined with established markers, synovial white blood cell count (Syn. WBC count) improved the accuracy in diagnosing chronic PJI in THA (sensitivity between 96% and 98%, and specificity between 98% and 100%). Synovial PTX3 demonstrated an excellent diagnostic potential in hip PJI, with a very high specificity (between 89% and 97%) irrespective of the diagnostic criteria for PJI. Both the CRP/Alb and CRP/Fib ratios demonstrated better sensitivity and specificity for diagnosing PJI than classical inflammatory markers (ESR, CRP). The diagnostic value of blood sample NGS was superior to that of drainage fluid NGS and bacterial culture. Most infected individuals could be identified by blood sample NGS. Furthermore, because of its high specificity, blood sample NGS can not only detect infectious bacteria but also differentiate infectious from noninfectious bacteria.

References

1. Luppi V, Regis D, Sandri A, Magnan B. Diagnosis of periprosthetic hip infection: a clinical update. Acta Biomed. 2023;94(S2):e2023095. https://doi.org/10.23750/abm.v94iS2.13792.
2. Lutro O, Mo S, Tjørhom MB, Fenstad AM, Leta TH, Bruun T, et al. How good are surgeons at disclosing periprosthetic joint infection at the time of revision, based on pre- and intra-operative assessment? A study on 16,922 primary total hip arthroplasties reported to the Norwegian Arthroplasty Register. Acta Orthop. 2024;95:67–72. https://doi.org/10.2340/17453674.2024.39914.
3. Fraval A, Zappley NR, Brown SA. Methylene blue infiltration as a method for distinguishing superficial and deep infections. J Arthroplasty. 2024;39(1):224–8. https://doi.org/10.1016/j.arth.2023.07.020.
4. Klemt C, Tirumala V, Smith EJ, Xiong L, Kwon YM. Complete blood platelet and lymphocyte ratios increase diagnostic accuracy of periprosthetic joint infection following total hip arthroplasty. Arch Orthop Trauma Surg. 2023;143(3):1441–9. https://doi.org/10.1007/s00402-021-04309-w.
5. Denyer S, Eikani C, Sheth M, Schmitt D, Brown N. Diagnosing periprosthetic joint infection: a validation study of blood cells ratio combinations. Bone Jt Open. 2023;4(11):881–8. https://doi.org/10.1302/2633-1462.411.BJO-2023-0094.R1.
6. Loppini M, Di Maio M, Avigni R, Leone R, Inforzato A, Grappiolo G, et al. Long pentraxin 3 as a new biomarker for diagnosis of hip and knee periprosthetic joint infections. J Clin Med. 2023;12(3):1055. https://doi.org/10.3390/jcm12031055.
7. McNally M, Sousa R, Wouthuyzen-Bakker M, Chen AF, Soriano A, Vogely HC, et al. The EBJIS definition of periprosthetic joint infection: a practical guide for clinicians. Bone Joint J. 2021;103-B(1):18–25.
8. Blom AW, Beswick AD, Burston A, Carroll FE, Garfield K, Gooberman-Hill R, et al. Infection after total joint replacement of the hip and knee: research programme including the INFORM RCT. Programme Grants Appl Res. 2022;10(10) https://doi.org/10.3310/HDWL9760.
9. Logroscino G, Fidanza A, Giusti I, Poppa G, Troianello L, Calafiore F, et al. Pentraxin 3, a new biomarker for the diagnosis and management of PJI in primary and revision hip arthroplasty. Acta Biomed. 2023;94(S2):e2023100. https://doi.org/10.23750/abm.v94iS2.13770.
10. Wu Y, Sun K, Liu R, Wu L, Zeng Y, Li M, et al. C-reactive protein/albumin and C-reactive protein/fibrinogen ratios for the diagnosis of periprosthetic joint infection in revision total joint arthroplasty. Int Immunopharmacol. 2023;115:109682. https://doi.org/10.1016/j.intimp.2023.109682.
11. Simon MJK, Beyersdorff J, Strahl A, Rolvien T, Rüther W, Niemeier A. Diagnostic value of open incisional biopsies in suspected, difficult-to-diagnose periprosthetic hip joint infection prior to revision surgery. Arch Orthop Trauma Surg. 2023;143(3):1663–70. https://doi.org/10.1007/s00402-022-04402-8.
12. Li C, Margaryan D, Perka C, Trampuz A. The role of biopsy in diagnosing infection after hip and knee arthroplasty: a meta-analysis. Arch Orthop Trauma Surg. 2023;143(4):1779–92. https://doi.org/10.1007/s00402-021-04323-y.
13. Zhang B, Li M, Liu Y, Zhang B, Liu Z, Chen X, et al. The diagnostic value of blood sample NGS in patients with early periprosthetic joint infection after total hip arthroplasty. Int Wound J. 2023;20(4):961–70. https://doi.org/10.1111/iwj.13943.

14. Suren C, Lazic I, Haller B, Pohlig F, von Eisenhart-Rothe R, Prodinger P. The synovial fluid calprotectin lateral flow test for the diagnosis of chronic prosthetic joint infection in failed primary and revision total hip and knee arthroplasty. Int Orthop. 2023;47(4):929–44. https://doi.org/10.1007/s00264-023-05691-3.
15. Wang Y, Wang R, Zhang X, Li L, Liu H, Chang Y, et al. Diagnostic efficiency of [68 Ga]Ga-DOTA-FAPI-04 in differentiating periprosthetic hip joint infection and aseptic failure. Eur J Nucl Med Mol Imaging. 2023;50(7):1919–28. https://doi.org/10.1007/s00259-023-06146-y.
16. Sun X, Zhang H, Liu Y, Lai Z, Zeng Y. Serum procalcitonin has no significance in the diagnosis of periprosthesis joint infection before total hip and knee replacement. Front Surg. 2023;10:1216103. https://doi.org/10.3389/fsurg.2023.1216103.
17. Cetik RM, Azboy I, Birinci M, Ozturkmen Y, Kalyenci AS, Atilla B. Predictive value of different glycemic control markers in total hip or knee arthroplasty: a prospective study. Acta Orthop Traumatol Turc. 2023;57(5):289–93. https://doi.org/10.5152/j.aott.2023.23037.

Revision Total Hip Arthroplasty for Periprosthetic Joint Infection

9

E. Carlos Rodríguez-Merchán
and Ricardo Fernández-Fernández

9.1 Introduction

Periprosthetic joint infection (PJI) is one of the most calamitous adverse events following total hip arthroplasty (THA), and comorbidities increase the risk [1]. Moreover, PJI represents a severe complication after THA and is associated with substantial morbidity [2]. Complications after revision THA (rTHA) can produce substantial morbidity and have an elevated mortality rate. Patient age and American Society of Anesthesiologists (ASA) physical status classification system score [3] are relevant determinants of mortality after rTHA [4]. The purpose of this chapter is to analyze the most recent data on rTHA for PJI.

9.2 Trends in rTHA for PJI

In 2023, Liukkonen et al. analyzed whether there was a temporal change in the demographics, especially regarding comorbidities, of individuals who have PJIs and were treated over a 13-year study period at a high-volume academic joint arthroplasty center. Besides, the surgical techniques utilized and the microbiology of the PJIs were evaluated [1]. Revisions ($N = 423$, 418 individuals) due to PJI of the hip carried out at their institution between 2008 and September 2021 were determined. All included PJIs fulfilled the 2013 International Consensus Meeting diagnostic criteria [5]. The surgeries were categorized into one of the following categories: debridement, antibiotics, and implant retention (DAIR), one-stage revision, and two-stage revision. Infections were classified as early, acute hematogenous, and chronic infections. There was no change in the median age of the individuals, but the proportion of ASA-class 4 individuals increased from 10.5% to 20%. The incidence of early infections increased from 0.11 per 100 primary THAs in 2008 to 1.09 in 2021. The incidence of one-stage revisions increased the most, rising from 0.10 per 100 primary THAs in 2010 to 0.91 per 100 primary THAs in 2021. Moreover, the proportion of infections caused by Staphylococcus aureus increased from 26.3% in 2008 to 2009 to 40% in 2020 to 2021 (Table 9.1). The comorbidity burden of PJI individuals increased during the study period. This increase might present a treatment challenge, as comorbidities are known to have a negative effect on PJI treatment results [1].

E. C. Rodríguez-Merchán (✉)
R. Fernández-Fernández
Department of Orthopedic Surgery, Hospital Universitario La Paz, Madrid, Madrid, Spain

E. C. Rodríguez-Merchán (ed.), *Advances in Periprosthetic Joint Infection*,
https://doi.org/10.1007/978-3-032-02945-4_9

Table 9.1 Trends in revision total hip arthroplasty (rTHA) for periprosthetic joint infection (PJI)

	Year 2018	Year 2021
Proportion of ASA-class 4 individuals	10.5%	20%
Incidence of early infections per 100 pTHAs	0.11	1.09
Incidence of one-stage revisions per 100 pTHAs	0.10	0.91
Proportion of infections caused by *Staphylococcus aureus*	26.3%	40%

ASA American Society of Anesthesiologists, *pTHA* primary total hip arthroplasty

9.3 One-Stage rTHA

9.3.1 Antibacterial Hydrogel Coating

In 2022, Pellegrini et al. performed a retrospective study to assess the results of one-stage rTHA following PJI in terms of eradication of the infection, improvement of pain, and joint function [6]. They hypothesized that this treatment strategy could lead to satisfying outcomes in selected individuals after preoperative microorganism isolation. Ten individuals experienced cementless one-stage rTHA with antibacterial hydrogel coating for the treatment of an infected THA. Inclusion criteria were: the presence of a known organism with known sensitivity, non-immunocompromised individuals with healthy soft tissues with minimal or moderate bone loss. Mean age at surgery was 69.4 years. Evaluation included objective examination, Harris hip score, visual analog scale pain score, and standard X-rays. At a mean follow-up of 3.1 years, none of the individuals had clinical or radiographic signs suggesting recurrent infection. Follow-up examination demonstrated substantial improvement of all variables compared with preoperative values. Radiographs did not exhibit progressive radiolucent lines or change in the position of the implant. One-stage rTHA with antibacterial hydrogel-coated implants represented a safe and efficacious technique, rendering infection eradication and satisfying subjective functional results in selected individuals [6].

9.3.2 Repeat One-Stage rTHA

According to Liechti et al. (2022), the result for a repeat one-stage rTHA after a failed one-stage exchange for infection remains unknown [7]. In their study, they reported the infection-free and all-cause revision-free survival of repeat one-stage rTHA, and investigated the association between the MSIS staging system [8] and further infection-related failure. They retrospectively analyzed all repeat one-stage rTHAs carried out after failed one-stage rTHA for infection. The final cohort included 32 individuals. The mean follow-up after repeat one-stage rTHA was 5.3 years. Patients were categorized according to the MSIS system, and their association with further infection was analyzed. A total of eight repeat septic revisions (25%) developed a further infection-related failure, and the 5-year infection-free survival was 81%. Nine (28%) experienced a further all-cause revision and the 5-year all-cause revision-free survival was 74%. Neither the MSIS classification of the host status nor the limb status was substantially associated with further infection-related failure. Liechti et al. found that repeat one-stage rTHA for PJI was associated with a favorable 5-year infection-free and all-cause revision-free survival. Moreover, the rate of infection control was encouraging when compared with the reported rates after repeat two-stage rTHA [7].

9.3.3 Cementless One-Stage rTHA

In 2022, Riemer et al. stated that cementless one-stage rTHA of chronic PJI by the "Cementless One-stage Revision of Infected Hip Arthroplasty (CORIHA)" protocol has been assessed positively with a 91% success rate. In their study, they wanted to assess the efficacy of cementless one-stage revision following the CORIHA protocol for early PJI in elective primary THA, regarding the risk of reoperation with exchange of implants [9]. They identified 18 individuals with early (less than 6 weeks postoperative) PJI after primary THA treated with one-stage cementless rTHA. Treatment followed the CORIHA protocol. Primary outcome was retention of implants at the most recent follow-up. Patients were followed for a minimum of 3 years. Mean follow-up time was 5 years. All individuals retained their implants, but two needed superficial soft tissue debridement due to persistent wound seepage. Cementless one-stage rTHA seemed to be an effective treatment of early PJI after primary THA and at least an equal choice of treatment compared with DAIR [9]. Figure 9.1 shows a case of cementless one-stage rTHA due to PJI.

9.3.4 One-Stage rTHA with Cemented Modular Stems for PJI with Massive Femoral Bone Loss

In a study with level 3 of evidence, Russo et al. (2023) analyzed survival and complications related to the use of cemented modular stems in one-stage septic rTHA with severe femoral bone loss [10]. A total of 150 individuals were included. The mean age was 68 years, and the mean follow-up was 105 months. Treatment was considered successful in 81.3% of cases. Individuals who experienced multiple prior surgeries showed a lower rate of treatment success. The main cause of failure was reinfection (11 of 28). Among cases that failed for aseptic reasons (17 of 28), loosening of the cemented modular stem was the cause of re-revision in two individuals (1.3%). The utilization of modular cemented stems is a viable alternative for septic one-stage rTHA associated with severe femoral bone loss. However, this technique is still characterized by a high rate of adverse events that might lead to further surgeries [10].

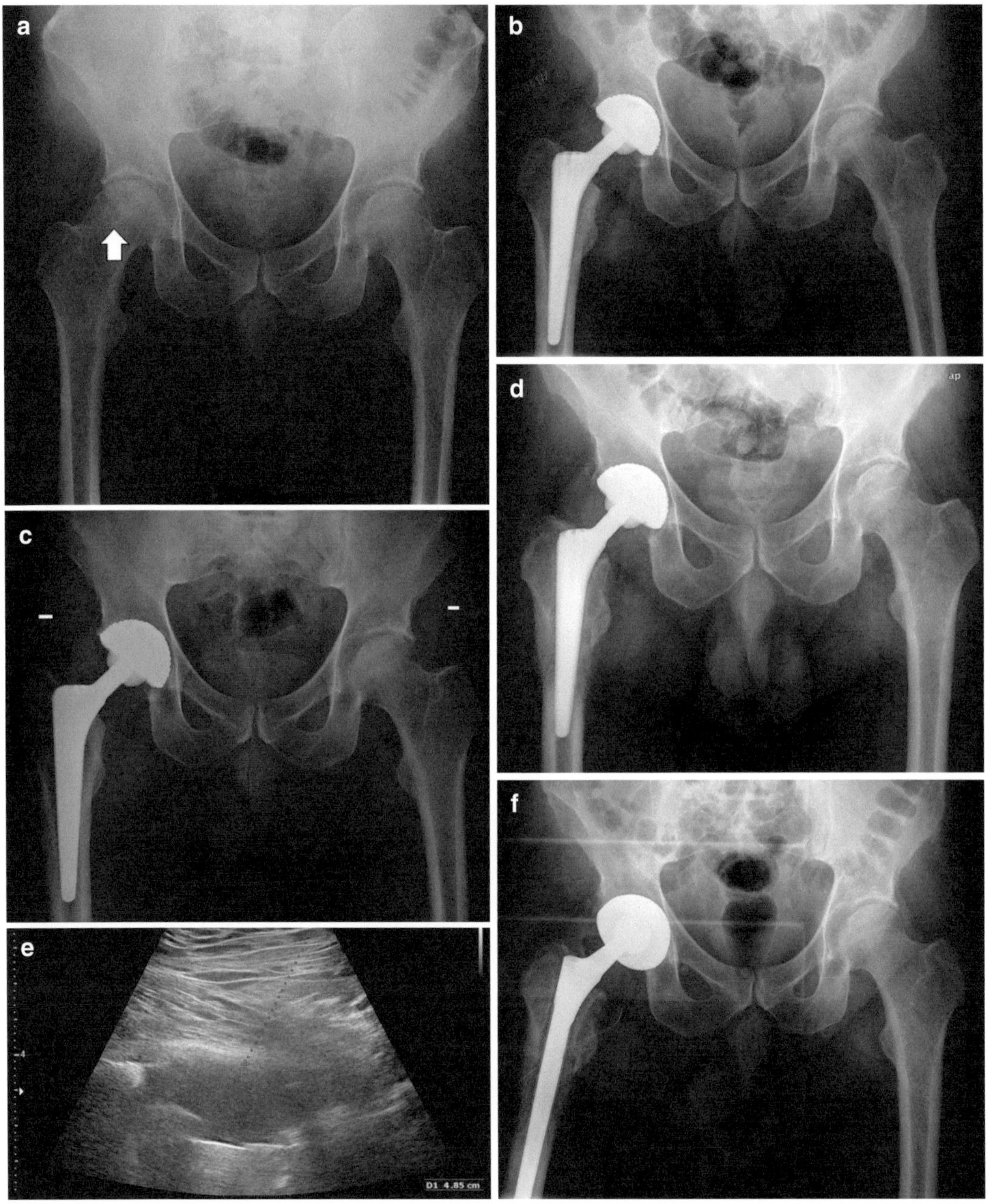

Fig. 9.1 A 56-year-old male patient underwent total hip replacement after being diagnosed with avascular necrosis of the right (white arrow) (**a**). A non-cemented total hip prosthesis with a ceramic-on-ceramic bearing was implanted (**b**). The patient initially showed favorable progress, remaining asymptomatic, pain-free, walking without crutches, and with a well-integrated prosthesis (**c**). Five years later, he began experiencing nocturnal thigh pain. The pain required him to walk with two crutches, and X-rays revealed peri-implant radiolucency and changes in femoral bone density (**d**). His recent history includes treatment for dental issues. Blood tests showed normal erythrocyte sedimentation rate with a high C-reactive protein level (77.9 mg/L, normal <5.0). An ultrasound-guided arthrocentesis was performed (**e**), with samples testing positive for methicillin-sensitive *Staphylococcus aureus*. A one-stage revision was decided upon, in which an uncemented dual-mobility acetabular cup (Avantage, Zimmer, Warsaw, IN) and an uncemented Wagner stem (Zimmer, Warsaw, IN) were implanted (**f**). One year after the revision, the patient is asymptomatic with normal lab values, and the implant shows bone ingrowth and is stable (**g**)

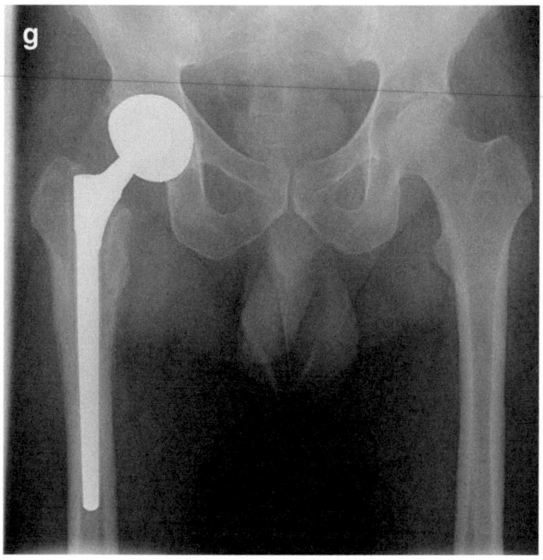

Fig. 9.1 (continued)

9.4 Two-Stage rTHA

9.4.1 Two-Stage rTHA with Commercial Polymethylmethacrylate (PMMA) Articulated Hip Spacer

Perez Alamino et al. affirmed in 2023 that orthopedic surgeons still fight against PJI and that two-stage rTHA is deemed the gold standard for chronic PJI for many authors, with success rates over 90%. This approach involves the removal of the prosthesis and the implantation of an antibiotic-impregnated cement spacer in the joint [11]. In their study, they evaluated the efficacy of a two-stage revision strategy utilizing a commercial prefabricated antibiotic-impregnated cement hip spacer for the treatment of hip PJI regarding monomicrobial and polymicrobial infections. They also evaluated risk factors for failure of two-stage rTHA. They performed a retrospective study on individuals that experienced rTHA between January 2002 and January 2018. They included adult individuals with a diagnosis of chronic hip PJI that experienced two-stage rTHA utilizing a prefabricated gentamicin-impregnated cement of PMMA hip spacer. They evaluated whether infections were monomicrobial or polymicrobial and assessed comorbidities. Treatment success was defined as eradication of the infection with no further procedures or mortality registered after the second stage. Persistence or recurrence of infection was deemed a failure of treatment. The final cohort consisted of 84 individuals treated with the same hip spacer: 60 (71.4%) monomicrobial, and 24 (28.6%) polymicrobial joint infections with an overall follow-up of 59 months. The overall success rate was 90.5%. Eight (9.5%) individuals failed. Smoking and body mass index (BMI) greater than 30 kg/m^2 were identified as independent risk factors for failure in multivariate analysis. This study suggested that prefabricated gentamicin-impregnated PMMA spacer was an effective tool for the treatment of PJI, accomplishing similar results whether the infections were monomicrobial or polymicrobial (Fig. 9.2). However, Perez Alamino et al. stated that randomized prospective studies were required to obtain more dependable conclusions [11].

9.4.2 Functional Results After rTHA in Individuals Treated With and Without an Antibiotic-Loaded Cement Spacer for PJI

In 2023, Fiore et al. stated that a staged revision with placement of a temporary antibiotic-loaded cement spacer after removal of the implant was the "gold standard" for management of chronic PJI. It enables local delivery of antibiotics, maintenance of limb length and mobility, and easier reimplantation. However, bacterial colonization of spacers and mechanical complications can also happen [12]. In their study, they assessed functional outcomes and infection control in two-stage rTHA PJI with and without a spacer. A retrospective review of 64 consecutive individuals was performed: 34 experienced two-stage revision utilizing a cement spacer (cohort A), and 30 experienced two-stage revision without a spacer (cohort B). At the final follow-up, functional assessment of individuals who underwent a THA,

Fig. 9.2 Two-stage revision total hip arthroplasty (rTHA) with commercial polymethylmethacrylate (PMMA) articulated hip spacer

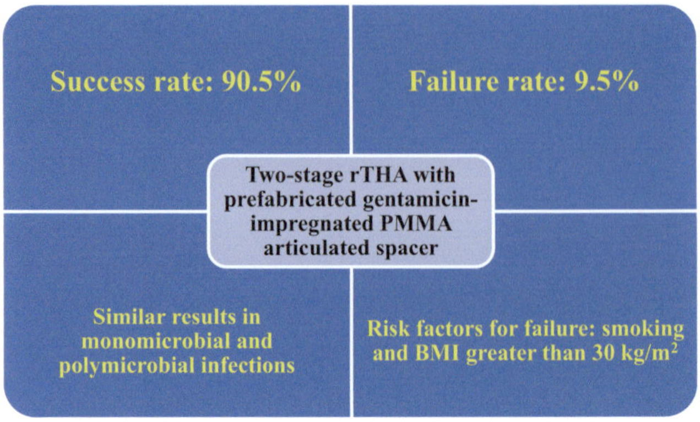

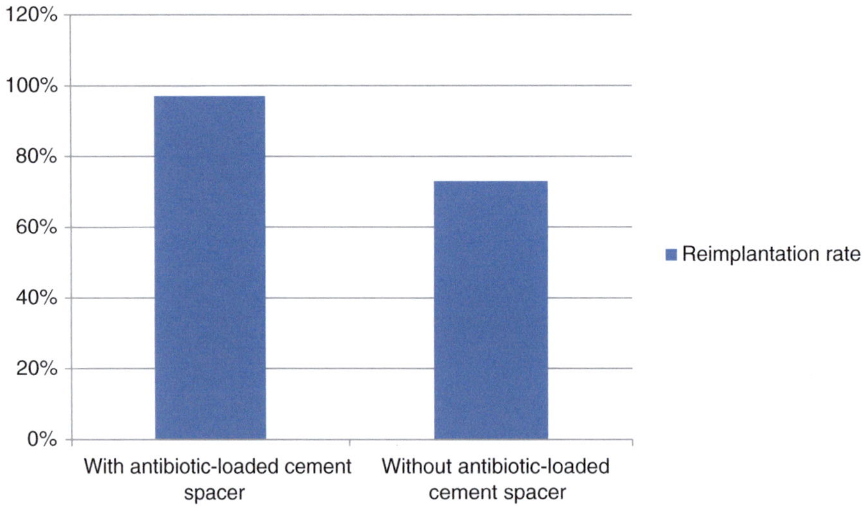

Fig. 9.3 Reimplantation rate after revision total hip arthroplasty (rTHA) in individuals treated with and without an antibiotic-loaded cement spacer for periprosthetic joint infection (PJI)

without PJI recurrence, was performed using the Harris hip score. Measurement of limb length and offset discrepancies was performed using anteroposterior pelvic X-rays. Most individuals in cohort B were older with more comorbidities preoperatively. Thirty-three individuals (97%) in cohort A experienced THA reimplantation compared with twenty-two individuals (73%) in cohort B (Fig. 9.3). No significant differences in limb length and offset were found. The outcomes of functional assessment performed during the final follow-up (mean, 41 months) demonstrated better function in individuals in cohort A (mean Harris hip score, 76.3 vs. 55.9). The utilization of antibiotic-loaded cement spacer appeared superior in terms of functional results and reimplantation rate [12].

9.4.3 Girdlestone Situation in the Interim Period

According to Adl Amini et al. (2023), most frequently spacers with or without antibiotics are implanted in a two-stage rTHA, even though not always indicated due to unknown pathogen, femoral and acetabular defects, or muscular insufficiency. A retrospective analysis (level 3 of evidence) of a prospectively collected database was performed, analyzing the treatment of 44

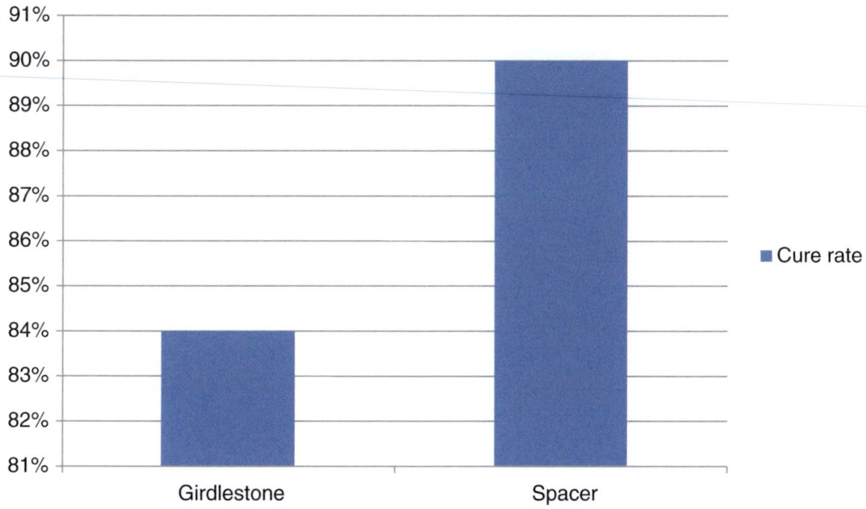

Fig. 9.4 Cure rate of revision total hip arthroplasty (rTHA) for periprosthetic joint infection (PJI): Girdlestone versus antibiotic-loaded cement spacer

consecutive cases with chronic PJI experiencing two-stage rTHA using a Girdlestone situation (GS) in the interim period between January 2015 and December 2018 [13]. Adl Amini et al. analyzed the general and age-group-specific success rate of management using GS. Moreover, they compared their findings with the literature on spacer implantation regarding common complications. In total, 21 women and 23 men at a mean age of 59.3 years were included. Age groups were divided into young, mid-age, and elderly. In most individuals, microbiology revealed *Staphylococcus epidermidis* in 39.1% of cases, followed by *Staphylococcus lugdunensis* and *Staphylococcus aureus* in 10.9% after THA explantation. For histology, Krenn and Morawietz type 2 (infectious type) was diagnosed in 40.9%, and type 3 (infectious and abrade-induced type) in 25% [14]. With GS, the total cure rate was 84% compared with 90% using a spacer as described in the literature (Fig. 9.4). Among age groups, the cure rate varied between 77.8% and 100%. Other adverse events, which only happened in the mid-age and elderly group, included the need for transfusion in 31%, and, one periprosthetic fracture was found in total (2%). According to Adl Amini et al., GS showed an acceptable cure rate at a minimum of 2 years when compared with the cure rate reported in the literature for spacers without major adverse events. For individuals with increased risks for treatment failure utilizing a spacer, GS appeared to be an alternative for chronic PJI when considering the success rate of management.

9.4.4 Custom-Made Articulating Spacer (CUMARS)

According to Wong et al. (2023), two-stage rTHA for PJI has been associated with poor patient tolerance, diminished patient mobility, and periarticular tissue contracture, leading to difficulty during second-stage reconstruction. The custom-made articulating spacer (CUMARS) was developed to provide an option that is better tolerated and to diminish the complexity of second-stage reconstruction. In their study, they detailed the treatment of an individual with PJI after THA with substantial periosteal reaction utilizing a CUMARS construct, which enabled prompt postoperative weight bearing, ultimate eradication of infection, restoration of femoral bone stock, and restraint of second-stage reconstruction [15].

9.4.5 New Intraoperatively Molded Articulating Spacer Design

In 2023, Cacciola et al. analyzed a new functional articulating hip spacer called "Spaceflex." A group of 56 individuals with chronic hip PJI experiencing two-stage rTHA utilizing a new intraoperatively molded articulating hip spacer design was analyzed. The rate of mechanical complications related to the spacer was low (5.8%). The rate of success of the two-stage procedure was 90.6%. PROMs also improved. Moreover, the reinfection rate was in line with other publications with different spacer designs [16].

9.4.6 Two-Stage rTHA: Cemented Versus Cementless

According to Hipfl et al. (2023), the influence of the previous fixation mode on the result of chronic PJI after THA is unclear. Besides, removal of cemented THA is challenging and residual cement may be associated with reinfection [17]. In their study, they compared the outcomes of two-stage revision for PJI in cemented and cementless THA. They analyzed 143 individuals experiencing two-stage rTHA for PJI. Thirty-six individuals with a fully cemented ($N = 6$), hybrid femur ($N = 26$), or hybrid acetabulum ($N = 4$) THA (cemented cohort) were matched 1:2 with a group of 72 individuals who experienced removal of a cementless THA (cementless cohort). Cohorts were matched by gender, age, number of previous surgeries, and history of infection treatment. Minimum follow-up was 2 years. Compared with PJI in cementless THA, individuals experiencing removal of cemented THA had increasingly severe femoral bone loss. Individuals in the cemented cohort had an increased risk of positive cultures during second-stage reimplantation (22% compared with 8%), higher rates of reinfection (22% compared with 7%), and all-cause revision (31% compared with 14%) compared with individuals experiencing two-stage revision of cementless THA (Fig. 9.5). Periprosthetic femoral fractures were more common in the cohort of individuals with previous cementation. Mean modified Harris hip score had been 37.5 in the cemented cohort and 39.1 in the cementless cohort, and these scores improved substantially in both cohorts. This study showed that chronic infection in cemented THA may be associated with increased bone loss, higher rates of reinfection and all-cause revision following two-stage rTHA [17]. Figure 9.6 shows a case of two-stage rTHA due to PJI.

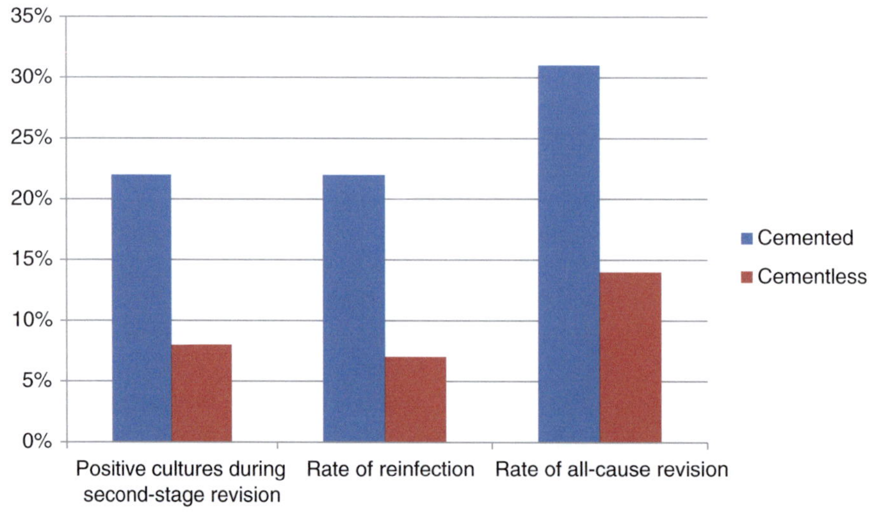

Fig. 9.5 Two-stage revision total hip arthroplasty (rTHA) for periprosthetic joint infection (PJI): cemented implant versus cementless implant

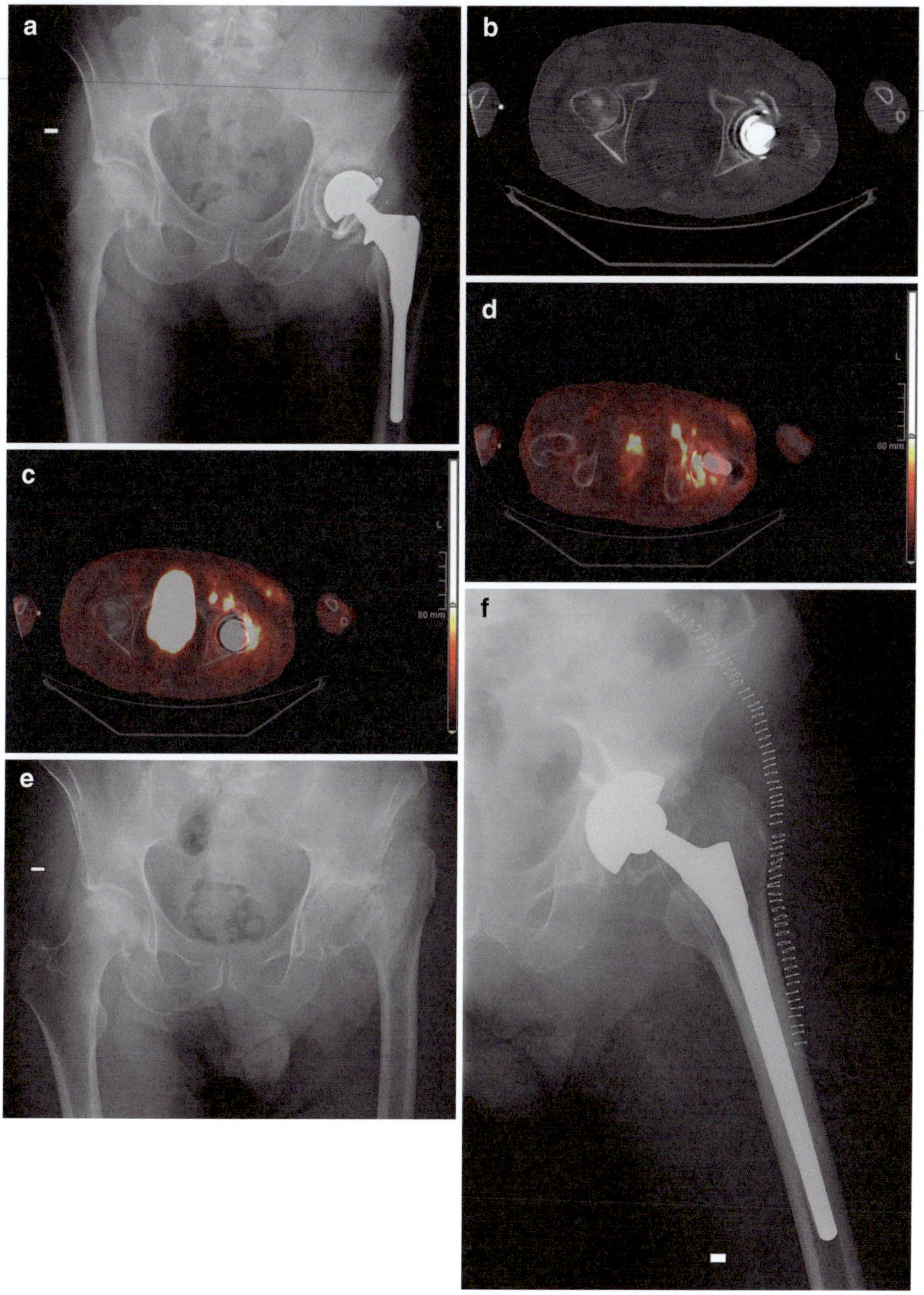

Fig. 9.6 A 72-year-old male with a history of immunodeficiency, currently on antiretroviral treatment, underwent a total hip replacement on the left side after a femoral neck fracture. He experienced several dislocations and underwent revision surgery 1 year later, receiving a cemented constrained acetabular cup. He was referred due to resting pain and walking pain, which forced him to use two crutches. Imaging studies showed loosening of the acetabular component with radiolucent lines, and blood tests indicated elevated acute phase reactants (**a**). A PET-CT scan showed uptake consistent with an infectious process related to his arthroplasty (**b–d**). An arthrocentesis was performed, and a methicillin-sensitive but quinolone- and clindamycin-resistant *Staphylococcus epidermidis* was cultured. A two-stage revision with a Girdlestone-type resection arthroplasty was decided (**e**). The same pathogen was cultured in all intraoperative samples. He was treated with intravenous cefazolin for 3 weeks, followed by 4 weeks of oral antibiotic therapy. After normalization of blood test values, he underwent re-implantation with a dual-mobility G7 acetabular cup (Zimmer-Biomet, Warsaw, IN) and a Wagner-type stem (Zimmer-Biomet, Warsaw, IN) (**f**). Six years post-revision, the implant remains well-integrated, and the patient is asymptomatic with normal blood test results (**g–i**)

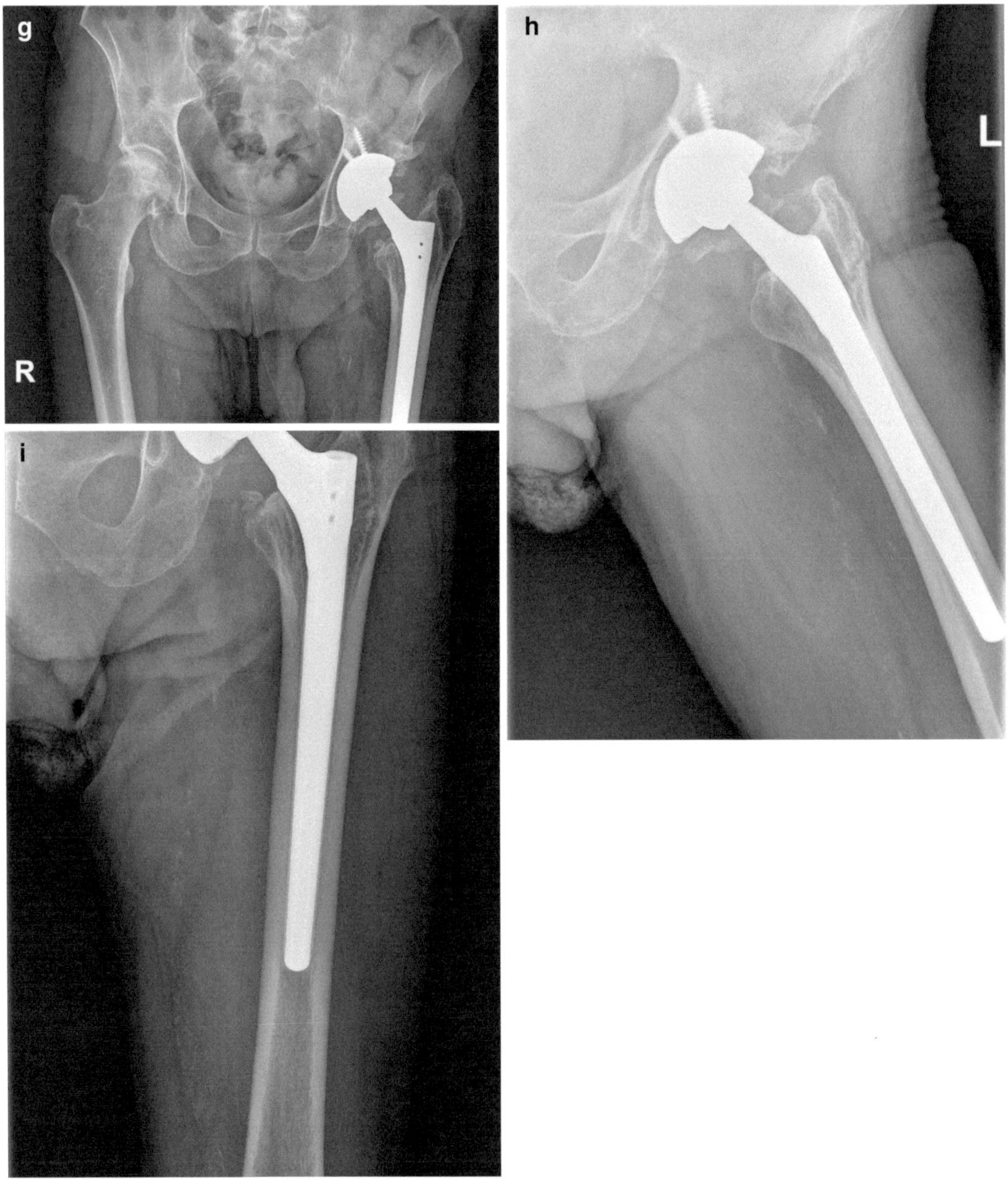

Fig. 9.6 (continued)

9.4.7 Optimal Reimplantation Timing

In 2024, Tsai et al. affirmed that the optimal timing for reimplantation for PJI has not been determined and varies from a few weeks to several months. In their study, they evaluated commendable time between implant removal and reimplantation in individuals who experienced two-stage exchange arthroplasty for PJI. They analyzed 361 individuals who were treated with two-stage exchange arthroplasty for hip and knee chronic PJI. In the final analysis, 27 (7.5%) had treatment failure. Factors related to treatment failure included interim spacer exchange, higher ESR level at reimplantation, and time to reimplantation. Performing rTHA from 16 to 20 weeks had the highest success rate. Reimplantation beyond 24 weeks had a lower success rate. However, no statistical significance when comparing each interval group was found [18].

9.5 Revision THA for *Enterobacter cloacae*–Associated PJI

In 2023, Ashkenazi et al. stated that while recent data suggested that *Enterobacter cloacae* was an emerging source of PJI, characteristics and results of *Enterobacter cloacae*–associated infections were rarely published. In their study, they presented and described the findings and results of *Enterobacter cloacae*–associated PJI in their center. The minimum follow-up was 2 years. Of 108 rTHAs, 12 individuals (11.1%) were diagnosed with *Enterobacter cloacae*–associated PJI. Most cases had a polymicrobial PJI ($N = 8$, 66.7%). Five *Enterobacter cloacae* strains (41.7%) were gentamicin-resistant. Six individuals (50%) experienced two or more revisions, while three of them (25%) needed four or more revisions until their PJI was resolved. When using the MSIS outcome score, the first surgical intervention was deemed successful (MSIS score levels 1 and 2) for five individuals (41.7%) and failed (levels 3 and 4) for seven individuals (58.3%) [2].

9.6 Re-rTHA: Modular Proximal Body Exchange

According to Harmer et al. (2023), modular fluted tapered stems (MFTSs) are commonly utilized in rTHA and render the option of exchanging the proximal modular portion to address future surgical problems without complete femoral revision. Between 1997 and 2019, they carried out 57 modular proximal body exchanges among 8079 rTHAs. In a study with level 4 of evidence, indications and results were documented at a mean follow-up of 3.4 years. Modular proximal body exchange was carried out on 47 of 1375 (3%) of MFTSs implanted. The indications for all 57 modular proximal body exchanges carried out during the study period were dislocation in 30 (53%), partial resection for PJI in 13 (23%), modular junction failure in 8 (14%), surgical exposure in 4 (7%), and concurrently with trochanteric osteotomy nonunion fixation in 2 (4%). At the final follow-up, subsequent re-revisions occurred in 10 of 30 (33%) of modular proximal body exchanges indicated for dislocation and in 5 of 13 of those indicated for PJI. One modular junction subsequently fractured after modular proximal body exchange [19].

9.7 Conclusions

Cementless one-stage rTHA seems to be an effective treatment of early (less than 6 weeks) PJI after primary THA and at least an equal choice of treatment compared with DAIR. Cemented modular stems in one-stage septic rTHA with severe femoral bone loss are successful in 81.3% of cases. The success rate of two-stage rTHA with commercial prefabricated gentamicin-impregnated PMMA articulated hip spacer is 90.5%. About 10% of individuals fail. Smoking and body mass index (BMI) greater than 30 kg/m^2 are independent risk factors for failure. Similar results are obtained in monomicrobial and polymicrobial infections. A comparison of two-stage rTHA for PJI with and without a spacer showed that the utilization of antibiotic-loaded cement spacer was superior in terms of reimplantation rate (97.1% vs. 73.3%). A comparison of two-stage rTHA for PJI with a spacer versus Girdlestone situation showed the total cure rate was 84.1% with Girdlestone versus 90.1% using a spacer as described in the literature.

References

1. Liukkonen RJ, Honkanen M, Reito AP, Skyttä ET, Karppelin M, Eskelinen AP. Trends in revision hip arthroplasty for prosthetic joint infection: a single-center study of 423 hips at a high-volume center between 2008 and 2021. J Arthroplast.

2023;38(6):1151–9. https://doi.org/10.1016/j.arth.2023.02.061.

2. Ashkenazi I, Morgan S, Snir N, Gold A, Dekel M, Warschawski Y. Outcomes of Enterobacter cloacae-associated periprosthetic joint infection following hip arthroplasties. Clin Orthop Surg. 2023;15(6):902–9. https://doi.org/10.4055/cios23102.
3. Doyle DJ, Hendrix JM, Garmon EH. American Society of Anesthesiologists classification. [Updated 2023 Aug 17]. In: StatPearls [Internet]. Treasure Island: StatPearls Publishing; 2024. Available from: https://www.ncbi.nlm.nih.gov/books/NBK441940/.
4. Jayasinghe G, Kumar R, Buckle C, Vinayakam P, Slack R. Patient mortality after total hip arthroplasty revision surgery. J Orthop. 2023;47:45–9. https://doi.org/10.1016/j.jor.2023.11.020.
5. Parvizi J, Gehrke T, Chen AF. Proceedings of the International Consensus on Periprosthetic Joint Infection. Bone Joint J. 2013;95-B(11):1450–2. https://doi.org/10.1302/0301-620X.95B11.33135.
6. Pellegrini A, Legnani C. High rate of infection eradication following cementless one-stage revision hip arthroplasty with an antibacterial hydrogel coating. Int J Artif Organs. 2022;45(1):113–7. https://doi.org/10.1177/0391398821995507.
7. Liechti EF, Neufeld ME, Soto F, Linke P, Busch SM, Gehrke T, et al. Favourable outcomes of repeat one-stage exchange for periprosthetic joint infection of the hip. Bone Joint J. 2022;104-B(1):27–33. https://doi.org/10.1302/0301-620X.104B1.BJJ-2021-0970.R1.
8. Blom AW, Beswick AD, Burston A, Carroll FE, Garfield K, Gooberman-Hill R, et al. Infection after total joint replacement of the hip and knee: research programme including the INFORM RCT. Programme Grants Appl Res. 2022;10(10):1–190. https://doi.org/10.3310/HDWL9760.
9. Riemer K, Lange J. Early periprosthetic hip joint infection managed by cementless one-stage revision – a case series. J Bone Jt Infect. 2022;7(1):43–50. https://doi.org/10.5194/jbji-7-43-2022.
10. Russo A, Camacho Uribe A, Abuljadail S, Bokhari A, Gehrke T, Citak M. Excellent survival rate of cemented modular stems in one-stage revision for periprosthetic hip infections with massive femoral bone loss: a retrospective single-center analysis of 150 cases. J Arthroplast. 2024;39(6):1577–82. https://doi.org/10.1016/j.arth.2023.12.006.
11. Perez Alamino L, Garabano G, Rodriguez JA, Cullari M, Del Sel H, Pesciallo CA. Effectiveness of two-stage revision with commercial polymethylmethacrylate articulated hip spacer: similar outcomes against monomicrobial and polymicrobial hip periprosthetic joint infections. J Bone Jt Infect. 2023;8(1):51–7. https://doi.org/10.5194/jbji-8-51-2023.
12. Fiore M, Rondinella C, Paolucci A, Morante L, De Paolis M, Sambri A. Functional outcome after reimplantation in patients treated with and without an antibiotic-loaded cement spacers for hip prosthetic joint infections. Hip Pelvis. 2023;35(1):32–9. https://doi.org/10.5371/hp.2023.35.1.32.
13. Adl Amini D, Wu CH, Perka C, Bäcker HC. Cure rate of infections is not an argument for spacer in two-stage revision arthroplasty of the hip. Arch Orthop Trauma Surg. 2023;143(4):2199–207. https://doi.org/10.1007/s00402-022-04463-9.
14. Krenn V, Morawietz L, Perino G, Kienapfel H, Ascherl R, Hassenpflug GJ, Thomsen M, Thomas P, Huber M, Kendoff D, Baumhoer D, Krukemeyer MG, Natu S, et al. Revised histopathological consensus classification of joint implant related pathology. Pathol Res Pract. 2014;210(12):779–86. https://doi.org/10.1016/j.prp.2014.09.017.
15. Wong R, Abbas AA, Ayob KA, Nasuruddin H, Selvaratnam V. Custom-made articulating spacer (CUMARS): the resolution of periosteal reaction and femur remodelling in periprosthetic hip infection. Cureus. 2023;15(7):e41669. https://doi.org/10.7759/cureus.41669.
16. Cacciola G, Giustra F, Bosco F, De Meo F, Bruschetta A, Cavaliere P. Two-stage revision in periprosthetic joint infection of the hip using a new intraoperatively molded articulating spacer design. J Clin Orthop Trauma. 2023;43:102223. https://doi.org/10.1016/j.jcot.2023.102223.
17. Hipfl C, Leopold V, Becker L, Pumberger M, Perka C, Hardt S. Two-stage revision for periprosthetic joint infection in cemented total hip arthroplasty: an increased risk for failure? Arch Orthop Trauma Surg. 2023;143(7):4481–90. https://doi.org/10.1007/s00402-022-04671-3.
18. Tsai ML, Herng-Shouh Hsu A, Wu CT, Lin PC, Tan TL, Kuo FC. Optimal reimplantation timing in two-stage exchange for periprosthetic joint infection: an observative cohort study in Asian population. BMC Musculoskelet Disord. 2024;25(1):28. https://doi.org/10.1186/s12891-023-07129-8.
19. Harmer JR, Hadley ML, Trousdale RT. Modular proximal body exchange for re-revision total hip arthroplasty: rarely utilized and moderately successful. J Arthroplast. 2023;38(7S):S229–34.e1. https://doi.org/10.1016/j.arth.2023.04.020.

Risk Factors of Periprosthetic Joint Infection in Total Knee Arthroplasty

10

E. Carlos Rodríguez-Merchán,
Hortensia De la Corte-Rodríguez,
and Alonso Moreno-García

10.1 Introduction

Periprosthetic joint infection (PJI) is the most serious and feared complication in total knee arthroplasty (TKA) and can have catastrophic effects (Fig. 10.1). The number of TKAs is rising, so infections could also be greater in the time to come [1].

PJI is a serious adverse event of primary TKA from the patient's point of view, and it is also expensive for health care systems. In 2010, the published incidence of PJI in the first 2 years after TKA was 1.55%, with an incidence of 0.46% between the second and tenth years. In 2022, it was reported that 1.41% of individuals needed revision TKA for PJI [2]. The purpose of this chapter is to analyze the most recent data on the risk factors of PJI in TKA.

E. C. Rodríguez-Merchán (✉) · A. Moreno-García
Department of Orthopedic Surgery, Hospital Universitario La Paz, Madrid, Madrid, Spain

H. De la Corte-Rodríguez
Department of Physical and Rehabilitation Medicine, Hospital Universitario La Paz, Madrid, Spain

E. C. Rodríguez-Merchán (ed.), *Advances in Periprosthetic Joint Infection*,
https://doi.org/10.1007/978-3-032-02945-4_10

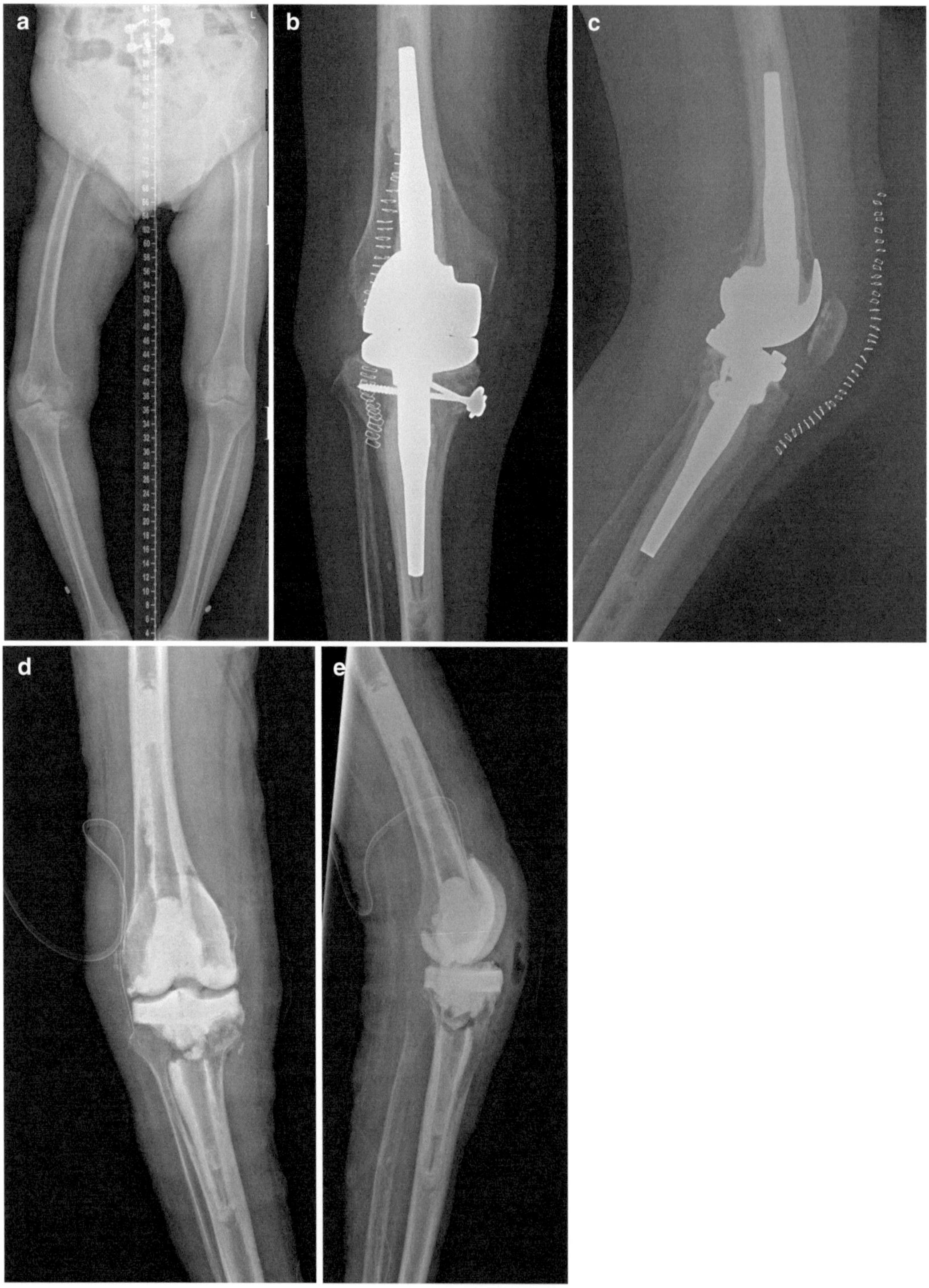

Fig. 10.1 Posttraumatic right knee osteoarthritis, with varus deformity and medial instability (**a**). A constrained implant was used, with the adjunct of an allograft on the medial metaphysis of the tibia. Anteroposterior (**b**) and lateral views (**c**). Ten months after the index surgery, the first stage (removal of the prosthesis and implantation of a cermented spacer) was performed due to *extended-spectrum beta-lactamase-producing Escherichia coli* PJI. Anteroposterior (**d**) and lateral views (**e**)

10.2 Risk Factors Associated with PJI After TKA

In a case-control study of individuals who experienced TKA, Blanco et al. (2020) tried to identify the most relevant risk factors associated with infection after a TKA. The study included 66 TKA PJI individuals and 66 control TKA individuals. Prolonged operative time (more than 90 minutes) and tourniquet time (more than 60 minutes) were the most relevant risk factors described. The utilization of non–antibiotic-loaded cement, obesity (BMI > 30), diabetes, high ASA grade, and blood transfusion requirement were also statistically significant risk factors for TKA PJI [1]. Risk factors that have been related to an increased risk of PJI are shown in Table 10.1. Preoperative intravenous tranexamic acid has been found to reduce the risk of delayed PJI [2].

In 2023, Weinstein et al. identified some patient and surgical factors of PJI happening early (≤3 months), delayed (between >3 and ≤12 months), and late (>12 months) after primary TKA [3]. They analyzed 79,367 individuals (median age of 65 years) in the overall cohort who experienced primary TKA, included 75,274 men (94.8%). A total of 1599 PJIs (2%) were found. The incidence rate of PJI was greater in the early (27 events per 10,000 person-months) and delayed stages (5 events per 10,000 person-months) versus the late postoperative stage (1 event per 10,000 person-

Table 10.1 Risk factors related to an increased risk of periprosthetic joint infection (PJI) in total knee arthroplasty (TKA)

Male sex
Younger age
Type II diabetes
Obesity class II
Hypertension
Hypoalbuminemia
Preoperative nutritional status as indicated by PNI and BMI
Rheumatoid arthritis
Posttraumatic osteoarthritis
Intraarticular injections prior to TKA
Previous multi-ligament knee surgery
Previous steroid therapy
Current tobacco use
Procedure type (bilateral)
LOS over 35 days
Patellar resurfacing
Prolonged operative time
Use of blood transfusions
Higher glucose variability in the postoperative phase
Discharge to convalescent care
Congestive heart failure
Chronic pulmonary illness
Preoperative anemia
Depression
Renal illness
Pulmonary circulation disorders
Psychoses
Metastatic tumor
Peripheral vascular illness
Valvular illness

PNI prognostic nutritional index, *BMI* body mass index, *LOS* length of stay

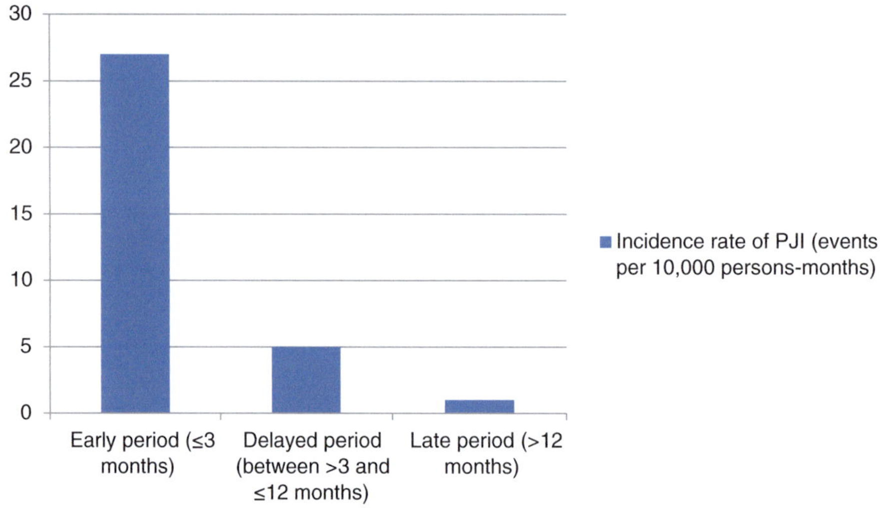

Fig. 10.2 Incidence rates of periprosthetic joint infection (PJI) during different time periods after primary total knee arthroplasty (TKA) implantation

months) (Fig. 10.2). *Staphylococcus aureus* was the most frequent bacterium isolated overall (33.2%); however, gram-negative infections were isolated in 15.4% of early PJIs. Hepatitis C virus infection, peripheral artery disease, and autoimmune inflammatory arthritis were associated with PJI across all postoperative stages. Diabetes, chronic kidney disease, and obesity ([body mass index] BMI ≥ 30) were not associated factors [3].

10.3 Risk Factors Associated with PJI After TKA in Patients Older than 80 Years

In a report with level 3 of evidence, Sodhi et al. (2020) studied the risk factors for surgical site infections (SSIs) at 90 days and PJIs at 2 years after surgery in individuals aged 80 years and older experiencing primary ($N = 275{,}717$) and revision TKA ($N = 28{,}779$). For primary TKA individuals, an increased risk of 90-day SSIs was associated with male sex, BMI greater than 25 kg/m^2, and other comorbidities. For revision TKA individuals, an increased risk of SSI was associated with iron-deficiency anemia [4].

10.4 Time Interval Between Knee Arthroscopy and Subsequent Primary TKA Is Associated with Increased Rates of PJI Following TKA

In a study with level 3 of evidence, Gu et al. (2021) found a time-dependent association between the timing of knee arthroscopy and adverse events following TKA, with the prevalence of revision surgery and PJI increasing as knee arthroscopy was performed closer to the time of TKA [5]. This study suggested that an interval of at least 36 weeks should be maintained between the two surgical procedures to minimize the risks of PJI and revision surgery. Data from 2006 to 2017 were collected from a national insurance database. Individuals who experienced knee arthroscopy within 1 year prior to primary TKA were stratified into the following groups based on stratum-specific likelihood ratio analysis: 0–15, 16–35, 36–43, and 44–52 weeks from the time of knee arthroscopy to TKA. In total, 130,128 individuals were analyzed; 6105 (4.7%) of those individuals experienced knee arthroscopy within 1 year before TKA and 124,023 (95.3%) experienced TKA without any previous knee surgery, including arthroscopy (the control cohort). Relative to the control cohort, the probability of experiencing revision surgery was substantially greater in individuals who experienced knee arthroscopy ≤15 weeks or 16–35 weeks before TKA. Individuals were at substantially increased risk for PJI if knee arthroscopy was performed ≤35 weeks before TKA [5].

10.5 Risk of PJI in Patients with TKA Undergoing Colonoscopy

In a study with level 3 of evidence, Shin et al. (2022) found that colonoscopy was associated with an increased PJI risk in TKA recipients, regardless of concomitant invasive colonoscopic procedures (biopsy, polypectomy, and mucosal or submucosal resection). In total, 45,612 and 211,841 individuals were matched in the colonoscopy and control groups, respectively. The colonoscopy cohort had greater 9-month and 1-year PJI risks from the index colonoscopy date than the matched controls [6].

10.6 Manipulation Under Anesthesia (MUA) Following Primary TKA Is Associated with Increased Rates of PJI

In 2023, Parkulo et al. found an increased incidence of revision surgery and PJI in individuals experiencing MUA due to stiffness following TKA [7]. They analyzed 142,440 individuals who had primary TKA from a national database and identified 3652 patients (2.6%) who experienced MUA. The incidence of MUA was higher in Black versus White individuals (4.1% versus 2.5%). Revision risk was significantly greater in the MUA cohort at 1-, 2-, and 5-year time points with a hazard ratio (HR) of 3.81, 3.90, and 3.22, respectively. One- and 2-year revision risk was substantially greater when MUA occurred at 6–12 months post-TKA compared with <3 months. Risk of PJI was substantially greater in the MUA cohort with an HR of 2.2, 2.2, and 2.1 at 1, 2, and 5 years, respectively [7].

10.7 Risk Factors for Revision due to PJI Following TKA

In 2023, Keemu et al. evaluated the risk factors for revision due to PJI following TKA based on the Finnish Arthroplasty Register. They found an increased risk for revision due to PJI when no incise drape was utilized. The use of drainage also increased the risk. Specializing in carrying out TKA diminished operative time and thereby also the PJI rate [8].

10.8 Prior Septic Arthritis Within 1 Year of TKA Is Associated with a High Risk for PJI

In 2023, Hameed et al. stated that a previous history of a septic knee might predispose individuals to a PJI after TKA [9]. In their study, an increased PJI risk in the first year after septic arthritis was found. The focus of the study was an evaluation of the incidence of TKA PJIs at various time intervals after the onset of a septic knee (0–3 months, 3–6 months, 6–9 months, and 9–12 months). They queried a national database to identify individuals who experienced a primary TKA between 2010 and 2021 (N = 1.9 million). Individuals who had a previous septic knee ipsilateral to the primary TKA were characterized (N = 4251) and were categorized into four specific groups based on the interval between the septic arthritis diagnosis and TKA: less than 3 months, 3–6 months, 6–9 months, and 9–12 months. A group of individuals who did not have a history of septic knee was utilized for comparison (N = 5000). All time groups were more likely to need revisions because of PJI, as compared to the comparison cohort. Substantial differences were shown among all time groups who had previous septic arthritis compared with individuals who did not have a history of septic arthritis. Therefore, orthopedic surgeons should be aware of the increased PJI risk after septic arthritis within the first year after TKA [9].

10.9 Tobacco and Cannabis Use Have a Synergistic Association on PJI Risk Following TKA

In 2023, Oster et al. evaluated tobacco, cannabis, and combined users who experienced primary TKA to determine 90-day to 2-year odds of PJI; odds of revision; and medical complications [10]. They queried a national, all-payer database of individuals experiencing primary TKA between 2010 and 2020. Individuals were stratified according to current use of tobacco products ($N = 30{,}000$), cannabis ($N = 400$), or a combination ($N = 3526$). A fourth cohort of TKA recipients who did not have tobacco or cannabis use was utilized as a matching group. Combined tobacco and cannabis use was associated with the highest rates of PJI after TKA. The odds of 90-day PJI risk among cannabis, tobacco, and combined users were 1.60, 2.14, and 3.39, respectively, as compared to the matched group. Co-users had the highest and substantially increased revision odds at 2 years after TKA. At 1 and 2 years following TKA, cannabis, tobacco, and co-users had higher rates of myocardial infarctions, respiratory failures, SSIs, and MUAs when compared to the matched group. Therefore, tobacco and cannabis use prior to primary TKA showed a synergistic association on PJI risk from 90 days through 2 years [10].

10.10 Conclusions

The following risk factors have been related to an increased risk of PJI: male sex, younger age, type II diabetes, obesity class II, hypertension, hypoalbuminemia, preoperative nutritional status as indicated by PNI and BMI, rheumatoid arthritis, post-traumatic osteoarthritis, intraarticular injections prior to TKA, previous multi-ligament knee surgery, previous steroid therapy, current tobacco use, procedure type (bilateral), length of stay over 35 days, patellar resurfacing, prolonged operative time, use of blood transfusions, higher glucose variability in the postoperative phase, and discharge to convalescent care. Other reported independent risk factors for PJI are congestive heart failure, chronic pulmonary illness, preoperative anemia, depression, renal illness, pulmonary circulation disorders, psychoses, metastatic tumor, peripheral vascular illness, and valvular illness. Preoperative intravenous tranexamic acid has been reported to diminish the risk of delayed PJI.

References

1. Blanco JF, Díaz A, Melchor FR, da Casa C, Pescador D. Risk factors for periprosthetic joint infection after total knee arthroplasty. Arch Orthop Trauma Surg. 2020;140(2):239–45. https://doi.org/10.1007/s00402-019-03304-6.
2. Rodriguez-Merchan EC, Delgado-Martinez AD. Risk factors for periprosthetic joint infection after primary total knee arthroplasty. J Clin Med. 2022;11(20):6128. https://doi.org/10.3390/jcm11206128.
3. Weinstein EJ, Stephens-Shields AJ, Newcomb CW, Silibovsky R, Nelson CL, O'Donnell JA, et al. Incidence, microbiological studies, and factors associated with prosthetic joint infection after total knee arthroplasty. JAMA Netw Open. 2023;6(10):e2340457. https://doi.org/10.1001/jamanetworkopen.2023.40457.
4. Sodhi N, Anis HK, Vakharia RM, Acuña AJ, Gold PA, Garbarino LJ, et al. What are risk factors for infection after primary or revision total joint arthroplasty in patients older than 80 years? Clin Orthop Relat Res. 2020;478(8):1741–51. https://doi.org/10.1097/CORR.0000000000001389.
5. Gu A, Fassihi SC, Wessel LE, Kahlenberg C, Ast MP, Sculco PK, et al. Comparison of revision risk based on timing of knee arthroscopy prior to total knee arthroplasty. J Bone Joint Surg Am. 2021;103(8):660–7. https://doi.org/10.2106/JBJS.20.00218.
6. Shin KH, Han SB, Song JE. Risk of periprosthetic joint infection in patients with total knee arthroplasty undergoing colonoscopy: a nationwide propensity score matched study. J Arthroplast. 2022;37(1):49–56. https://doi.org/10.1016/j.arth.2021.09.015.
7. Parkulo TD, Likine EF, Ong KL, Watson HN, Smith LS, Malkani AL. Manipulation following primary total knee arthroplasty is associated with increased rates of infection and revision. J Arthroplast. 2023;38(3):567–572.e1. https://doi.org/10.1016/j.arth.2022.09.027.
8. Keemu H, Alakylä KJ, Klén R, Panula VJ, Venäläinen MS, Haapakoski JJ, et al. Risk factors for revision

due to prosthetic joint infection following total knee arthroplasty based on 62,087 knees in the Finnish Arthroplasty Register from 2014 to 2020. Acta Orthop. 2023;94:215–23. https://doi.org/10.2340/17453674.2023.12307.

9. Hameed D, Bains SS, Chen Z, Dubin JA, Delanois RE, Mont MA, et al. Prior septic arthritis within one year of knee arthroplasty is associated with a high risk for infection. J Arthroplast. 2023;38(5):925–929.e1. https://doi.org/10.1016/j.arth.2022.11.020.

10. Oster B, Hameed D, Bains SS, Delanois RE, Johnson AJ, Nace J, et al. Tobacco and cannabis use have a synergistic association on infection risk following total knee arthroplasty. J Arthroplast. 2023;38(10):2137–41. https://doi.org/10.1016/j.arth.2023.04.053.

11 Prevention of Periprosthetic Joint Infection in Total Knee Arthroplasty

E. Carlos Rodríguez-Merchán,
Hortensia De la Corte-Rodríguez,
and Alonso Moreno-García

11.1 Introduction

According to Dobson and Reed rates of periprosthetic joint infection (PJI) in primary total knee arthroplasty (TKA) range between 0.3% and 1.9%, and up to 10% in revision cases. Substantial morbidity is associated with this disastrous complication. The economic burden on healthcare systems is extensive and the personal cost to the affected individual is vast [1]. We perform careful skin antisepsis and povidone-iodine lavage prior to TKA. Then an impervious stockinet and sterile drapes are placed (Fig. 11.1). The purpose of this chapter is to analyze the most recent data on the prevention of PJI in TKA.

E. C. Rodríguez-Merchán (✉) · A. Moreno-García
Department of Orthopedic Surgery, Hospital Universitario La Paz, Madrid, Madrid, Spain

H. De la Corte-Rodríguez
Department of Physical and Rehabilitation Medicine, Hospital Universitario La Paz, Madrid, Spain

E. C. Rodríguez-Merchán (ed.), *Advances in Periprosthetic Joint Infection*,
https://doi.org/10.1007/978-3-032-02945-4_11

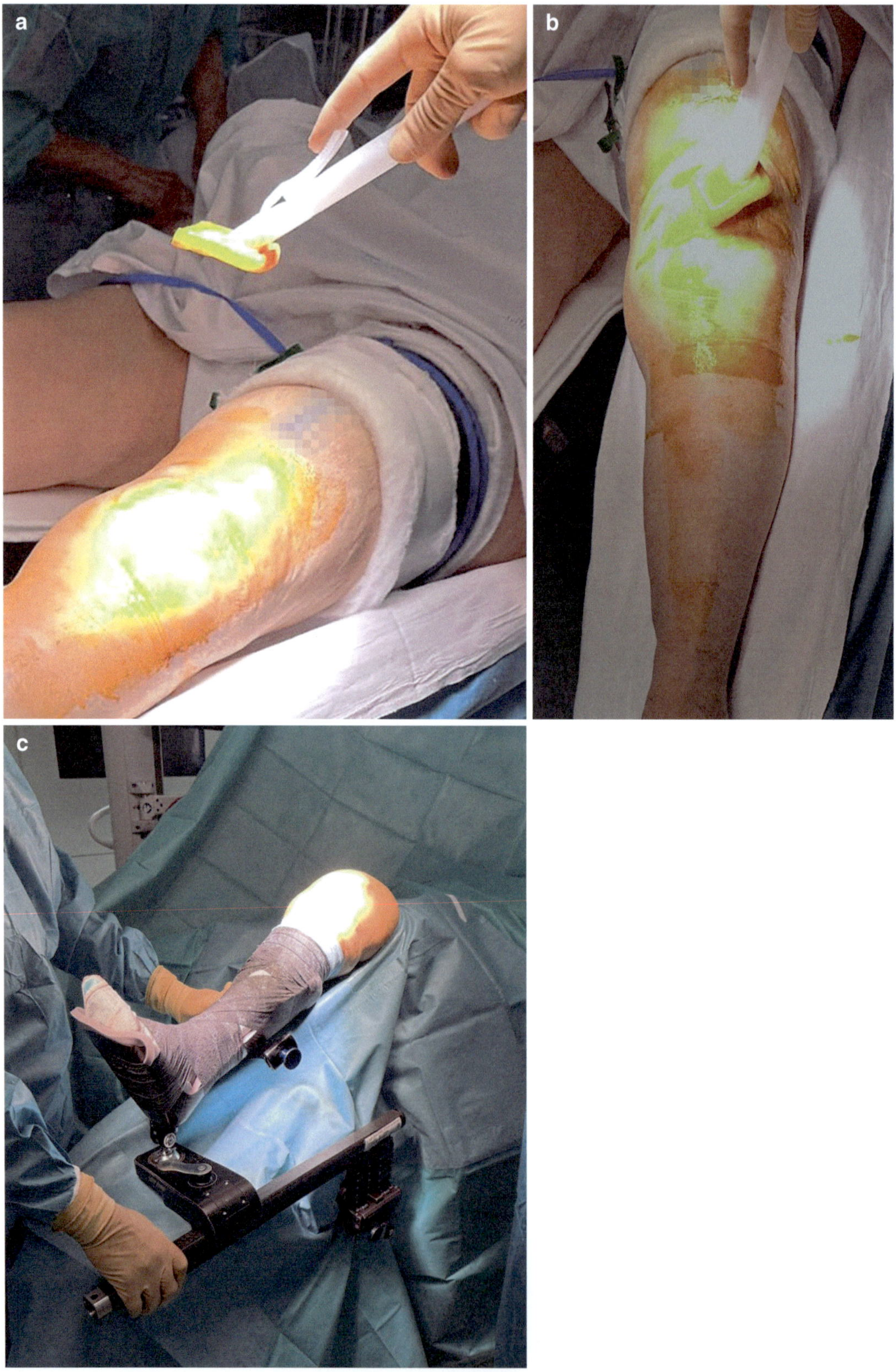

Fig. 11.1 Careful skin antisepsis and povidone-iodine lavage previous to total knee arthroplasty (**a**, **b**); an impervious stockinet and sterile drapes are placed, and the surgical site preparation is finished (**c**)

11.2 Multifaceted Strategy for the Prevention of Infection in Primary TKA

The risk of surgical site infection (SSI) and PJI is related to surgical factors and patient factors such as age, body mass index (BMI), comorbidities, and lifestyle. Reducing the risk of SSI in primary TKA requires a multifaceted approach that is shown in Table 11.1 [1]. In a study with level 4 of evidence published in 2022, Indelli et al. reported the results of a survey distributed among The European Knee Associates (EKA), the American Association of Hip and Knee Surgeons (AAHKS) International Committee, and the Arthroplasty Society in Asia (ASIA) members and their affiliated arthroplasty surgeons. The survey consisted of 20 single and multiple-response questions focused on PJI prevention approaches at three perioperative periods: preoperatively, intraoperatively, and postoperatively. Three hundred and ninety-four arthroplasty surgeons from six different continents completed the survey. Table 11.2 summarizes the results of the survey

Table 11.1 Multifaceted strategy for the prevention of infection in primary total knee arthroplasty (TKA)

Preoperative patient bacterial decolonization
Screening and avoidance of anemia
Perioperative patient warming
Skin antisepsis
Povidone-iodine wound lavage
Antibacterial-coated sutures
Potential effects of blood transfusion, laminar flow, and protective hoods and suits

Table 11.2 Periprosthetic joint infections (PJI) prevention after primary total knee arthroplasty (TKA): results of a survey distributed among The European Knee Associates (EKA), the American Association of Hip and Knee Surgeons (AAHKS) International Committee, and the Arthroplasty Society in Asia (ASIA) members and their affiliated arthroplasty surgeons

Preoperative	Intraoperative	Postoperative
PJI risk stratification: 40.6% routinely set thresholds (e.g., BMI, HgbA1C) to be met to qualify for surgery, 36.5% only review past medical history; 9.1% use machine learning to personalize PJI risk.	*Antibiotic prophylaxis in high-risk patients*: 43.4% use single antibiotic for 24 hours; 21.3% use double antibiotic for 24 hours; 14.2% use single/double antibiotic for 7 days postoperatively.	*Routine monitoring of PJI serologic markers*: 42% only in symptomatic patients; 34.2% do not; 20.8% in all patients.
BMI limit: 36% no limit; 15.4% BMI <35; 30.9% BMI <40; 17.2% BMI <45.	*Skin cleansing*: 68.7% at home (45.6% chlorhexidine sponge; 11.9% clippers).	*Serologic markers to rule in/out PJI*: 95.9% CRP; 71% ESR; 60.6% WBC.
Nutritional status: 55.3% do not screen; among those who screen their patients (44.7%), albumin is the single most used marker (86.3%).	*Intraoperative skin disinfection*: 46.9% single chlorhexidine; 25% double chlorhexidine-povidone-iodine; 15.4% single povidone-iodine.	*Synovial fluid test to rule in/out PJI*: 79.6% culture/sensitivity; 69.5% WBC count; 31.4% CRP.
Hyperglycemia/diabetes: 83.3% check this comorbidity; 88.1% use HgbA1C as single best screening test.	*Tranexamic acid (TXA) to reduce bleeding/SSI*: 96% yes (51% double IV dose, 35.2% single IV dose, 23.6% intraarticular injection).	
MRSA nasal colonization: 63.7% do not test; 28.9% test all patients; 7.4% test selectively.	*Surgical suction drain*: 52% do not use drains; 19.7% use a drain <24 hours.	
	Intraarticular lavage: 64.9% use only saline; 28.1% use dilute povidone-iodine.	
	Antibiotic local delivery to prevent PJI: 82.4% use antibiotic-added cement.	

BMI body mass index, *HgbA1C* glycated hemoglobin, *CRP* C-reactive protein, *ESR* Erythrocyte sedimentation rate, *WBC* white blood cells, *SSI* surgical site infection, *IV* intravenous, *MRSA* methicillin-resistant *Staphylococcus aureus*

[2]. The survey showed that important differences still existed in the employment of PJI preventive measures across different geographic areas.

11.3 Antibiotic Prophylaxis

11.3.1 Cefazolin Remains the Linchpin for Preventing Acute PJI Following Primary TKA

In 2022, Buchalter et al. affirmed that vancomycin and clindamycin frequently substitute cefazolin as the preoperative antibiotic prophylaxis in primary TKA, particularly in the framework of established allergy to penicillin. Besides, Buchalter et al. stated that topical povidone-iodine lavage and vancomycin powder (VIP) were adjuncts that might further widen antimicrobial coverage [3]. In their study, Buchalter et al. compared the risk of acute PJI in primary TKA individuals who received cefazolin and VIP with those who received a non-cephalosporin alternative and VIP. This was a retrospective cohort study of 11,550 primary TKAs carried out between 2013 and 2019. The primary outcome was PJI occurring within 90 days of surgery. Individuals were stratified into two cohorts (cefazolin vs non-cephalosporin) based on their preoperative antibiotic. All individuals also received the VIP protocol at wound closure. In all, 10,484 knees (90.8%) received cefazolin, while 1066 knees (9.2%) received a non-cephalosporin antibiotic (either vancomycin or clindamycin) as preoperative prophylaxis. The rate of PJI in the cefazolin cohort (0.5%) was substantially lower than the rate of PJI in the non-cephalosporin cohort (1%). The odds ratio of developing a PJI was increased in the non-cephalosporin group compared to the cefazolin group. In spite of the utilization of topical irrigant solutions and the addition of local antibiotics, the utilization of a non-cephalosporin perioperative antibiotic continues to be associated with a greater risk of TKA PJI compared to cefazolin [3].

11.3.2 Topical Vancomycin Powder

According to Yavuz et al. (2020), vancomycin powder (VP) had been used to prevent PJI. However, studies analyzing the effectiveness of VP to prevent infection in primary TKA were very rare [4]. In a study with level 3 of evidence, Yavuz et al. investigated the effectiveness of VP utilization to prevent PJI in TKA. Between 2012 and 2016, 976 consecutive individuals who experienced primary TKA were included in the study. Individuals were divided into two cohorts. There were 474 individuals (48.6%) in the VP cohort and 502 individuals in the control cohort (51.4%). Except for VP, all procedures were the same in both cohorts. In the VP cohort, 2 g of VP was poured into the joint just before the fascia was closed. Average follow-up was 53.2 months. Infection was found in 4 (0.84%) of 474 individuals in the VP cohort and 5 (0.99%) of 502 individuals in the control cohort. There was no statistically significant difference between cohorts in terms of infection rates. *Staphylococcus aureus* was encountered in 2 individuals in the VP cohort. Two individuals had *Staphylococcus aureus* and one individual had *Pseudomonas aeruginosa* in the control cohort. There was no statistically significant difference between cohorts in terms of demographic parameters. Intrawound VP administration did not change the infection rates in primary TKA. The VP administration for preventing PJI was not advised in primary TKA [4]. In a systematic review with level 3 of evidence published in 2021, Wong et al. concluded that topical vancomycin (VP) should not be utilized in routine primary TKA [5].

11.3.3 Vancomycin Powder and Dilute Povidone-Iodine Lavage (VIP)

In 2021, Buchalter et al. found that VIP diminished early primary TKA PJI frequency in both the high-risk and all-risk groups compared with the pre-VIP group by 44.6% and 56.4%, respectively (1.01% versus 0.56% versus 0.44%). Besides, after introducing VIP to all-risk TKA individuals, compared with high-risk TKA individuals, the relative risk of PJI dropped an additional 21.4%, but this finding did not reach statistical significance (0.56% versus 0.44%). There were no demographic differences between the three VIP PJI groups [6]. In a systematic review and meta-analysis published in 2024, Martin et al. found that intraarticular VP and povidone-iodine lavage caused a substantial decrease in PJI in primary and revision TKA [7].

11.3.4 Extended Oral Antibiotic Prophylaxis

According to Carender et al. (2021), extended oral antibiotic prophylaxis (EOAP) after primary TKA and total hip arthroplasty (THA) in individuals with BMI ≥40 kg/m^2 might diminish the rate of early PJI; however, existing data were limited [8]. In their study, they examined rates of wound complications and PJI in individuals with BMI ≥40 kg/m^2 treated with and without EOAP after surgery. EOAP was given 7–14 days after surgery. Wound complications and PJI were analyzed at 90 days postoperatively. In total, 650 cases (205 THAs and 445 TKAs) were studied. Mean age was 58 years and 62% were women. Mean BMI was 44 kg/m^2. EOAP was prescribed in 177 cases (27%). At 90 days, there was no difference between prophylaxis and non-prophylaxis cohorts in the rate of wound complications (11% versus 8%) or PJI (1.7% versus 0.6%). Increased operative time and diabetes mellitus were associated with increased risk of 90-day wound complications. No patient factors were associated with increased risk of PJI at 90 days postoperatively. EOAP after primary TKA did not diminish rates of wound complications or early PJI in a morbidly obese patient population [8].

In 2024, Dasari et al. stated that there was growing interest in extended antibiotic prophylaxis (EAP) after total joint arthroplasty (TJA); however, the benefit of EAP remained controversial. In a meta-analysis of the literature, both oral and intravenous antibiotic protocols were included in the EAP group [9]. They compared outcomes of primary and aseptic revision THA and TKA individuals who were treated with either ≤24 hours of postoperative antibiotic prophylaxis (standard of care [SoC]) or >24 hours of EAP. The primary outcome was PJI. Individuals treated with EAP were 35% less likely to develop PJI relative to the SoC. When analyzing primary TJA, individuals treated with EAP were 39% and 40% less likely to develop a PJI for TJA and THA, respectively. There was no substantial difference for primary TKA. When analyzing aseptic revision TJA, EAP led to a 36% and 47% decrease in the likelihood of a PJI for aseptic revision TJA and aseptic revision TKA, respectively; no benefit was found for aseptic revision THA. This meta-analysis showed that individuals treated with EAP were less likely to develop a PJI relative to those treated with the SoC for all TJA, primary TJA, primary THA, aseptic revision TJA, and aseptic revision TKA. There was no substantial difference encountered between EAP and SoC for primary TKA or aseptic revision THA [9].

11.3.5 Regional Prophylactic Antibiotics by Intraosseous Injection

In a study with level 3 of evidence published in 2021, Parkinson et al. affirmed that recent studies had shown that the administration of regional prophylactic antibiotics by intraosseous (IO) injection accomplished tissue concentrations around the knee that were 10- to 15-fold higher than intravenous (IV) delivery of prophylactic antibiotics [10]. They analyzed whether the utilization of regional prophylactic antibiotics for primary TKA would result in a lower risk of PJI. A retrospective comparative study of all 1906 TKAs (725 IO, 1181 IV) over a 5-year period (January 2013 to December 2017) was carried out to establish the risk of early PJI. The minimum follow-up was 12 months. Both groups had similar ages, BMI, and American Society of Anesthesiologists (ASA) grades; however, a greater proportion of individuals in the IO group were smokers, while a greater proportion of individuals were diabetic in the IV group. The utilization of regional prophylactic antibiotics by the IO technique resulted in a lower PJI risk than IV prophylactic antibiotics (0.1% compared with 1.4%). Surgeons should contemplate administering regional prophylactic antibiotics in primary TKA to diminish the risk of early PJI [10].

11.3.6 Addition of a Single-Dose Gentamicin

According to Ashkenazi et al. (2023), first-generation cephalosporins are utilized as antibiotic prophylaxis in TJA individuals. However, this regimen does not address Gram-negative bacteria causing PJI. They also stated that previous publications had suggested that the addition of an aminoglycoside as antibiotic prophylaxis in THA diminished SSI [11]. In their study, they investigated if the addition of a single-dose gentamicin, administered preoperatively, was associated with lower rates of infection in TKA individuals. In a retrospective study, they analyzed individuals who experienced primary TKA as treatment for osteoarthritis, with a minimum 1-year follow-up. The mean age was 69.9, the mean BMI was 29.7, and most individuals had an ASA score of 2–3 (92.9%). Individuals were stratified based on the perioperative antibiotic prophylaxis they received: cefazolin with the addition of gentamicin (case cohort) or cefazolin (control cohort). The primary study endpoints were rates of PJI and SSI, which were compared between cohorts. The final study population consisted of 1590 individuals, 1008 (63.4%) in the control cohort and 582 (36.6%) in the case cohort. The total infection rate for individuals that received gentamicin dropped by 34%; however, this finding did not reach statistical significance [1.3% (control) versus 0.86% (case)]. The same drop was found after subdivision of infections to PJI (0.5% versus 0.34%, 32% drop) and SSI (0.8% versus 0.52%, 35% drop). A single dose of gentamicin administered preoperatively to a standard antibiotic prophylaxis was not associated with a substantial lower rate of PJI [11].

11.4 Intravenous Administration of Tranexamic Acid

In a systematic review and meta-analysis with level 3 of evidence, Imanishi et al. assessed the effectiveness of intravenous administration of tranexamic acid (TXA) in preventing PJI and surgical site infection (SSI) in individuals who experienced TKA and THA. Treatment with intravenous TXA substantially diminished the frequency of overall infection, including PJI, SSI, and other infections (OR 0.55; 95% CI 0.49–0.62) ($p < 0.00001$), and that of PJI alone (OR 0.53; 95% CI 0.47–0.59) ($p < 0.00001$). TXA reduced the incidence of overall infection in individuals who experienced TKA (OR 0.55; 95% CI 0.43–0.71) ($p < 0.00001$) [12].

11.5 Encouragement, Education, Exercise, Employment, and Evaluation (5E) Rehabilitation Nursing Model

In 2024, Weng et al. explored the effects of 5E rehabilitation nursing on the prevention of PJI after TKA. Participants were 80 TKA postoperative individuals who were randomly divided into two cohorts: the intervention cohort, the 5E cohort, with 40 individuals and the control cohort, with 40 individuals. The control cohort received routine nursing, while the 5E group received 5E rehabilitation nursing. Compared to the control cohort, the incidence of PJI at 90 days after surgery was significantly lower in the 5E cohort (0% versus 17.5%) [13].

11.6 Application of Machine Learning in the Prevention of PJI Following TKA

In a systematic review published in 2023 by Chong et al., the potential application of machine learning (ML) for the prevention of PJI was analyzed. It was found that ML might be a favorable alternative to manual methods in the prevention of PJI following TKA. It helped in preoperative health optimization, preoperative surgical planning, early diagnosis of infection, early application of appropriate antibiotics, and prediction of clinical results [14].

11.7 Conclusions

There is no single intervention that will eliminate infection risk for TKA individuals. Undoubtedly, some individuals are more prone than others to infection, but even the healthiest are at risk. Based on current evidence, TKA surgeons should utilize many strategies in their practice to diminish the risk of SSI, although debate exists as to what constitutes best practice. Infection prevention in TKA needs a multifaceted approach that includes patient bacterial decolonization, avoidance of anemia, blood transfusion, perioperative patient warming, laminar flow, space suits, careful skin antisepsis, povidone-iodine wound lavage, and triclosan-coated sutures. A recent survey has shown that important differences still exist in the employment of PJI preventive measures across different geographic areas.

References

1. Dobson PF, Reed MR. Prevention of infection in primary THA and TKA. EFORT Open Rev. 2020;5(10):604–13. https://doi.org/10.1302/2058-5241.5.200004.
2. Indelli PF, Iannotti F, Ferretti A, Valtanen R, Prati P, Pérez Prieto D, et al. Recommendations for periprosthetic joint infections (PJI) prevention: the European Knee Associates (EKA)-International Committee American Association of Hip and Knee Surgeons (AAHKS)-Arthroplasty Society in Asia (ASIA) survey of members. Knee Surg Sports Traumatol Arthrosc. 2022;30(12):3932–43. https://doi.org/10.1007/s00167-021-06742-1.
3. Buchalter DB, Nduaguba A, Teo GM, Kugelman D, Aggarwal VK, Long WJ. Cefazolin remains the linchpin for preventing acute periprosthetic joint infection following primary total knee arthroplasty. Bone Jt Open. 2022;3(1):35–41. https://doi.org/10.1302/2633-1462.31.BJO-2021-0051.R1.
4. Yavuz IA, Oken OF, Yildirim AO, Inci F, Ceyhan E, Gurhan U. No effect of vancomycin powder to prevent infection in primary total knee arthroplasty: a retrospective review of 976 cases. Knee Surg Sports Traumatol Arthrosc. 2020;28(9):3055–60. https://doi.org/10.1007/s00167-019-05778-8.
5. Wong MT, Sridharan SS, Davison EM, Ng R, Desy NM. Can topical vancomycin prevent periprosthetic joint infection in hip and knee arthroplasty? A systematic review. Clin Orthop Relat Res. 2021;479(8):1655–64. https://doi.org/10.1097/CORR.0000000000001777.
6. Buchalter DB, Kirby DJ, Teo GM, Iorio R, Aggarwal VK, Long WJ. Topical vancomycin powder and dilute povidone-iodine lavage reduce the rate of early periprosthetic joint infection after primary total knee arthroplasty. J Arthroplast. 2021;36(1):286–90.e1. https://doi.org/10.1016/j.arth.2020.07.064.
7. Martin VT, Zhang Y, Wang Z, Liu QL, Yu B. A systematic review and meta-analysis comparing intrawound vancomycin powder and povidone iodine lavage in the prevention of periprosthetic joint infection of hip and knee arthroplasties. J Orthop Sci. 2024;29(1):165–76. https://doi.org/10.1016/j.jos.2022.11.013.
8. Carender CN, DeMik DE, Glass NA, Noiseux NO, Brown TS, Bedard NA. Do extended oral postoperative antibiotics prevent early periprosthetic joint infection in morbidly obese patients undergoing primary total joint arthroplasty? J Arthroplast. 2021;36(8):2716–21. https://doi.org/10.1016/j.arth.2021.03.018.
9. Dasari SP, Kanumuri SD, Yang J, Manner PA, Fernando ND, Hernandez NM. Extended prophylactic antibiotics for primary and aseptic revision total joint arthroplasty: a meta-analysis. J Arthroplast. 2024;39(9S2):S476–87. https://doi.org/10.1016/j.arth.2024.01.014.
10. Parkinson B, McEwen P, Wilkinson M, Hazratwala K, Hellman J, Kan H, et al. Intraosseous regional prophylactic antibiotics decrease the risk of prosthetic joint infection in primary TKA: a multicenter study. Clin Orthop Relat Res. 2021;479(11):2504–12. https://doi.org/10.1097/CORR.0000000000001919.
11. Ashkenazi I, Amzallag N, Snir N, Morgan S, Garceau S, Kotz L, et al. Does addition of gentamicin for antibiotic prophylaxis in total knee arthroplasty reduce the rate of periprosthetic joint infection? Arch Orthop Trauma Surg. 2023;143(8):5255–60. https://doi.org/10.1007/s00402-022-04744-3.
12. Imanishi K, Kobayashi N, Kamono E, Yukizawa Y, Takagawa S, Choe H, et al. Tranexamic acid administration for the prevention of periprosthetic joint infection and surgical site infection: a systematic review and meta-analysis. Arch Orthop Trauma Surg. 2023;143(11):6883–99. https://doi.org/10.1007/s00402-023-04914-x.

13. Weng H, Zhang Q, Ding L, Shen J, Shen D, Xiong P, et al. Prevention of periprosthetic infection after orthopedic knee replacement based on 5E rehabilitation nursing model. Altern Ther Health Med. 2024;30(12):92–9. PMID: 38430180.
14. Chong YY, Chan PK, Chan VWK, Cheung A, Luk MH, Cheung MH, et al. Application of machine learning in the prevention of periprosthetic joint infection following total knee arthroplasty: a systematic review. Art. 2023;5(1):38. https://doi.org/10.1186/s42836-023-00195-2.

Antibiotic Prophylaxis in Total Knee Arthroplasty: Its Role in Decreasing Periprosthetic Joint Infection Rates

12

E. Carlos Rodríguez-Merchán, Juan S. Ruiz-Pérez, and Primitivo Gómez-Cardero

12.1 Introduction

Intravenous (IV) antibiotic prophylaxis is commonly used in total joint arthroplasty (TJA) in order to decrease periprosthetic joint infection (PJI) rates. However, there are still many unresolved questions today, such as which IV antibiotic or combination of antibiotics is the most advisable, what is the role of prolonged use of oral antibiotics after TJA, or the role of intraosseous antibiotics [1–4]. The aim of this chapter is to analyze the most recent advances on the above-mentioned topics.

12.2 Intravenous (IV) Prophylaxis

With respect to IV prophylaxis, there are currently several topics of great interest that are discussed below:

12.2.1 Antibiotic Prophylaxis Regimens in Use for Elective Primary TJA

In 2023, Mabrouk et al. stated that prophylactic antibiotic regimens for elective primary total hip arthroplasty (THA) and total knee arthroplasty (TKA) varied widely across hospitals in the United Kingdom (UK) [1]. In a study aimed to determine antibiotic prophylaxis regimens in use for elective primary TJA across the UK, identify variations in antibiotic prophylaxis regimens and their influence on the risk of PJI in the first-year post-index procedure, and assess adherence to international consensus guidance (the 2018 Philadelphia Consensus Guidance) [5]. Mabrouk et al. found that the primary option and dosing of the prophylactic antimicrobial regimens differed widely. The two most utilized regimens were combined teicoplanin and gentamicin, and cefuroxime followed by two or three doses of cefuroxime eight-hourly, advised by 24 hospitals (22.02%) each. The alternative option and dosing of the prophylactic antimicrobial regimen also differed widely across the 83 centers with data accessible. Prophylaxis regimens across some hospitals fail to cover the likeliest causes of surgical site infection (SSI). Five centers (4.6%) advised co-amoxiclav, which confers no *Staphylococcus* coverage, while 33 hospitals (30.3%) advised cefuroxime, which confers no *Enterococcus* coverage. Inadequate adherence to 2018 Philadelphia Consensus Guidance was encountered, with 67 centers (61.5%) not including a cephalosporin in their guidance [1].

E. C. Rodríguez-Merchán (✉) · J. S. Ruiz-Pérez
P. Gómez-Cardero
Department of Orthopedic Surgery, Hospital Universitario La Paz, Madrid, Madrid, Spain

E. C. Rodríguez-Merchán (ed.), *Advances in Periprosthetic Joint Infection*,
https://doi.org/10.1007/978-3-032-02945-4_12

12.2.2 Extended Prophylactic Antibiotics for Primary and Aseptic Revision TJA

In a systematic review and meta-analysis published in 2024 by Dasari et al., they compared outcomes of primary and aseptic revision THA and TKA individuals who were treated with either ≤24 hours of postoperative antibiotic prophylaxis (standard of care) or >24 hours of extended antibiotic prophylaxis (EAP). There were 18 studies with a total of 19,153 individuals included [2]. There was considerable variation in antibiotic prophylaxis protocols, with first-generation cephalosporins being the most commonly implemented antibiotic for both cohorts. Patients treated with EAP were 35% less likely to develop PJI relative to the standard of care. When examining primary TJA, patients treated with EAP were 39% and 40% less likely to develop a PJI for TJA and THA, respectively. There was no significant difference for primary TKA. When examining aseptic revision TJA, EAP led to a 36% and 47% reduction in the probability of a PJI for aseptic revision TJA and aseptic revision TKA, respectively; there was no observed benefit for aseptic revision THA. This meta-analysis demonstrated that patients treated with EAP were less likely to develop a PJI relative to those treated with the standard of care for all TJA, primary TJA, primary THA, aseptic revision TJA, and aseptic revision TKA. There was no significant difference observed between EAP and standard of care for primary TKA or aseptic revision THA [2].

12.2.3 Documented Penicillin Allergies Should Not Avert Utilization of Preoperative Cefazolin in THA and TKA

According to Kurcz et al. (2023), perioperative cefazolin administration for TJA is a first-line antibiotic advised by the American Academy of Orthopedic Surgeons (AAOS) guidelines for the prevention of PJIs. In a study, Kurcz et al. analyzed the clinical viability of giving individuals with a documented penicillin allergy a perioperative full-strength cefazolin "test dose" under anesthesia [6]. The study was a retrospective chart review of 2451 TJAs from a high-volume arthroplasty orthopedic surgeon over a 5-year period. This surgeon routinely gave individuals with a documented penicillin allergy a full-strength cefazolin test dose while under anesthesia instead of administering a second-line antibiotic. The primary outcomes assessed were allergic reaction and postoperative infection. Cefazolin was given to 87.1% of all individuals ($N = 1990$) and 46% of individuals with a penicillin allergy ($N = 143$). The total rate of allergic reactions among all individuals was 0.5% ($N = 11$). Only one individual with a documented penicillin allergy who received cefazolin had an allergic reaction. The reaction was not severe and did not need any additional management. In individuals who had no reported allergies and received cefazolin, 0.3% ($N = 6$) had an allergic reaction. There was no statistically significant difference in the rate of allergic reaction when comparing individuals with and without a penicillin allergy. Individuals receiving cefazolin had an overall PJI rate of 3% ($N = 57$) versus those individuals receiving antibiotics other than cefazolin who sustained a 6% PJI rate ($N = 16$), which was statistically significant (Fig. 12.1). Therefore, this study found that the use of a full-strength test dose of cefazolin in individuals with a documented penicillin allergy is a possible, safe, and effective way of increasing the rate of cefazolin administration and thus reducing the risk of PJIs [6].

12.2.4 Addition of Vancomycin to Beta-lactam Prophylaxis in Adult Individuals Without Known Methicillin-Resistant *Staphylococcus aureus* (MRSA) Colonization

In 2023, Peel et al. stated that the addition of vancomycin to beta-lactam prophylaxis in TJA might diminish SSIs; however, the efficacy and safety were unclear. In a multicenter, double-blind,

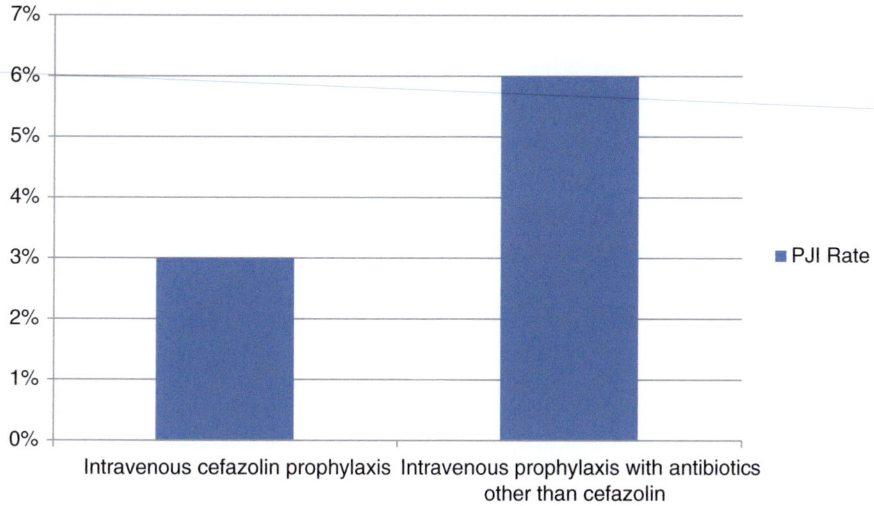

Fig. 12.1 Rates of periprosthetic joint infection (PJI): individuals receiving intravenous cefazolin prophylaxis versus individuals receiving intravenous prophylaxis with antibiotics other than cefazolin

superiority, placebo-controlled trial, Peel et al. randomly assigned adult individuals without known MRSA colonization undergoing TJA to receive 1.5 g of vancomycin or normal saline placebo, in addition to cefazolin prophylaxis [7]. The primary outcome was SSI within 90 days after surgery. A total of 4239 individuals experienced randomization. Among 4113 individuals in the modified intention-to-treat population (2233 undergoing TKA, 1850 undergoing THA, and 30 undergoing total shoulder arthroplasty—TSA), SSIs occurred in 91 of 2044 individuals (4.5%) in the vancomycin cohort and in 72 of 2069 individuals (3.5%) in the placebo cohort (relative risk, 1.28). Among individuals undergoing TKA, SSIs occurred in 63 of 1109 individuals (5.7%) in the vancomycin cohort and in 42 of 1124 individuals (3.7%) in the placebo cohort (relative risk, 1.52). Among individuals experiencing THA, SSIs happened in 28 of 920 individuals (3%) in the vancomycin cohort and in 29 of 930 individuals (3.1%) in the placebo cohort (relative risk, 0.98). Complications occurred in 35 of 2010 individuals (1.7%) in the vancomycin cohort and in 35 of 2030 individuals (1.7%) in the placebo cohort, including hypersensitivity reactions in 24 of 2010 individuals (1.2%) and 11 of 2030 individuals (0.5%), respectively (relative risk, 2.20), and acute kidney injury in 42 of 2010 individuals (2.1%) and 74 of 2030 individuals (3.6%), respectively (relative risk, 0.57). Therefore, the addition of vancomycin to cefazolin prophylaxis was not superior to placebo for the prevention of SSIs in TJA among individuals without known MRSA colonization [7].

12.2.5 Does Addition of Gentamicin for Antibiotic Prophylaxis in TKA Diminish the Rate of PJI?

According to Ashkenazi et al. (2023), although first-generation cephalosporins are utilized as antibiotic prophylaxis in TJA individuals, this regimen does not address Gram-negative bacteria causing PJI. In a study, Ashkenazi et al. investigated if the addition of a single-dose gentamicin, administered preoperatively, was associated with lower rates of infection in TKA individuals [8]. In a retrospective study, they analyzed patients who experienced primary TKA as treatment for osteoarthritis, with a minimum 1-year follow-up. The mean age was 69.9, the mean body mass index (BMI) was 29.7, and most individuals had American Society of Anesthesiology (ASA) score of 2–3 (92.9%). Individuals were stratified based on the perioperative antibiotic prophylaxis they received: cefazolin with the addition of gentamicin (case cohort) or cefazolin (control cohort). The primary study endpoints were rates of PJI and SSI, which were compared between cohorts. The final study population consisted of 1590 individuals, 1008 (63.4%) in the control cohort and 582 (36.6%) individuals in the case cohort. The total infection rate for individuals that received gentamicin dropped by 34%; however, this finding did not reach statistical significance [1.3% (control) versus 0.86% (case)]. The same drop was seen after subdivision of infections into PJI (0.5% versus 0.34%, 32% drop) and SSI (0.8% versus 0.52%, 35% drop). Therefore, a single dose of gentamicin administered preoperatively to a standard antibiotic prophylaxis was not associated with a statistically significant lower rate of PJI [8].

12.2.6 No Difference in Risk of Revision due to Infection Between Clindamycin and Cephalosporins as Antibiotic Prophylaxis in Cemented Primary TKAs

In 2023, Pawloy et al. stated that systemic antibiotic prophylaxis with clindamycin, which was often utilized in penicillin- or cephalosporin-allergic individuals, has been associated with a higher risk of surgical revision for deep PJI than cloxacillin in primary TKA. In a study, Pawloy et al. investigated whether clindamycin increases the risk of surgical revisions due to PJI compared with cephalosporins in primary cemented TKA [9]. Data from 59,081 TKAs in the Norwegian Arthroplasty Register (NAR) 2005–2020 were included. 2655 (5%) received clindamycin and 56,426 (95%) received cephalosporins. Of the TKAs included, 1.3% ($N = 743$) were revised for PJI. 96% ($N = 713$) had received cephalosporins and 4% ($N = 30$) clindamycin for perioperative prophylaxis. Comparing cephalosporins and clindamycin, at 3-month follow-up, the adjusted hazard ratio rate (HRR) for PJI was 0.7, at 1 year, 0.9, and at 5 years, 0.9. Analysis utilizing propensity score matching demonstrated similar outcomes. Moreover, comparing cefalotin (reference) and cefazolin, HRR was 1 at 3 months and 1 at 1-year follow-up. Therefore, Pawloy et al. found no difference in risk of revision for PJI when utilizing clindamycin compared with cephalosporins in primary cemented TKAs. It appeared safe to continue the utilization of clindamycin in penicillin- or cephalosporin-allergic individuals [9].

12.2.7 Bone Penetration of Intravenous Flucloxacillin and Gentamicin as Antibiotic Prophylaxis During THA and TKA

In 2017, Torkington et al. investigated the bone penetration of intravenous antibiotic prophylaxis with flucloxacillin and gentamicin during THA and TKA, and their efficacy against *Staphylococcus aureus* and *Staphylococcus epidermidis* [10]. Bone samples from the femoral head, neck, and acetabulum were collected from 18 individuals experiencing THA and from the femur and tibia in 21 individuals during TKA. The concentration of both antibiotics in the samples was analyzed utilizing high-performance liquid chromatography. Penetration was expressed as a percentage of venous blood concentration. The efficacy against common infecting organisms was measured against both the minimum inhibitory concentration 50, and the more stringent epidemiological cutoff value for resistance (ECOFF). The bone penetration of gentamicin was higher than flucloxacillin. Relative to ECOFF, flucloxacillin concentrations were effective against *Staphylococcus aureus* and *Staphylococcus epidermidis* in all THAs and 20 (95%) TKAs. Gentamicin concentrations were effective against *Staphylococcus epidermidis* in all bone samples. Gentamicin was effective against *Staphylococcus aureus* in 11 (61.1%) femoral neck samples in THA. Effective concentrations of gentamicin against *Staphylococcus aureus* were only accomplished in four (19%)

femoral and six (29%) tibial samples in TKA. Flucloxacillin and gentamicin were found to penetrate bone during THA and TKA. Gentamicin was effective against *Staphylococcus epidermidis* in both THA and TKA, while levels were subtherapeutic against *Staphylococcus aureus* in most TKAs. Bone penetration of both antibiotics was less in TKA than THA, and this may relate to the utilization of a tourniquet. Using this antibiotic combination, effective cover against the two common infective organisms was accomplished in all THAs and all but one TKA [10].

12.2.8 Perioperative Antibiotic Prophylaxis in TJA: A Single Dose Is as Effective as Multiple Doses

In 2019, Tan et al. compared the efficacy of a single dose of prophylactic antibiotics with that of multiple doses of antibiotics for prevention of PJI in individuals undergoing TJA in a study with level 3 of evidence [11]. A retrospective study of 20,682 primary TJAs performed from 2006 to 2017 was carried out. Individuals who received a single dose of prophylactic antibiotics ($N = 4523$) were compared with individuals who received multiple doses of antibiotics ($N = 16{,}159$). The overall PJI rate was 0.60% (27 of 4523) for individuals who received a single dose of antibiotics compared with 0.88% (142 of 16,159) for those who received multiple doses. There was no difference in the PJI rate between individuals who received a single dose of antibiotics and those who received multiple doses. Moreover, multiple doses did not show any additional benefit for individuals with a high preoperative risk of PJI. This study supported the notion that the administration of additional antibiotics following skin closure might not be needed for primary TJA, regardless of the patient's preoperative risk of PJI [11].

12.2.9 Incomplete Administration of Intravenous Vancomycin Prophylaxis Is Common and Associated with Increased Infectious Complications After Primary THA and TKA

According to Feder et al. (2021), vancomycin is frequently utilized as antimicrobial prophylaxis in individuals undergoing THA and TKA. Besides, vancomycin requires longer infusion times to avoid associated side effects. In a study, Feder et al. hypothesized that vancomycin infusion was frequently begun too late and that delayed infusion may predispose individuals to increased rates of SSIs and PJIs [12]. They reviewed clinical data for all primary THA and TKA individuals at their hospital between 2013 and 2020 who received intravenous vancomycin usage primary perioperative gram-positive antibiotic prophylaxis. Feder et al. estimated the duration of infusion prior to incision or tourniquet inflation, with a cutoff of 30 minutes defining appropriate administration. Individuals were divided into two cohorts: (1) adequate administration and (2) incomplete administration. Surgical factors and quality results were compared between cohorts. Feder et al. reviewed 1047 primary THAs and TKA individuals (524 THAs and 523 TKAs). The indication for intravenous vancomycin usage was allergy (61%), MRSA (17%), both allergy and colonization (14%), and other (8%). 50.4% of individuals started infusion >30 minutes preoperatively (cohort A), and 49.6% started infusion <30 minutes preoperatively (cohort B). Cohort B had significantly higher rates of readmissions for infectious causes (3.6 versus 1.3%). This included a statistically significant increase in confirmed PJIs (2% versus 1%) (Fig. 12.2). Regression analysis confirmed <30 minutes of vancomycin infusion as an independent risk factor for PJI when controlling for comorbidities (odds ratio 5.22). Therefore, it seemed that late infusion of

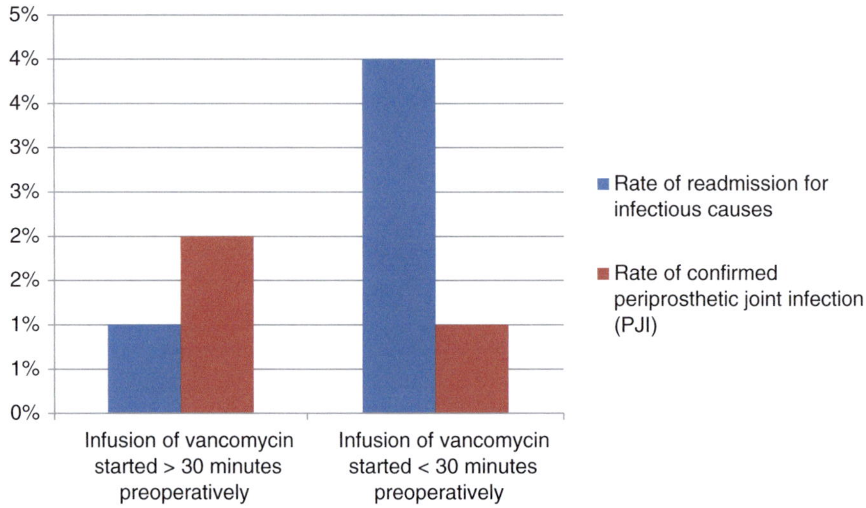

Fig. 12.2 Rate of readmission for infectious causes and rate of confirmed periprosthetic joint infection (PJI): individuals who started vancomycin infusion >30 minutes preoperatively versus those who started vancomycin infusion <30 minutes preoperatively

vancomycin was frequent and associated with increased rates of infectious causes for readmission and PJI [12].

12.2.10 Timing and Duration of Antibiotic Prophylaxis Are Associated with the Risk of Infection After THA and TKA

In 2022, Badge et al. stated that antibiotic prophylaxis involving timely administration of adequately dosed antibiotic was considered effective to diminish the risk of SSI after THA and TKA. They also affirmed that cephalosporins provided effective prophylaxis, although evidence regarding the optimal timing and dosage of prophylactic antibiotics was inconclusive. In their study, Badge et al. examined the association between cephalosporin prophylaxis dose, timing, and duration, and the risk of SSI after THA and TKA. A prospective multicenter cohort study was performed. Data were analyzed for 1838 individuals. There were 264 SSIs comprising 63 deep SSIs (defined as requiring intravenous antibiotics, readmission, or reoperation) and 161 superficial SSIs (defined as requiring oral antibiotics) experienced by 249 (13.6%) individuals within 365 days of surgery. It was concluded that ensuring adequate, weight-adjusted dosing and early, preoperative delivery of prophylactic antibiotics might diminish the risk of SSI in THA and TKA, while the duration of prophylaxis beyond 24 hours was unnecessary [13].

12.3 Intraosseous Antibiotics

12.3.1 Intraosseous Vancomycin in THA

In 2023, Harper et al. stated that literature has shown that intraosseous (IO) infusions were capable of rendering increased local concentrations compared to those administered via IV access. Successes while utilizing the technique for antibiotic prophylaxis administration in TKA prompted consideration for use in THA however; no study existed for the utilization of IO vancomycin in THA. Harper et al. performed a single-blind randomized control trial from December 2020 to May 2022 [3]. Twenty individuals were randomized into 1 of 2 cohorts: IV vancomycin

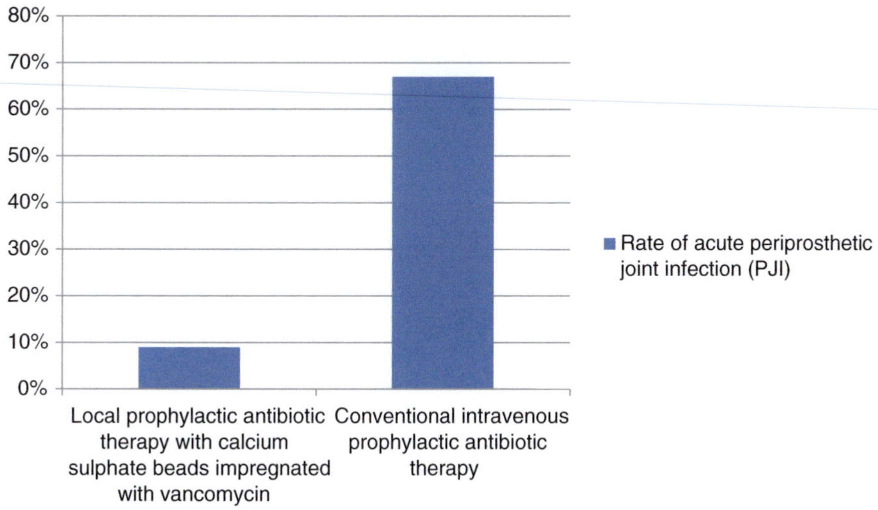

Fig. 12.3 Rate of acute periprosthetic joint infection (PJI): local prophylactic antibiotic therapy with calcium sulphate beads impregnated with vancomycin versus conventional intravenous prophylactic antibiotic therapy

(15 mg/kg) given routinely, or IO vancomycin (500 mg/100 cc of NS) injected into the greater trochanter during incision. Serum vancomycin levels were taken at incision and closure. Soft tissue vancomycin levels were collected from local tissues (at start and end of case). A statistically significant reduction in serum vancomycin levels was found when comparing IO to IV vancomycin at both the start and at the end of the procedure. All local tissue samples had higher concentrations of vancomycin in the IO cohort. This study showed the utility of IO vancomycin in primary THA with increased local tissue and decreased systemic concentrations. With positive findings in an area without tourniquet utilization, IO might be considered for antibiotic delivery for alternative procedures [3].

12.3.2 Decrease in Acute PJIs Incidence with Vancomycin-Loaded Calcium Sulfate Beads in Individuals with Non-modifiable Risk Factors

In a clinical trial with level 2 of evidence published in 2022 by de LaChica et al., the incidence of PJI after local or IV antibiotic prophylaxis was assessed [14]. The aim of their study was to compare the PJI incidence in a population with non-modifiable risk factors after local prophylaxis with vancomycin-loaded calcium sulfate beads versus a control cohort. A total of 83 individuals were assessed, inclusion criteria included individuals over 60 years of age, with at least one main risk factor for PJI who experienced THA or TKA. Cases were randomized, and the intervention cohort received local prophylactic antibiotic therapy with calcium sulfate beads impregnated with vancomycin; conventional IV prophylactic antibiotic therapy was administered for the control cohort. Acute PJI was encountered in 27 individuals (68%) in the control cohort and 4 (9%) in the intervention cohort (Fig. 12.3) [14].

12.4 Extended Oral Antibiotic Prophylaxis

In a study with level 3 of evidence published in 2023 by Villa et al., they investigated whether extended oral antibiotic prophylaxis (EOAP) (>24 hours, $N = 93$) reduced PJI rates after aseptic first-time revision THA and TKA when compared to standard prophylaxis (≤24 hours, $N = 85$). They performed a retrospective review of 178 consecutive revisions. There were no significant differences in demographics. However, skin-to-skin operative time was significantly higher in the EOAP cohort (123 minutes versus 98 minutes). Mean follow-up was 849 days (range, 15–1671). Postoperative PJI rates were not significantly different: 2.2% EOAP prophylaxis versus 3.5% standard prophylaxis [15].

In a review of the literature published in 2024 by Weiner et al., it was stated that while the role and benefit of perioperative IV antibiotics in individuals experiencing TJA was well-established, oral antibiotic utilization in TJA remained a controversial topic. Weiner et al. stated extended oral antibiotic prophylaxis (EOAP) utilization in high-risk primary, aseptic revision, and exchange TJA for infection might be useful in reducing PJI rates. When prescribing oral antibiotics either as EOAP or for draining wounds, patient factors, type of surgery, and type of infectious organisms should be considered in order to optimally avert and manage PJI. It is important to maintain antibiotic stewardship by administering the proper duration, dose, and type of antibiotics (Tables 12.1 and 12.2) [16].

In 2024, Bundschuh et al. compared 3-month PJI rates in all individuals experiencing primary or aseptic revision TJA with or without EOAP. In total, 2982 consecutive primary (*N* = 2677) and aseptic revision (*N* = 305) TJAs were retrospectively reviewed (level 3 of evidence) [4]. Beginning January 2020, all individuals received 7 days of 300 mg oral cefdinir twice daily immediately postoperatively. Rates of PJI at 3 months were compared between individuals who received or did not receive EOAP. Rates of PJI at 3 months in individuals undergoing primary and aseptic revision TJA were significantly lower in those receiving EOAP compared to those who did not (0.41 versus 1.13%). After primary TJA, lower PJI rates were found with EOAP utilization (0.23 versus 0.74%; odds ratio 3.85). Following aseptic revision TJA, PJI rates trended toward a significant decrease with the EOA compared to without (1.88 versus 4.83%, respectively; odds ratio 2.71). All individuals experiencing primary or aseptic revision TJA who received extended oral antibiotic prophylaxis (EOAP) were 3.85 and 2.71 times less likely, respectively, to develop PJI at 3 months compared to those without EOAP. However, Bundschuh et al. stated that future studies were required to establish if these results were maintained at postoperative time periods beyond 3 months following primary TJA [4].

In 2024, Mohiuddin et al. compared PJI rates in aseptic revision THA (rTHA) performed with EOAP with PJI rates in published studies of aseptic rTHA patients not receiving EOAP [17].

Table 12.1 Common side effects of antibiotics used in total joint arthroplasty (TJA)

Oral antibiotics	Side effects
Amoxicillin	Skin rash, anaphylaxis, *Clostridium difficile*–associated diarrhea
Amoxicillin-clavulanate	Skin rash, anaphylaxis, *Clostridium difficile*–associated diarrhea
Cefadroxil	Skin rash, anaphylaxis, *Clostridium difficile*–associated diarrhea
Cephalexin	Skin rash, anaphylaxis, *Clostridium difficile*–associated diarrhea
Ciprofloxacin	Hepatotoxicity, Achilles tendinitis/ruptures, neuropathy, *Clostridium difficile*–associated diarrhea
Clindamycin	*Clostridium difficile*–associated diarrhea
Cotrimoxazole	Leucopenia/anemia, skin rash
Doxycycline	Skin hyperpigmentation, hepatotoxicity
Levofloxacin	Hepatotoxicity, Achilles tendinitis/rupture, neuropathy, *Clostridium difficile*–associated diarrhea
Linezolid	Thrombocytopenia/anemia, serotonin syndrome with tricyclic antidepressants, myelosuppression, optic neuritis, peripheral neuropathy
Minocycline	Skin hyperpigmentation, hepatotoxicity
Penicillin	Skin rash, anaphylaxis, *Clostridium difficile*–associated diarrhea
Rifampin	Hepatotoxicity, skin rash, gastrointestinal upset, drug interactions, interstitial nephritis, cytopenia

Table 12.2 Extended oral antibiotic prophylaxis (EOAP) in total joint arthroplasty (TJA)

	Oral antibiotics	Oral dose (mg = milligrams; h = hours)	Duration of dose
EOAP following primary or aseptic revision TJA			
	Amoxicillin-clavulanate	1000 mg/12 h	7 days
	Cephalosporins (cefadroxil and cephalexin)	500 mg/12 h, 500 mg/6 h	7 days; 7–14 days
	Ciprofloxacin	500 mg/12 h	7 days; 7–14 days
	Clindamycin	300 mg/8 h	7 days; 7–14 days
	Cotrimoxazole	800/160 mg/12 h	7 days; 7–14 days
	Doxycycline	100 mg/12 h	7 days; 7–14 days
EOAP following successful exchange for PJI			
	Cephalexin	500/6 h	>4 weeks; 6 months
	Cotrimoxazole	800/160 mg/12 h	>4 weeks; 6 months
	Doxycycline	100 mg/12 h	>4 weeks; 3–6 months
	Fluoroquinolones (ciprofloxacin and levofloxacin)	500 mg/12 h	>4 weeks; 6 months
	Linezolid	600 mg/12 h	>4 weeks; 6 months
	Rifampin (combination therapy)	300 mg/8 h	6 months
Oral prophylaxis used to treat draining wounds or peri-incisional erythema			
	Amoxicillin-clavulanate	NA	Mean 16.5 days
	Cephalexin	NA	NA
	Clindamycin	NA	NA

PJI periprosthetic joint infection, *NA* not available

Prospectively documented data on 127 consecutive aseptic rTHAs were retrospectively reviewed. Evidence-based perioperative infection prevention protocols were utilized, and all individuals were discharged on a 7-day EOAP. Superficial and deep infections at 30 and 90 days postoperatively and at mean latest follow-up of 27.8 months were statistically compared with all US studies reporting the prevalence of PJI after aseptic rTHA. Complications related to EOAP within 120 days of the index procedure were also reported. No superficial or deep infections were found at 30 and 90 days postoperatively when 7-day postdischarge EOAP was utilized. Superficial and deep infection rates were 1.57% (two individuals) and 3.15% (four individuals) at mean latest follow-up, respectively. Comparisons with published 30-day PJI rates of 1.37% and 1.85% were not statistically significant. Two of four comparisons with published 90-day PJI rates of 3.43% and 5.74% were statistically different. The deep PJI rate of 3.15% at mean latest follow-up was significantly lower than two of three published rates at equivalent follow-up including 10.10% and 9.12%. No antibiotic-related complications were observed within 120 days of the index procedure. Study findings possibly support the utilization of EOAP after aseptic rTHA to prevent catastrophic PJI with revision implants, indicating that the efficacy of EOAP cannot be definitively ruled-in or ruled-out based on available evidence [17].

12.5 Recommendations for Antibiotic Prophylaxis in TJA Surgery

In North America, cephalosporins with a broad range of antibacterial activities against Gram-positive and Gram-negative bacteria are used as first-line prophylaxis [18–20] (Table 12.3).

However, in the United Kingdom, the most commonly used first-line prophylaxis is a combination of flucloxacillin plus gentamicin, which is to reduce the incidence of *Clostridium difficile*–associated colitis purportedly driven by high cephalosporin use. Glycopeptides (vancomycin) are considered for patients who are carriers of MRSA or who have an anaphylactic reaction to penicillin. However, they only cover Gram-positive bacteria, thus they are often combined with an aminoglycoside (gentamicin). Decisions on using single versus dual-agent prophylaxis should depend on local epidemiology, and resistant rates addressing particular needs [21, 22].

Table 12.3 Recommendations for antibiotic prophylaxis in total joint arthroplasty (TJA) surgery

Cefazolin or cefuroxime [19]
Clindamycin or vancomycin if confirmed penicillin allergy [19]
Intravenous start within 1 hour of incision (within 2 hours for vancomycin) [19]
Infuse completely before tourniquet inflation [19]
If weight >80 kg, double dose for cefazolin [19]
Additional dose if operating time exceeds 2–4 hours (6–12 hours for vancomycin) or there is "significant" blood loss [19]
Duration should not exceed 24 hours postoperative [19]
Dosage: 2 g cefazolin; 1.5 g cefuroxime; 15 mg/kg vancomycin [20]

12.6 Conclusions

There is considerable variation in antibiotic prophylaxis protocols with intravenous (IV) first-generation cephalosporins being the most commonly implemented antibiotic to prevent periprosthetic joint infection (PJI). Individuals treated with IV extended antibiotic prophylaxis (EAP) are less likely to develop a PJI relative to those treated with the standard of care for all total joint arthroplasty (TJA), primary TJA, primary total hip arthroplasty (THA), aseptic revision TJA, and aseptic revision total knee arthroplasty (TKA). Multiple doses add no additional benefit for individuals with a high preoperative risk of PJI. It seems safe to use clindamycin in penicillin- or cephalosporin-allergic individuals. Late infusion of vancomycin is frequent and associated with increased rates of infectious causes for readmission and PJI. Ensuring adequate, weight-adjusted dosing and early, preoperative delivery of prophylactic antibiotics might diminish the risk of surgical site infection (SSI) in THA and TKA, while the duration of prophylaxis beyond 24 hours is unnecessary.

Intraosseous (IO) vancomycin might be considered for primary THA. Local prophylaxis with calcium sulfate beads diminished the incidence of acute PJI in individuals with non-modifiable risk factors undergoing THA and TKA compared to conventional prophylaxis with a relative risk of 0.13.

All individuals experiencing primary or aseptic revision TJA who received extended oral antibiotic prophylaxis (EOAP) were 3.85 and 2.71 times less likely, respectively, to develop PJI at 3 months compared to those without EOAP. The utilization of EOAP after aseptic rTHA can be supported to prevent catastrophic PJI with revision implants. However, the efficacy of EOAP cannot be definitively ruled-in or ruled-out based on available evidence.

References

1. Mabrouk A, Abouharb A, Stewart G, Palan J, Pandit H. National variation in prophylactic antibiotic use for elective primary total joint replacement. Bone Joint Open. 2023;4(10):742–9. https://doi.org/10.1302/2633-1462.410.BJO-2023-0055.R1.

2. Dasari SP, Kanumuri SD, Yang J, Manner PA, Fernando ND, Hernandez NM. Extended prophylactic antibiotics for primary and aseptic revision total joint arthroplasty: a meta-analysis. J Arthroplast. 2024;39(9S2):S476–87. https://doi.org/10.1016/j.arth.2024.01.014.
3. Harper KD, Park KJ, Brozovich AA, Sullivan TC, Serpelloni S, Taraballi F, et al. Otto Aufranc award: intraosseous vancomycin in total hip arthroplasty – superior tissue concentrations and improved efficiency. J Arthroplast. 2023;38(7S):S11–5. https://doi.org/10.1016/j.arth.2023.04.028.
4. Bundschuh KE, Muffly BT, Ayeni AM, Heo KY, Khawaja S, Tocio AJ, et al. Should all patients receive extended oral antibiotic prophylaxis? Defining its role in patients undergoing primary and aseptic revision total joint arthroplasty. J Arthroplast. 2024;39(9S2):S117–21.e4. https://doi.org/10.1016/j.arth.2024.01.012. Epub 2024 Jan 11.
5. Schwartz EM, Parvizi J, Gehrke T, Aiyer A, Battenberg A, Brown SA, et al. 2018 International consensus meeting on musculoskeletal infection: research priorities from the general assembly questions. J Orthop Res. 2019;37(5):997–1006. https://doi.org/10.1002/jor.24293.
6. Kurcz BP, Allan DG, Nestler AJ, Lister EL, Yarnell WC, Delfino KR, et al. Documented penicillin allergies should not preclude use of preoperative cefazolin in hip and knee arthroplasty. J Am Acad Orthop Surg. 2023;31(2):e107–17. https://doi.org/10.5435/JAAOS-D-22-00122.
7. Peel TN, Astbury S, Cheng AC, Paterson DL, Buising KL, Spelman T, et al. ASAP Trial Group. Trial of vancomycin and cefazolin as surgical prophylaxis in arthroplasty. N Engl J Med. 2023;389(16):1488–98. https://doi.org/10.1056/NEJMoa2301401.
8. Ashkenazi I, Amzallag N, Snir N, Morgan S, Garceau S, Kotz L, et al. Does addition of gentamicin for antibiotic prophylaxis in total knee arthroplasty reduce the rate of periprosthetic joint infection? Arch Orthop Trauma Surg. 2023;143(8):5255–60. https://doi.org/10.1007/s00402-022-04744-3.
9. Pawloy K, Fenstad AM, Leta T, Hallan G, Gjertsen JE, Dale H, et al. No difference in risk of revision due to infection between clindamycin and cephalosporins as antibiotic prophylaxis in cemented primary total knee replacements: a report from the Norwegian Arthroplasty Register 2005–2020. Acta Orthop. 2023;94:404–9. https://doi.org/10.2340/17453674.2023.16907.
10. Torkington MS, Davison MJ, Wheelwright EF, Jenkins PJ, Anthony I, Lovering AM, et al. Bone penetration of intravenous flucloxacillin and gentamicin as antibiotic prophylaxis during total hip and knee arthroplasty. Bone Joint J. 2017;99-B(3):358–64. https://doi.org/10.1302/0301-620X.99B3.BJJ-2016-0.
11. Tan TL, Shohat N, Rondon AJ, Foltz C, Goswami K, Ryan SP, et al. Perioperative antibiotic prophylaxis in total joint arthroplasty: a single dose is as effective as multiple doses. J Bone Joint Surg Am. 2019;101(5):429–37. https://doi.org/10.2106/JBJS.18.00336.
12. Feder OI, Yeroushalmi D, Lin CC, Galetta MS, Meftah M, Lajam CM, et al. Incomplete administration of intravenous vancomycin prophylaxis is common and associated with increased infectious complications after primary total hip and knee arthroplasty. J Arthroplast. 2021;36(8):2951–6. https://doi.org/10.1016/j.arth.2021.03.035.
13. Badge H, Churches T, Xuan W, Naylor JM, Harris IA. Timing and duration of antibiotic prophylaxis is associated with the risk of infection after hip and knee arthroplasty. Bone Joint Open. 2022;3(3):252–60. https://doi.org/10.1302/2633-1462.33.BJO-2021-0181.R1.
14. de Lachica JCV, Reyes SSS, Ureña JAP, Fragoso MAR. Decrease in acute periprosthetic joint infections incidence with vancomycin-loaded calcium sulfate beads in patients with non-modifiable risk factors. A randomized clinical trial. J ISAKOS. 2022;7(6):201–5. https://doi.org/10.1016/j.jisako.2022.08.002.
15. Villa JM, Pannu TS, Braaksma W, Higuera CA, Riesgo AM. Extended oral antibiotic prophylaxis after aseptic total hip or knee arthroplasty revisions: a preliminary report. J Arthroplast. 2023;38(1):141–5. https://doi.org/10.1016/j.arth.2022.08.003.
16. Weiner TR, El-Najjar DB, Herndon CL, Wyles CC, Cooper HJ. How are oral antibiotics being used in total joint arthroplasty? A review of the literature. Orthop Rev (Pavia). 2024;16:92287. https://doi.org/10.52965/001c.92287.
17. Mohiuddin A, Rice J, Ziemba-Davis M, Meneghini RM. Infection rates after aseptic revision total hip arthroplasty with extended oral antibiotic prophylaxis. J Am Acad Orthop Surg. 2024;32(10):472–80. https://doi.org/10.5435/JAAOS-D-23-00750.
18. de Beer J, Petruccelli D, Rotstein C, et al. Antibiotic prophylaxis for total joint replacement surgery: results of a survey of Canadian orthopedic surgeons. Can J Surg. 2009;52(6):E229–34. PMID: 20011156.
19. Bratzler DW, Houck PM. Surgical infection prevention guidelines writers workgroup; American Academy of Orthopedic Surgeons. Antimicrobial prophylaxis for surgery: an advisory statement from the National Surgical Infection Prevention Project. Clin Infect Dis. 2004;38(12):1706–15. https://doi.org/10.1086/421095.
20. The French Society of Anesthesia and Resuscitation. Recommendations for the practice of antibiotic prophylaxis in surgery. Current status 1999 [Article in French]. Chirurgie. 1999;124(4):441–7. PMID: 10546400.

21. Hickson CJ, Metcalfe D, Elgohari S, Oswald T, Masters JP, Rymaszweska M, et al. Prophylactic antibiotics in elective hip and knee arthroplasty: an analysis of organisms reported to cause infections and national survey of clinical practice. Bone Joint Res. 2015;4(11):181–9. https://doi.org/10.1302/2046-3758.411.2000432.

22. Bosco JA, Prince Rainier RT, Catanzano AJ, Stachel AG, Phillips MS. Expanded Gram-negative antimicrobial prophylaxis reduces surgical site infections in hip arthroplasty. J Arthroplast. 2016;31(3):616–21. https://doi.org/10.1016/j.arth.2015.09.051.

13 Open Debridement, Antibiotic, and Implant Retention (DAIR) for Periprosthetic Joint Infection in Total Knee Arthroplasty

E. Carlos Rodríguez-Merchán, Juan S. Ruiz-Pérez, and Primitivo Gómez-Cardero

13.1 Introduction

Periprosthetic joint infection (PJI) is the most frequent cause of failure following total knee arthroplasty (TKA) [1]. According to Chaiyanit et al., debridement, antibiotics, and implant retention (DAIR) is the advised management for acute hematogenous PJI after TKA. Nevertheless, DAIR is associated with an elevated rate of unsuccessful results [2]. Besides, Boyle et al. (2020) reported that published clinical results have varied for DAIR for PJI in TKA [3]. The purpose of this chapter is to analyze the most recent data on the role of open DAIR for PJI in TKA.

13.2 Trends in Utilization of DAIR for Infection After TKA

According to Boyle et al. (2020), little was known in 2020 regarding trends in utilization of DAIR [3]. They thus assessed the percentage of DAIR utilization for TKA and total hip arthroplasty (THA) PJI over a decade and clinical factors associated with these trends. A retrospective study of primary TKAs and THAs was conducted using Medicare data from 2005 to 2014 via the PearlDiver database platform. *Procedural Technology and International Classification of Diseases, Ninth Edition* codes identified individuals who experienced a surgical revision for PJI, and whether the revision was a DAIR, as well as associated clinical factors, including the timing from the index arthroplasty. The proportion of revision TKAs and THAs performed using DAIR was 27% and 12% across all years, respectively. This proportion varied by year for TKAs and THAs, with a linear trend toward increasing relative utilization of DAIR calculated as 1.4% and 0.9% per year. DAIR for TKA and THA performed within 90 days increased at a faster rate, 3.4% and 2.1% per year. Trends over time in TKA DAIRs exhibited an association with the Elixhauser Comorbidity Index (ECI), with the 0–5 group increasing at 2% per year and in individuals older than 85 years. Therefore, this study showed that the proportion of revision arthroplasty cases for PJI managed with DAIR had been increasing over time in the United States, with the most significant increase seen within 90 days from index arthroplasty. Age, gender, and ECI had a minimal association with this trend, except in the TKA population older than 85 years and in those with a very low ECI score [3].

E. C. Rodríguez-Merchán (✉) · J. S. Ruiz-Pérez
P. Gómez-Cardero
Department of Orthopedic Surgery, Hospital Universitario La Paz, Madrid, Madrid, Spain

E. C. Rodríguez-Merchán (ed.), *Advances in Periprosthetic Joint Infection*,
https://doi.org/10.1007/978-3-032-02945-4_13

13.3 Success Rates of DAIR in Infected TKAs

In 2021, Zhu et al. analyzed the success of DAIR in a large group of TKA PJIs and evaluated the utility of current classification systems in predicting DAIR outcomes in early postoperative, late hematogenous, and chronic PJIs [1]. In a multicenter review over 15 years, 230 patients experienced DAIR for first-episode PJI following primary TKA. Patients were followed up for an average of 6.9 years. The overall success rate of DAIR was 53.9%. On receiver operating characteristic analysis, 3 months (area under the curve = 0.63) and 1-year implant age (area under the curve = 0.66) cut-offs were similarly predictive of results. DAIR was successful in 64% of "early" PJIs (implant <1 year) versus 38% of "late hematogenous" PJIs (implant >1 year) (Fig. 13.1). For late PJIs (implant >1 year), *Staphylococcus aureus* and gram-negative infections were risk factors for DAIR failure. Therefore, this study showed that DAIR had a high failure percentage in all PJIs that occurred more than a year post-primary TKA, particularly when caused by *Staphylococcus aureus* or gram-negative bacteria. The age of implant was an important predictor of DAIR results [1].

In 2022, Walkay et al. retrospectively reviewed all individuals who experienced DAIR for PJI at their center between 2010 and 2018 [4]. Individuals who experienced revision surgery as an index procedure, arthroscopic washout, and those with less than 2 years of follow-up were excluded. Treatment failure was defined as revision arthroplasty for recurrence of infection within 2 years of the index procedure. Of the 60 individuals (40 knees, 20 hips) who experienced DAIR, 18 (13 knees, 5 hips) needed revision arthroplasty within 2 years, which accounted for a success rate of 70%. Predictive factors for revision were American Society of Anesthesiologists (ASA) score of greater than 2, body mass index (BMI) >35, C-reactive protein (CRP) >200 mg/L, and *Staphylococcus aureus* growth (Fig. 13.2). The 5-year survival rate for DAIR was 70%, which remained constant after 2 years from DAIR. The conclusions of this study were that the success rate of DAIR in PJI was 70% which was comparable to similar studies in the literature; that ASA >2, BMI >35, CRP >200, and *Staphylococcus aureus* growth were predictors for DAIR failure; and that implant survival rate and duration were better following DAIR in early-onset PJI [4].

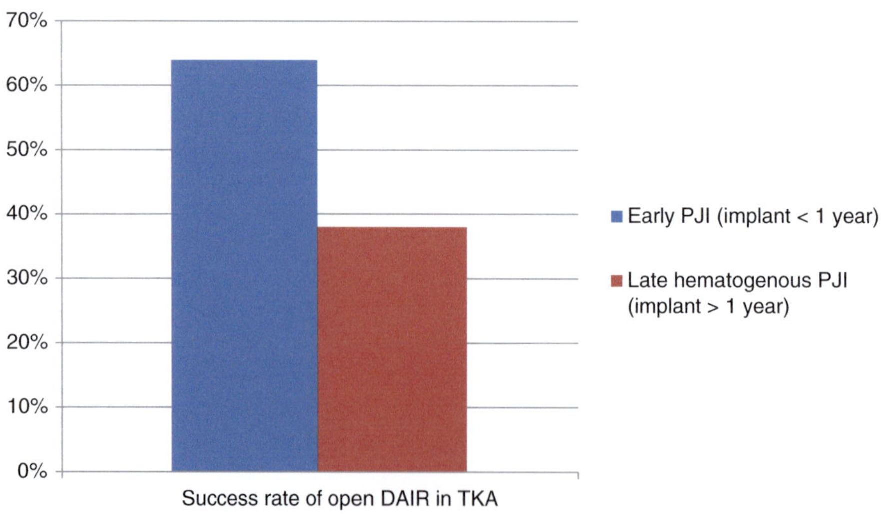

Fig. 13.1 Success rate of open DAIR (debridement, antibiotic, and implant retention) in periprosthetic joint infection (PJI) after total knee arthroplasty (TKA): "early" PJI versus "late hematogenous" PJI

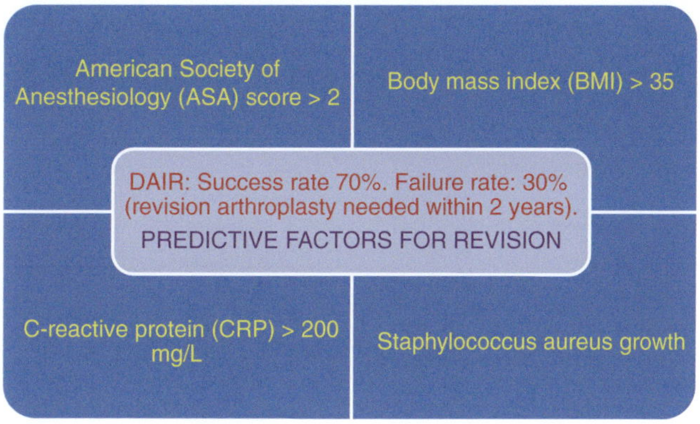

Fig. 13.2 Success rate of open DAIR (debridement, antibiotic, and implant retention) and predictive factors for revision arthroplasty in periprosthetic joint infection (PJI) after total knee arthroplasty (TKA)

In a systematic review published by Hulleman et al. in 2023, they found that current literature suggested that DAIR was a valid management alternative for early infections after revision TKA with success rates of 50–70%. Repeat DAIR exhibited success rates of around 50%. However, Hulleman concluded that further research was required for predicting successful (repeat/two-stage) DAIRs in larger cohorts, antibiotic regimes, and the cost-effectiveness of a second DAIR after revision TKA [5].

In 2023, Rahardja et al. analyzed the success rate of DAIR for PJI in a large prospective group of individuals experiencing TKA. The ability of different PJI classification systems to predict success was evaluated [6]. One hundred eighty-nine newly diagnosed knee PJIs were managed with DAIR between July 2014 and December 2017. Individuals were prospectively followed up for 2 years. A strict definition of success was utilized, requiring the patient to be alive with documented absence of infection, no ongoing antibiotics, and the index prosthesis in place. Success was compared against the Coventry (early PJI ≤1 month), International Consensus Meeting (early ≤90 days), Auckland (early <1 year), and Tsukayama (early ≤1 month, hematogenous >1 month with <7 days symptoms, chronic >1 month with >7 days symptoms) classifications. DAIR success was 45% and was highest in early PJIs defined according to the Coventry, the International Consensus Meeting, and the Auckland classification. Success was lower in both hematogenous and chronic infections. This study showed that the time since primary TKA is an important predictor of DAIR success. Success was highest in infections occurring <1 month after primary TKA and progressively diminished as the time since primary TKA increased [6].

In a study with level III of evidence (2024), van Engen et al. stated that controversy surrounds DAIR in the treatment of acute PJI, and that information regarding DAIR's rate of infection resolution is variable with little investigation of functional results. They identified 191 DAIR cases from 2008 to 2020. Median follow-up for all 191 cases was 5.9 years. Survivorship without subsequent operation for infection was 84% at 1 year, 82% at 2 years, and 79% at 5 years (Fig. 13.3). Knee and mental health results in successful DAIR procedures were similar to uncomplicated TKA. DAIR's success rate was 79% in treating acute PJI at 5 years [7]. Figure 13.4 shows a case of chronic *Streptococcus pyogenes* infection of knee prosthesis (rotational hinge design) treated by extensive synovectomy, debridement, implant retention, and lavage with Bactisure solution.

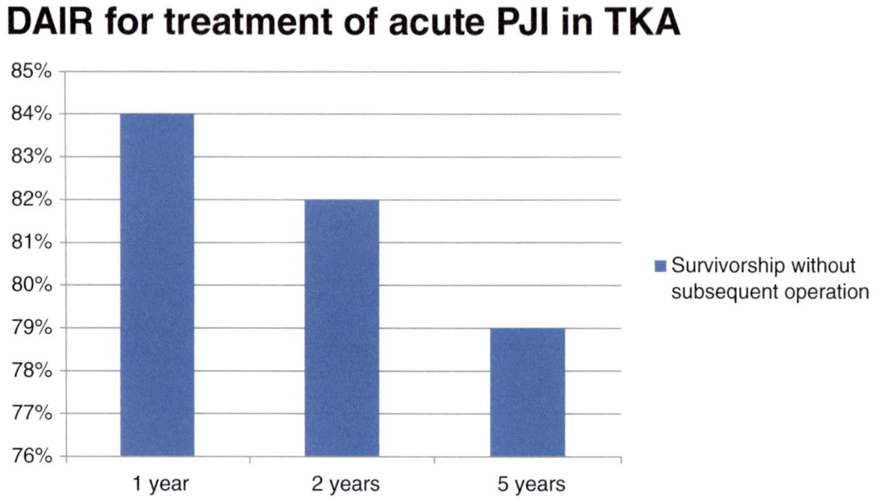

Fig. 13.3 Survivorship without subsequent operation for periprosthetic joint infection (PJI) of open DAIR (debridement, antibiotic, and implant retention) in total knee arthroplasty (TKA)

Fig. 13.4 Chronic *Streptococcus pyogenes* infection of knee prosthesis (rotational hinge design) treated by extensive synovectomy, debridement, implant retention and lavage with Bactisure solution: (**a**) image showing chronic fistula with involvement of the knee extensor apparatus (red arrow); (**b**) intense osteolysis in the medial area of the femoral prosthetic component (black arrow); (**c**) intense osteolysis also in the lateral area of the femoral component (black arrow); (**d**) image after completion of surgery

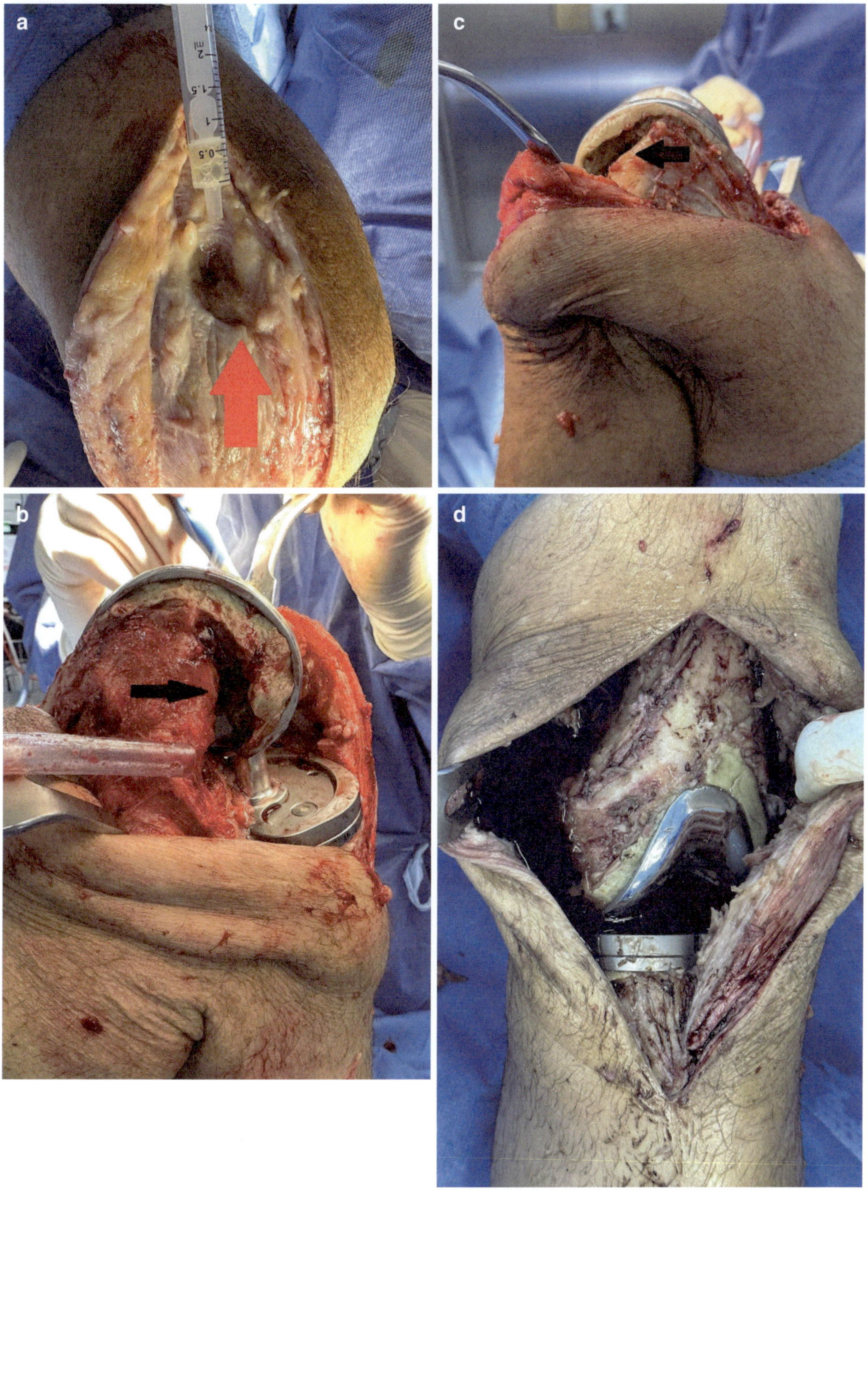
a
b
c
d

13.4 Morbid Obesity Is a Risk Factor for Infection Recurrence After DAIR for PJI in TKA

In 2020, Katakam et al. stated that although morbid obesity was a proven risk factor for PJI following THA and TKA, little was known regarding the infection control rate of this group following DAIR [8]. Therefore, they studied the infection control rate following DAIR in a morbidly obese individual group compared to a nonobese individual group and noticed the relationship between time from diagnosis to management and risk of DAIR failure. Results of all DAIR procedures were retrospectively reviewed across four hospitals. Those with a BMI of at least 40 kg/m^2 were matched 2:1 on the basis of patient age, sex, date of surgery, and presence of staphylococcal species in culture to a group of individuals with a BMI of <30 kg/m^2. The morbidly obese cohort experienced a higher management failure rate (57.9%) compared to the nonobese cohort (36.8%). Morbid obesity and major depressive disorder/generalized anxiety disorder diagnosis substantially increased the risk of failure, with hazard ratios of 1.82 and 2.09, respectively. Morbidly obese individuals who underwent DAIR within 48 hours of symptom presentation did not face an increased risk of reinfection compared to nonobese individuals. This study suggested that morbidly obese individuals faced an increased risk of DAIR failure; nevertheless, this risk can be lessened if DAIR was performed within 48 hours of symptom onset [8].

13.5 DAIR Combined with Direct Intraarticular Antibiotic Infusion in Individuals with Acute Hematogenous PJI of the Knee

In 2021, Chaiyanit et al. stated that since 2007, direct intraarticular antibiotic infusion, which can yield a high intraarticular antibiotic concentration, had been utilized in combination with DAIR to improve management results among individuals in their hospital [2]. In their study, they evaluated the results of DAIR combined with direct intraarticular antibiotic infusion in individuals who presented with acute hematogenous PJI after TKA. They reviewed the information of all individuals diagnosed with acute hematogenous PJI after primary TKA (from 2008 to 2015) who underwent DAIR combined with direct intraarticular antibiotic infusion. In total, 15 knees in 12 individuals were semi-urgently treated with this approach. The mean follow-up time was 93.3 (minimum: 56) months, and the longest follow-up time was 11 years. Two individuals (N = 3 knees) had a well-functioning, noninfected prosthesis 6 and 10 years after the procedure. Two individuals (N = 2 knees) had reinfection 2 and 5 years after surgery, and they needed a two-stage revision. None of the individuals were lost to follow-up. Finally, 13 (86.6%) of 15 infected knees were successfully managed with this approach. DAIR combined with direct intraarticular antibiotic infusion seemed to be an efficacious management strategy for acute hematogenous PJI after TKA [2].

13.6 Results of DAIR for PJI in TKA Supplemented with the Use of Intraosseous Antibiotics

In 2021, Kildow et al. assessed if the addition of a single dose of intraosseous (IO) administration of vancomycin at the time of DAIR would improve results [9]. A retrospective case series of 35 PJI TKA individuals, with a median age of 67 years, who experienced DAIR combined with IO vancomycin (500 mg), was carried out with a minimum 12 months' follow-up. A total of 26 individuals with primary implants were managed for acute perioperative or acute hematogenous infections. Besides, nine individuals were treated for chronic infections with components that were deemed unresectable. Primary outcome was defined by no reoperations for infection, nor clinical signs or symptoms of PJI. Mean follow-up for acute infection was 16.5 months (12.1–24.2) and 15.8 months (12–24.8) for chronic infections with unresectable components. Overall nonrecurrence rates for acute infection were 92.3% (24/26) but only 44.4% (4/9) for chronic infections with unresectable components. Most individuals endured on suppressive oral antibiotics. Musculoskeletal Infection Society (MSIS) host grade was a substantial indicator of failure. The addition of IO vancomycin at the time of DAIR was demonstrated to be safe with improved outcomes compared to those in the current literature (2021) utilizing standard DAIR without IO antibiotic administration. However, use of this technique in chronic infections should be used with caution. While these outcomes are encouraging, this technique needs longer follow-up prior to widespread adoption [9].

13.7 Timing of DAIR for Early Postsurgical Knee PJI Does Not Affect 1-Year Re-revision Rates

In 2021, van der Ende et al. stated that the timing between the primary TKA and the DAIR is probably a determinant for its successful result. However, the optimal timing of a DAIR and the chance of success still remain unclear [10]. In their study, they analyzed the risk of re-revision within 1 year after a DAIR procedure and assessed the timing of the DAIR in primary THA and TKA. They used information from the Dutch Arthroplasty Register (LROI) and selected all primary THA and TKA in the period 2007–2016 that experienced a DAIR within 12 weeks after primary procedure. A DAIR was defined as a revision for infection in which only modular parts were exchanged. A DAIR was defined as successful if not followed by a re-revision within 1 year after DAIR; 207 DAIRs were carried out in less than 4 weeks after THA, of which 16 (8%) underwent a complete revision within 1 year. DAIR procedures carried out between 4 and 12 weeks (N = 98) had a failure rate of 9% (N = 9). After TKA 126 DAIRs were carried out in less than 44 weeks, of which 11 (9%) underwent a complete revision within 1 year; 83 DAIRs were carried out between 4 and 12 weeks, of which 14 (17%) were revised. In conclusion, there was no substantial difference in 1-year re-revision rate after a DAIR procedure by timing of the DAIR procedure for THA and TKA based on Dutch registry information [10].

13.8 DAIR: What Predicts Success or Failure?

According to Toh et al. (2021), there is limited literature on predictive prognostic factors for DAIR [11]. Therefore, they analyzed outcomes of DAIR and studied the predictive prognostic factors. They retrospectively reviewed 106 DAIRs. Failure was defined as requiring the removal of TKA implants. Predictive factors that might impact the success of DAIR treatment, such as age, gender, BMI, ethnicity, ASA score, comorbidities, preoperative ESR and CRP, symptom duration, time between TKA and DAIR, cultures, rifampicin use, polyethylene liner change, and antibiotic duration were analyzed. The success rate of DAIR was 69.8%. In successful cases, mean time from DAIR to mortality was longer than in failures (61.6 versus 9.75 months). Methicillin-sensitive *Staphylococcus aureus* (MSSA) PJI was a substantial predictor for failure of DAIR. Higher preoperative ESR correlated to failure. In successful cases, mean ESR was 75.4, whereas mean ESR in failures was 116. An ESR >107.5 predicted failure with a sensitivity of 51.5 and specificity of 85.2. ESR >107.5 correlated to failure. Repeat DAIRs were strongly correlated to failure. In conclusion, DAIR failure was associated with earlier time to mortality. Repeat DAIRs, elevated ESR >107.5, and *Staphylococcus aureus* PJI were associated with management failure and two-stage revision was advised [11].

13.9 DAIR: Does Chronicity of Symptoms Matter?

In 2021, Tarity et al. stated that chronic infection was generally considered a contraindication to DAIR; however, results stratified by chronicity had not been well documented [12]. A retrospective review of all DAIR cases carried at a single center from 2008 to 2015 was conducted. Chronicity of PJI was categorized as acute postoperative, chronic, or acute hematogenous. Failure after DAIR, defined as re-revision for infection recurrence with the same organism, was assessed among the three chronicity cohorts at 90 days as well as at a minimum 2-year follow-up. Overall, 248 individuals experiencing DAIR for THA or TKA PJI were included. Categorization of PJI was acute (acute postoperative) in 59 cases (24%), chronic in 54 cases (22%), and acute hematogenous in 135 cases (54%). DAIR survivorship was 47% (range 0.3–10 years). Overall, there were 118 (47.6%) treatment failures after DAIR with a minimum of 2-year follow-up. There was no difference in failure rate between THA and TKA individuals. Individuals infected with *Staphylococcus* are at a higher risk of failure for all DAIR procedures regardless of chronicity category. Identification of microbial species before performing DAIR might be more clinically relevant than stratification according to chronicity category when considering management alternatives [12].

13.10 DAIR After Revision Arthroplasty: Antibiotic Mismatch, Timing, and Repeated DAIR Associated with Poor Outcome

In 2022, Veermane et al. (2022) stated that the result of DAIR after revision arthroplasty had not been reported [13]. They analyzed 88 individuals who experienced DAIR within 90 days of revision THA or revision TKA between 2012 and 2019. The overall success rate of DAIR, with respect to the retention of components and the cure of infection, was 68% after 2 years. DAIR carried out with an interval of >30 days after the index revision procedure, a repeated DAIR within 90 days, and the use of an immunosuppressive agent were associated with a substantially diminished success rate. In the culture-positive cohort, a mismatch between the antibiotic treatment and the susceptibility of the organism was associated with a substantially lower success rate. DAIR seemed to be an acceptable form of surgical treatment for individuals with a suspected early PJI after revision THA or revision TKA. DAIRs carried out after a prolonged interval, multiple DAIRs, and antibiotic mismatches were substantially associated with an increased risk of failure. Optimization of the host immune response and the prevention of antibiotic mismatch are modifiable factors that might improve the result [13].

13.11 DAIR in Treating Chronic PJI After TKA Using Continuous Local Antibiotic Perfusion Therapy

Zenke et al. (2024) investigated the results of DAIR combined with continuous local antibiotic perfusion (CLAP) for chronic PJI after TKA [14]. Six individuals (male; one case, female; five cases, mean age 79.5 years experienced CLAP for chronic PJI after TKA. Minimum follow-up was 1 year. Two of six patients had a recurrence of infection at 5 weeks and 5 months after initial CLAP and needed repeat CLAP treatment, but all individuals could preserve their components. The organisms responsible for the flare-ups were MSSA in three cases, *Klebsiella pneumonia* in one case each, and unknown pathogens in one case. CLAP therapy for all individuals was administered eight times in six cases. Adverse events included one case of reversible acute kidney injury during CLAP in an individual with recurrent infection. DAIR with CLAP for chronic post-TKA infection could be a useful treatment alternative to preserve components and allow the infection to subside, provided the implant is not markedly loosened [14].

13.12 Validation of a Classification System for Optimal Application of DAIR in PJIs Following TKA

In 2024, Tseng et al. evaluated a new scoring system's accuracy in predicting DAIR success (Table 13.1) [15]. 119 TKA individuals

Table 13.1 Israeli Orthopedic Association (IOA) novel classification system

Parameter	Subparameter	Definition/examples	Score
1. Acuteness	Acute	Acute or late acute hematogenous infection: <3 weeks of symptoms after onset	2
	Subacute	Late subacute infection: 3–4 weeks of symptoms	4
	Chronic	Chronic infection: >4 weeks after onset of symptoms	6
2. Bacteria	Normal	Single bacteria, MSSE, MSSA	1
	Moderately resilient bacteria	MRSA, MRSE	2
	Resilient bacteria	Vancomycin-resistant *Enterococci*, polyorganism, *Fungi*	3
3. Host	Normal/mildly compromised	CCI (0–1)	1
	Moderately compromised	CCI (2–3)	2
	Severely compromised	CCI (>4)	3

From Tseng et al. [15], licensed under CC-BY 4.0
Total score is summed from each parameter
MRSA Methicillin-resistant *Staphylococcus aureus*, *MRSE* Methicillin-resistant *Staphylococcus epidermidis*, *MSSE* Methicillin-sensitive *Staphylococcus epidermidis*, *MSSA* Methicillin-sensitive *Staphylococcus aureus*, *CCI* Charlson Comorbidity Index

(2008–2019) diagnosed with PJI who experienced DAIR were included for analysis. Mean follow-up was 2.5 years with an average age of 65.5 years, BMI of 31.9 kg/m^2, and Charlson Comorbidity Index (CCI) of 3.04. Successful infection eradication occurred in 75.6% of individuals. The classification system showed 61.1% sensitivity, 72.4% specificity, and 87.3% positive predictive value (PPV) when the DAIR cutoff was a score less than 6. For a cutoff of less than 8, sensitivity was 100%, specificity was 37.9%, and PPV was 83.3%. To date, there is no consensus on a classification system predicting DAIR success. This novel scoring system, with high PPV, shows promise. However, further refinement is crucial for enhanced predictive accuracy [15].

13.13 Conclusions

In a study, DAIR for PJI of primary TKA was successful in 64% of "early" PJIs (implant <1 year) versus 38% of "late hematogenous" PJIs (implant >1 year). For late PJIs (implant >1 year), *Staphylococcus aureus* and gram-negative infections were risk factors for DAIR failure. In other study, DAIR success after PJI of primary TKA was 45% and was highest in early PJIs. Success was lower in both hematogenous and chronic infections.

Some authors have found a success rate of 70% after DAIR in PJI after primary TKA. ASA >2, BMI >35, CRP >200, and *Staphylococcus aureus* growth were predictors for DAIR failure; they also found that implant survival rate and duration were better following DAIR in early-onset PJI.

In a study the succes rate was 79% in treating acute PJI after primary TKA at 5 years. Other authors found a success rate of DAIR of 69.8%. MSSA PJI was a substantial predictor of failure of DAIR. ESR >107.5 correlated to failure. Repeat DAIRs were strongly correlated to failure.

Current literature suggests that DAIR is a valid management alternative for early infections after revision TKA, with success rates of 50–70%. Repeat DAIR exhibits success rates of around 50%.

References

1. Zhu MF, Kim K, Cavadino A, Coleman B, Munro JT, Young SW. Success rates of debridement, antibiotics, and implant retention in 230 infected total knee arthroplasties: implications for classification of periprosthetic joint infection. J Arthroplast. 2021;36(1):305–10.e1. https://doi.org/10.1016/j.arth.2020.07.081.
2. Chaiyakit P, Meknavin S, Hongku N, Onklin I. Debridement, antibiotics, and implant retention

combined with direct intra-articular antibiotic infusion in patients with acute hematogenous periprosthetic joint infection of the knee. BMC Musculoskelet Disord. 2021;22(1):557. https://doi.org/10.1186/s12891-021-04451-x.
3. Boyle KK, Kapadia M, Landy DC, Henry MW, Miller AO, Westrich GH. Utilization of debridement, antibiotics, and implant retention for infection after total joint arthroplasty over a decade in the United States. J Arthroplast. 2020;35(8):2210–6. https://doi.org/10.1016/j.arth.2020.03.029.
4. Walkay S, Wallace DT, Balasubramaniam VSC, Maheshwari R, Changulani M, Sarungi M. Outcomes of debridement, antibiotics and implant retention (DAIR) for periprosthetic joint infection in a high-volume arthroplasty centre. Indian J Orthop. 2022;56(8):1449–56. https://doi.org/10.1007/s43465-022-00655-y.
5. Hulleman CWJ, de Windt TS, Veerman K, Goosen JHM, Wagenaar FBM, van Hellemondt GG. Debridement, antibiotics and implant retention: a systematic review of strategies for treatment of early infections after revision total knee arthroplasty. J Clin Med. 2023;12(15):5026. https://doi.org/10.3390/jcm12155026.
6. Rahardja R, Zhu M, Davis JS, Manning L, Metcalf S, Young SW. Success of debridement, antibiotics, and implant retention in prosthetic joint infection following primary total knee arthroplasty: results from a prospective multicenter study of 189 cases. J Arthroplast. 2023;38(7 Suppl 2):S399–404. https://doi.org/10.1016/j.arth.2023.04.024.
7. Van Engen MG, Carender CN, Glass NA, Noiseux NO. Outcomes after successful debridement, antibiotic, and implant retention therapy for periprosthetic joint infection in total knee arthroplast. J Arthroplast. 2024;39(2):483–9. https://doi.org/10.1016/j.arth.2023.08.015.
8. Katakam A, Melnic CM, Bedair HS. Morbid obesity is a risk factor for infection recurrence following debridement, antibiotics, and implant retention for periprosthetic joint infection. J Arthroplast. 2020;35(12):3710–5. https://doi.org/10.1016/j.arth.2020.07.005.
9. Kildow BJ, Patel SP, Otero JE, Fehring KA, Curtin BM, Springer BD, et al. Results of debridement, antibiotics, and implant retention for periprosthetic knee joint infection supplemented with the use of intraosseous antibiotics. Bone Joint J. 2021;103-B(6 Supple A):185–90. https://doi.org/10.1302/0301-620X.103B6.BJJ-2020-2278.R1.
10. van der Ende B, van Oldenrijk J, Reijman M, Croughs PD, van Steenbergen LN, Verhaar JAN, et al. Timing of debridement, antibiotics, and implant retention (DAIR) for early post-surgical hip and knee prosthetic joint infection (PJI) does not affect 1-year re-revision rates: data from the Dutch Arthroplasty Register. J Bone Joint Infect. 2021;6(8):329–36. https://doi.org/10.5194/jbji-6-329-2021.
11. Toh RX, Yeo ZN, Liow MHL, Yeo SJ, Lo NN, Chen JY. Debridement, antibiotics, and implant retention in periprosthetic joint infection: what predicts success or failure? J Arthroplast. 2021;36(10):3562–9. https://doi.org/10.1016/j.arth.2021.05.023.
12. Tarity TD, Gkiatas I, Nocon AA, Jones CW, Carli AV, Sculco PK. Irrigation and debridement with implant retention: does chronicity of symptoms matter? J Arthroplast. 2021;36(11):3741–9. https://doi.org/10.1016/j.arth.2021.07.018.
13. Veerman K, Raessens J, Telgt D, Smulders K, Goosen JHM. Debridement, antibiotics, and implant retention after revision arthroplasty: antibiotic mismatch, timing, and repeated DAIR associated with poor outcome. Bone Joint J. 2022;104-B(4):464–71. https://doi.org/10.1302/0301-620X.104B4.BJJ-2021-1264.R1.
14. Zenke Y, Motojima Y, Ando K, Kosugi K, Hamada D, Okada Y, et al. DAIR in treating chronic PJI after total knee arthroplasty using continuous local antibiotic perfusion therapy: a case series study. BMC Musculoskelet Disord. 2024;25(1):36. https://doi.org/10.1186/s12891-024-07165-y.
15. Tseng J, Oladipo V, Dandamudi S, Jones CM, Levine BR. Validation of a classification system for optimal application of debridement, antibiotics, and implant retention in prosthetic joint infections following total knee arthroplasty: a retrospective review. Antibiotics (Basel). 2024;13(1):48. https://doi.org/10.3390/antibiotics13010048.

Revision Total Knee Arthroplasty for Periprosthetic Joint Infection

14

E. Carlos Rodríguez-Merchán,
Carlos A. Encinas-Ullán,
and Primitivo Gómez-Cardero

14.1 Introduction

According to Lazic et al., total knee arthroplasty (TKA) is a successful treatment for osteoarthritis with good clinical results. Periprosthetic joint infection (PJI) in TKA has a low incidence between 0.5% and 3% [1]. PJI is a devastating adverse event following TKA [2]. Revision total knee arthroplasty (rTKA) is challenging to carry out in individuals with PJI due to the difficulty of eliminating the infection and potential for bone and ligamentous deficits [3]. There are two basic ways to resolve PJI after TKA: one-stage exchange and two-stage exchange. The purpose of this chapter is to analyze the most recent data on the role of rTKA for PJI.

14.2 Individuals with Synovial Fluid WBC Counts of at Least 934 and PMN% of 52% or More Should Not Experience Reimplantation but Rather a Repeat Debridement, as Their Risk of Persistent or Recurrent PJI Seems Prohibitively High

In a study with level 3 of evidence published in 2021 by Ascione et al. it was stated that although synovial fluid can be used to diagnose PJI effectively, only the cutoff values adopted at the time of PJI diagnosis have been standardized, and few data are currently available about the effective-

E. C. Rodríguez-Merchán (✉) · C. A. Encinas-Ullán
P. Gómez-Cardero
Department of Orthopedic Surgery, Hospital Universitario La Paz, Madrid, Madrid, Spain

E. C. Rodríguez-Merchán (ed.), *Advances in Periprosthetic Joint Infection*,
https://doi.org/10.1007/978-3-032-02945-4_14

ness of synovial fluid examination before definitive reimplantation [4]. They studied what were the most appropriate thresholds for synovial fluid white blood cell (WBC) counts and polymorphonuclear percentage (PMN%) in a patient group experiencing definitive reimplantation after an uninterrupted course of antibiotic therapy for chronic PJI. They also studied what was the predictive value of synovial WBC and PMN% threshold compared with previously proposed thresholds. In all, 101 individuals with PJI were assessed for inclusion from January 2016 to December 2018. Nineteen percent (19 of 101) of individuals were excluded because of the presence of a chronic inflammatory disease, acute/late hematogenous infection, low amount of synovial fluid for laboratory investigations or infection persistence after spacer placement, and adequate antibiotic therapy. Finally, 81% (82 of 101) of individuals with a median age of 74 years experiencing two-stage revision for chronic TKA infection, who were followed up for a period of 96 weeks or more, were included in the study. The individuals did not discontinue antibiotic treatment prior to reimplantation and were managed for 15 days after reimplantation if intraoperative cultures were negative. No individual remained on suppressive treatment after reimplantation. Synovial fluid was aspirated aseptically with a knee spacer in place to assess the cell counts prior to reimplantation. Thirteen percent (11 of 82) of individuals had persistent or recurrent infection, defined as continually elevated erythrocyte sedimentation rate (ESR) or C-reactive protein (CRP) levels coupled with local signs and symptoms or positive cultures. The synovial fluid WBC counts and PMN% from the 11 individuals with persistent or recurrent PJI were compared with the 71 individuals who were believed to be free of PJI. Receiver operating characteristic (ROC) curve analyses evaluated the predictive value of the parameters, and the areas under the curves (AUCs) were assessed. The sensitivities, specificities, and positive and negative predictive values were determined for the WBC count and PMN%. Individuals with persistent or recurrent infection had higher median WBC counts (471 cells/µL versus 1344 cells/µL) and PMN% (36% versus 61%) than did individuals believed to be free of PJI. ROC curve analysis identified the best threshold values to be a WBC count of 934 cells/µL or more (sensitivity 0.82, specificity 0.82 as well as a PMN% of at least 52% (sensitivity 0.82 and specificity 0.78. Ascione et al. encountered no difference between the AUCs for the WBC count and the PMN% (0.87 versus 0.84). Comparing the sensitivities and specificities of the synovial fluid WBC count and PMN% proposed by other authors, Ascione et al. encountered that a PMN% of more than 52% showed better predictive value than previously reported. Based on these findings, Ascione et al. believed that individuals with WBC counts of at least 934 and PMN% of 52% or more should not experience reimplantation but rather a repeat debridement, as their risk of persistent or recurrent PJI seemed prohibitively high. The accuracy of the proposed cutoffs was better than previously published [4].

14.3 One-Stage Exchange

In a meta-analysis published in 2023, Peddada et al. found that the all-cause revision surgery rate was 11.8% for single-stage rTKA [5]. According to Razii et al. (2021), two-stage rTKA has traditionally been deemed the gold standard of management for established infection, but increasing evidence is emerging in support of one-stage exchange for selected individuals [2]. In their study, they tried to determine the results of single-stage rTKA for PJI, with mid-run follow-up. A total of 84 individuals, with a mean age of 68 years (36–92), experienced single-stage rTKA for confirmed PJI between 2006 and 2016. In all, 37 individuals (44%) were treated for an infected primary TKA, while the majority presented with infected revisions: 31 had experienced one previous revision (36.9%) and 16 had multiple prior revisions (19.1%). Contraindications to single-stage exchange included systemic sepsis, large osseous or soft-tissue loss, extensor mechanism failure, or if primary wound closure was unlikely to be accomplishable (Fig. 14.1). Individuals were not

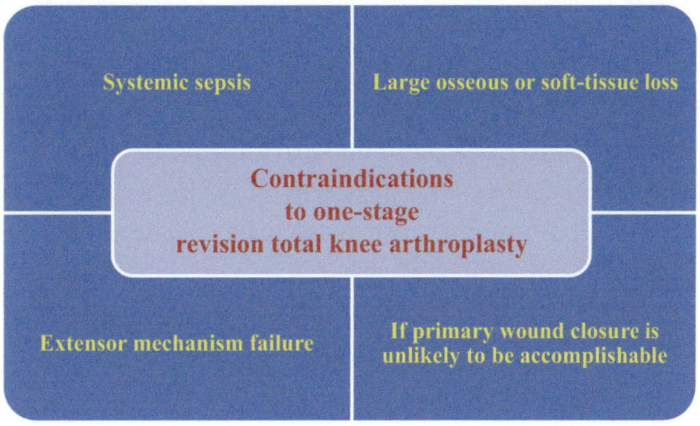

Fig. 14.1 Contraindications to one-stage revision total knee arthroplasty

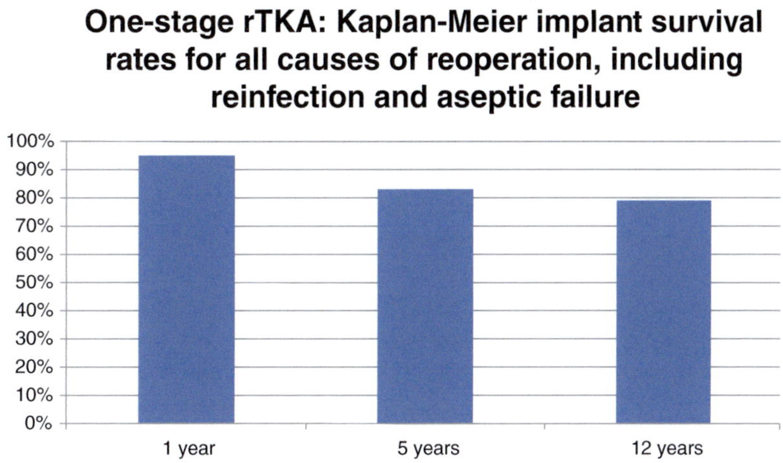

Fig. 14.2 One-stage revision total knee arthroplasty (rTKA): Kaplan-Meier implant survival rates for all causes of reoperation at 1 year (95%), 5 years (83%), and 12 years (79%), including infection and aseptic failure

excluded for culture-negative PJI or the presence of a sinus. Overall, 76 individuals (90.5%) were infection-free at a mean follow-up of 7 years, with eight reinfections (9.5%). Culture-negative PJI was not related to a higher reinfection percentage. However, there was a substantially higher rate of recurrence in individuals with polymicrobial infections. The mean Oxford Knee Score (OKS) improved from 18.7 before surgery to 33.8 at 6 months postoperatively. The Kaplan-Meier implant survival rate for all causes of reoperation, including reinfection and aseptic failure, was 95% at 1 year, 83% at 5 years, and 79% at 12 years (Fig. 14.2). It seemed that one-stage exchange, utilizing a strict debridement protocol and multidisciplinary input, was an efficacious management alternative for the infected TKA [2].

In 2021, Pellegrini et al. assessed the results of one-stage rTKA in terms of eradication of the infection, improvement of pain, and knee function [6]. Between 2009 and 2016, 20 individuals experienced one-stage rTKA for the management of a PJI. Inclusion criteria were as follows: individuals non-immunocompromised with minimal or moderate bone loss, known organisms with known sensitivity. After a mean follow-up of 6.2 years (range, 2–10 years), none of the individuals had signs suggesting recurrent infection. Follow-up examination showed substantial improvement of all variables compared to preoperative values. One-stage revision surgery rendered infection eradication and satisfying subjective functional results for infected TKA in selected individuals. One-stage rTKA was a valuable resource to approach PJIs in selected individuals whose infecting microorganism and sensitivity are determined prior to surgery. In order to succeed, strict inclusion criteria should be applied, as only non-immunocompromised individuals with healthy soft tissues with minimal or moderate bone loss are eligible for one-stage rTKA [6].

In 2023, Ji et al. assessed the mid-run survival of varus-valgus constrained (VVC) implants utilized in one-stage rTKA for chronic PJI [3]. The study included 132 patients with chronic PJI who experienced one-stage revision utilizing a VVC implant. The average follow-up was 51.6 months. Five-year survival analysis was carried out to set recurrent infection and mechanical failure as the end point. Hospital for Special Surgery (HSS) as functional results were assessed preoperatively and at the latest follow-up. A total of 12 individuals (9.1%) experienced retreatment for reinfection (nine individuals) and mechanical failure (three individuals). The overall 5-year revision-free survival was 82.7%, the infection-free survival was 91.1%, and the mechanical failure-free survival was 98.3%. The preoperative Hospital for Special Surgery (HSS) knee score improved from 35.6 points before surgery to 76.8 points at the latest follow-up. Adverse events were found in 20 individuals (15.2%), which included aseptic osteolysis in 4 cases, acceptable flexion instability in 3 cases, arthrofibrosis in 2 individuals, hematomas in 2 cases, calf intermuscular venous thrombosis in 6 individuals, and femoral stem tip pain in 3 cases. This was the first study to report the results of one-stage rTKA utilizing VVC implants for knee PJI. Improved functional results and good mid-run survival were shown at an average follow-up of 51.6 months [3].

In a study with level 4 of evidence published in 2021, Ohlmeier et al. stated that in spite of the growing number of studies reporting on PJI, there was little information on one-stage exchange arthroplasty for the revision of infected rotating-hinge prostheses, which can be among the most difficult PJI presentations to manage [7]. Between January 2011 and December 2017, 101 individuals with infected rotating-hinge knee prostheses were treated. All individuals who experienced a one-stage exchange utilizing another rotating-hinge implant were potentially eligible for the study. During that period, Ohlmeier et al. generally utilized a one-stage approach when managing PJIs. Eighty-three percent (84 of 101) of individuals were treated with one-stage exchange, and the remainder were treated with two-stage exchange. Of the 84 treated with one-stage exchange, eight individuals died of unrelated causes and were therefore excluded, one individual declined to participate in the study, and another eight individuals were lost before the minimum study follow-up of 2 years or had incomplete datasets, leaving 80% (67 of 84) for analysis in the study. The included study population consisted of 60% males (40 of 67) with a mean age of 64 years and a mean body mass index (BMI) of 30 kg/m^2. The mean number of prior surgeries was four on the affected knee. Fifteen percent (10 of 67) of knees had a preoperative joint communicating sinus tract, and 66% (44 of 67) had experienced a prior PJI on the affected knee. The antimicrobial regimen was individually adapted for the organism cultured. The mean follow-up duration was 6 years. Kaplan-Meier survivorship analysis was carried out utilizing the endpoints of survivorship free from repeat revision for infection and survivorship free from all-cause revision. The functional result was evaluated utilizing the OKS (on a 12–60-point scale, with lower scores representing less pain and greater function), obtained by interviewing individuals for the study at their most recent follow-up visit. Preoperative scores were not obtained. The Kaplan-Meier analysis showed an overall survivorship free from reoperation for any cause of 75% at the mean follow-up of 6 years postoperatively. Survivorship free from any repeat operative procedure for infection was 90% at 6 years. The mean postoperative OKS was 37 points. With an overall revision rate of about 25% at 6 years and the limited functional results based on the poor OKSs, individuals should be counseled to have modest expectations concerning postoperative pain and function level after one-stage exchange of an infected rotating-hinge arthroplasty. However, individuals might be informed about a reasonable chance of PJI eradication and may opt for this approach as a means to try to avert high transfemoral amputation or knee arthrodesis [7].

In 2024, Liechti et al. stated that rotating or pure hinge knee prostheses are frequently utilized in PJI [8]. In their study, they described the outcomes of both hinge knee prostheses after one-stage septic exchange. One hundred sixty-seven one-stage septic exchanges of a primary unconstrained TKA to a cemented hinge prosthesis (117 rotating and 50 pure hinge TKAs) carried out between 2008 and 2017 were analyzed. Exclusion criteria were stem extensions or augments utilized in primary TKA, history of extensor mechanism reconstruction, and a follow-up less than 2 years after surgery. At 5 years, the all-cause revision-free survival was 77%. Thirty-one individuals (19%) had further revision for aseptic reasons. In the rotating hinge cohort, the mechanical failure rate was more than twice as high as in the pure hinge cohort (13% versus 6%), substantially influenced by higher body weight. At a mean follow-up of 6.7 years, 21 (13%) individuals had a reinfection and experienced a further surgery. Reinfection rates did not differ between the two cohorts. The use of hinge TKA in the revision of PJI showed favorable 5-year infection-free and all-cause revision-free survival rates of 91% and 77%, respectively. This study showed poorer outcomes of the rotating hinge design [8].

14.4 Two-Stage Exchange

According to Warth et al. (2020), in the setting of chronic or age-indeterminate TKA infection, a two-staged approach had been traditionally the preferred method of treatment over single-stage reimplantation or DAIR (debridement, antibiotics, and implant retention). The two-stage treatment method was preferred in North America and had shown better overall success than the single-stage techniques. Additionally, the two-stage method was the preferred treatment for difficult-to-treat pathogens and for individuals who had already experienced a previous revision procedure. An articulating prefabricated antibiotic spacer had entered the armamentarium of two-stage revision knee surgery, and had shown comparable outcomes to custom and static spacers in terms of the primary objective of infection control [9].

In 2020, Bongers et al. stated that two-stage revision was the most frequently carried out revision procedure of a (suspected) PJI after TKA. The reported outcomes of this treatment have shown large variability between studies, ranging from 0% to 40% failure [10]. The objectives of Bongers et al. were to determine long-run reinfection rate; re-revision rates for any reason; and the reinfection rate of individuals with positive cultures at reimplantation. They prospectively followed and retrospectively reviewed 113 consecutive two-stage rTKAs, carried out between 2003 and 2013, with a minimum follow-up of 2 years. Diagnosis of PJI was based on the major MSIS criteria for PJI. After a mean follow-up of 94 months (range 24–172 months), infection recurred in 23 cases (23%). Of these, nine cases (9%) were defined as relapse (same microorganism as index revision) and in 14 cases another causative was found (14%). In 11 individuals, DAIR of the prosthesis successfully eradicated the reinfection. After overall follow-up 17 individuals (17%) experienced re-revision surgery: 11 individuals (11%) due to an infection and 6 individuals (6%) for aseptic reasons. The conclusion was that treatment of a (suspected) infection of a TKA by a two-stage revision had acceptable outcomes based on re-revision and reinfection rates in the long run (>5 years), resembling the short-run outcomes (<2 years). Reinfection rates were higher in cases with positive cultures at reimplantation [10].

According to Theil et al., megaprosthetic distal femoral reconstruction (DFR) is a limb-salvage procedure to address bone loss following two-stage revision for PJI [11]. In a study with level 4 of evidence they analyzed the survival of DFR compared to hinged TKA. It was hypothesized that DFR was associated with a poorer survival. In this study, 97individuals who experienced two-stage revision of chronic knee PJI were included. Among these, 41 were DFR. The diagnosis of PJI was established utilizing the MSIS criteria. Implant survival was estimated utilizing the Kaplan-Meier method and compared with the log-rank test as well as multivariate Cox regression at a minimum follow-up period of 24 months. The median follow-up period was 59 months. Overall, 24% (23/97) of individuals needed revision surgery for infection. The infection-free survival of rotating hinge revision TKA was 93% at 5 years compared to 50% for DFR. In multivariate analysis, the risk factors for reinfection were DFR reconstruction, length of megaprosthesis, and higher BMI. 10% (4/41) of individuals experiencing DFR underwent amputation to treat recurrent infection. Megaprosthetic DFR as part of a two-stage exchange for PJI was a salvage treatment that had a high risk for reinfection compared to non-megaprosthetic TKA [11].

In 2022, Christiner et al. stated that two-stage rTKA was the gold standard for treatment and eradication of knee PJI, but the literature was limited on the results of repeat two-stage TKA after PJI recurrence [12]. This study presented the results of a repeat two-stage revision TKA and investigated potential factors contributing to success or failure. A retrospective study was performed analyzing all two-stage rTKA carried out between 2005 and 2020. Twenty cases experienced repeat two-stage revision TKA. Patient results and factors contributing to treatment success or failure were analyzed. PJI was diagnosed according to Musculoskeletal Infection Society (MSIS) criteria. Of the 20 cases, 14 were classified as failed treatment (70%) due to a failure to eradicate infection, further surgical intervention, or death. In this group, there were no statistically significant differences between the cohorts regarding factors contributing to treatment success or failure. In the success cohort, patient-reported functional results were variable. This study showed that individuals experiencing a repeat two-stage TKA had very poor results. This study did not identify any factors that predicted failure [12].

In 2023, Puetzler et al. affirmed that the two-stage rTKA was a common treatment alternative for chronic PJI and that the time to reimplantation (TTR) published in the literature varies substantially from a few days to several hundred days. They performed a systematic review of the literature and hypothesized that longer TTR could be associated with worse infection control after the second stage. Eleven studies investigating TTR as a potential risk factor for reinfection met the inclusion criteria. The cutoff points above which TTR was regarded as "long" ranged from 4 to 18 weeks. No study found a benefit for long TTR. In all studies, similar or even better infection control was found for short TTR. However, the optimal TTR was not yet defined [13].

In 2023, Steinicke et al. stated that two-stage revision was a frequently chosen technique to manage chronic PJI. However, treatment of recurrent infection after a two-stage exchange remained debated and the result of a repeat two-stage procedure was unclear [14]. They investigated the success rates of repeat two-stage exchange revision arthroplasty and analyzed possible risk factors for failure. They retrospectively identified 55 individuals (23 hips, 32 knees) who were treated with repeat resection arthroplasty and planned delayed reimplantation for recurrent PJI between 2010 and 2019 after a prior two-stage revision. The minimum follow-up was 1 year, with a median follow-up time of 34 months; 78% (43/55) experienced reimplantation after a repeat implant removal. Of those who completed the second-stage surgery, 37% (16/43) experienced additional revision for infection and 14% (6/55) experienced amputation. The reinfection-free implant survivorship amounted to 77% after 1 year and 38% after 5 years. Individuals with a higher comorbidity score were less likely to experience second-stage reimplantation (median 5 versus 3). Moreover, obese individuals and diabetics had a higher risk of further infection. Most frequently, cultures yielded polymicrobial growth at the repeat two-stage exchange (27%, 15/55) and at re-reinfection (32%, 9/28). Pathogen persistence was found in 21% (6/28) of re-reinfected individuals. The success rates after repeat two-stage exchange arthroplasty were low [14].

In 2023, Senel et al. assessed the factors influencing the clinical results of individuals experiencing two-stage rTKA for PJI [15]. Forty-nine individuals were retrospectively assessed. Forty-four individuals met the inclusion criteria. After a mean follow-up of 48.8 months, reinfection was detected in five out of 44 individuals (10.4%). No substantial difference was observed regarding clinical and functional (C&F) KSS results when comparing time intervals between the two stages, whether they were shorter or longer than 10 weeks. However, better range of motion (ROM) results were obtained in individuals with less than 10 weeks between stages. The relationship between spacer type, ROM, and C&F KSS was not found to be significant. Particularly, the addition of 4 g of teicoplanin to the cement shortened the time between the two stages. Senel et al. concluded that CRP and ESR levels can be deemed safe parameters for diagnosis, reimplantation timing, and follow-up. The utilization of dynamic spacers or reimplantation carried out within 10 weeks after the first stage was associated with better ROM results. Besides, the addition of teicoplanin to the cement shortened the duration of antibiotic therapy [15].

In 2024, Tsai et al. affirmed that the optimal timing for reimplantation for PJI had not been established and varied from a few weeks to several months. In their study, they evaluated the commendable time between implant removal and reimplantation in individuals who experienced two-stage exchange arthroplasty for PJI [16]. They retrospectively reviewed 361 individuals who were managed with two-stage exchange arthroplasty for hip and knee chronic PJI between January 2000 and December 2018. All patients were followed for a minimum of 1 year. In the final analysis, 27 (7.5%) had treatment failure. Factors related to treatment failure including interim spacer exchange, higher ESR level at reimplantation, and TTR. Performing revision arthroplasty surgery from 16 to 20 weeks had the highest successful rate. The reimplantation over 24 weeks had a lower successful rate. However, no statistical significance in comparing each interval group was found. This study emphasized the importance of timely reimplantation in accomplishing successful results. Factors such as ESR levels, spacer exchange, and the duration of TTR influenced the likelihood of management failure in two-stage exchange arthroplasty for hip and knee PJI [16].

According to Thomas et al. (2024), the use of antibiotic-impregnated cement during 2-stage revision arthroplasty for PJI poses a risk of renal complications following spacer insertion [17]. The mean incidences of spacer-related acute kidney injury (AKI) across total hip arthroplasty (THA), TKA, and THA + TKA groups were 4.2%, 14%, and 27%, respectively. The most frequent patient-related risk factors for AKI were underlying chronic kidney disease or high baseline creatinine, low preoperative hemoglobin, and blood transfusion requirement. Spacer-related risk factors included high antibiotic dosage (>3.6 g/cement batch) and antibiotic type. While most recovered without complication, select individuals needed hemodialysis for acute management (2 THA, 18 THA + TKA) and/or developed chronic kidney disease (8 TKA, 8 THA). Orthopedic surgeons should be cognizant of this serious complication and should closely monitor at-risk individuals for AKI following antibiotic-loaded spacer insertion [17].

In a study with level 4 of evidence published in 2024, Lee et al. affirmed that the cause of early septic failure after two-stage exchange rTKA for chronic PJI and the factors affecting it were not well known. In their study, they tried to determine the surgical results and the risk factors for early septic failure after two-stage rTKA for chronic PJI. They analyzed 151 individuals who experienced two-stage exchange rTKA for chronic PJI and who had a minimum 3-year follow-up, were analyzed. Early septic failures happened within 3 years after reimplantation in 48 individuals (31.8%). Male individuals, fungus or mycobacterial infection, and positive culture at reimplantation were independently associated with an increased risk of early septic failure after two-stage exchange rTKA despite normal CRP values before reimplantation [18].

In a study with level 3 of evidence published in 2024, Puetzler et al. investigated the TTR during two-stage revision utilizing static spacers regarding management success and function in individuals with chronic PJI of the knee [19]. One hundred sixty-three individuals (median age 72 years, 72 women) who experienced two-stage exchange for chronic knee PJI between 2012 and 2020 were retrospectively analyzed (based on the 2011 MSIS criteria). When TTR exceeded 94 days, the adjusted hazard of reinfection was increased 2.8-fold. The reinfection-free rate was 67% after 2 years and 33% after 5 years for a longer TTR compared to 89% and 80% at 2 and 5 years, respectively, for a shorter TTR. Overall survival and the number of aseptic revisions did not differ between the longer TTR and shorter TTR cohorts. Although a long TTR is sometimes unavoidable in clinical practice, surgeons should be aware of a potentially higher risk of reinfection [19]. Figures 14.3 and 14.4 show two cases

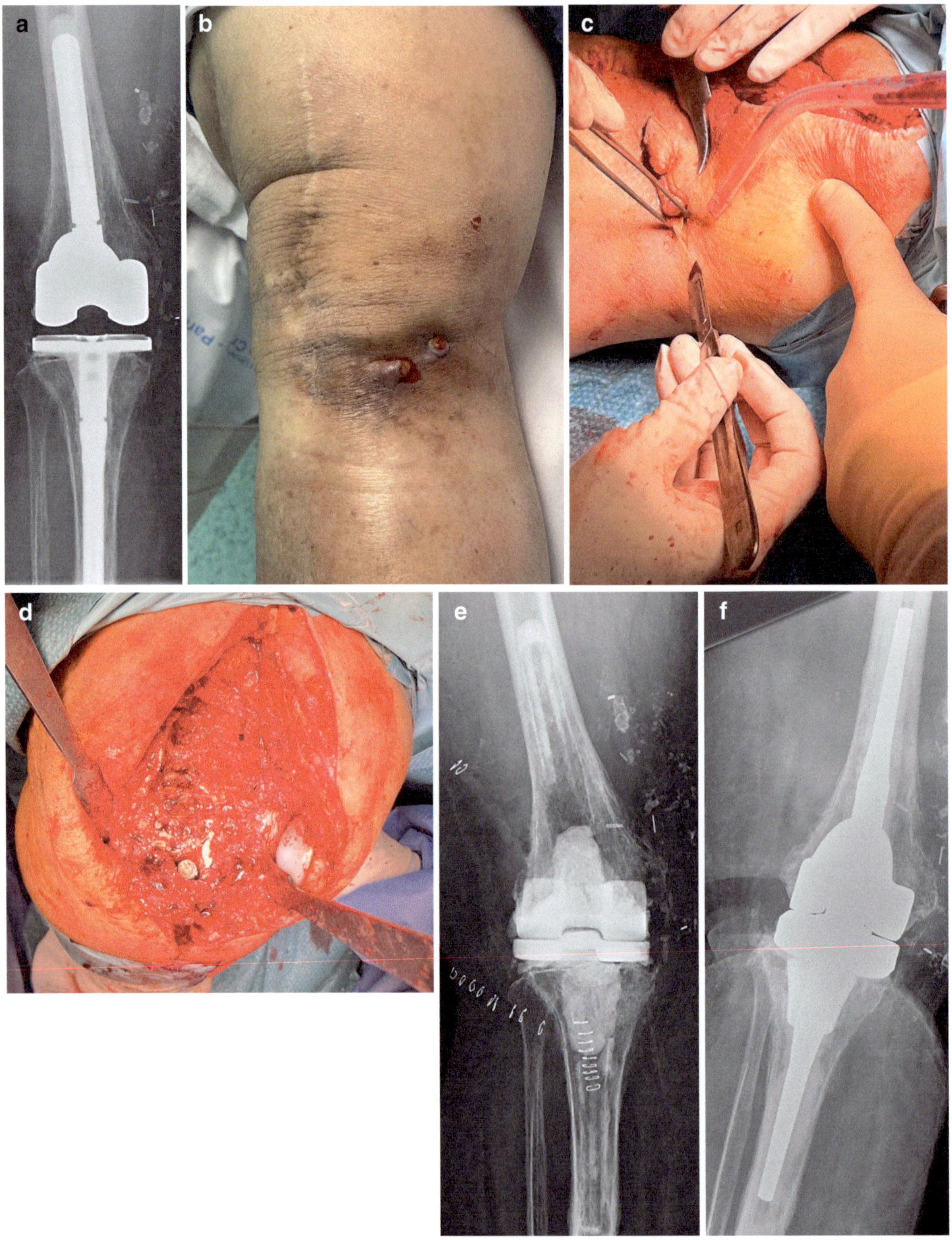

Fig. 14.3 Periprosthetic joint infection (PJI) of a Legacy Constrained Condylar Knee (LCCK) prosthesis that was treated by two-stage revision total knee arthroplasty (rTKA) with a rotating-hinge design: (**a**) anteroposterior (AP) radiograph before the first stage of rTKA (septic loosening); (**b**) the patient had two fistulas; (**c**) resection of the fistulous tracts was performed; (**d**) first stage of rTKA (removal of the infected implant); (**e**) first stage of rTKA (placement of articulating spacer with antibiotics); (**f**) second stage of rTKA (implantation of a rotating-hinge design with supplement and tibial cone)

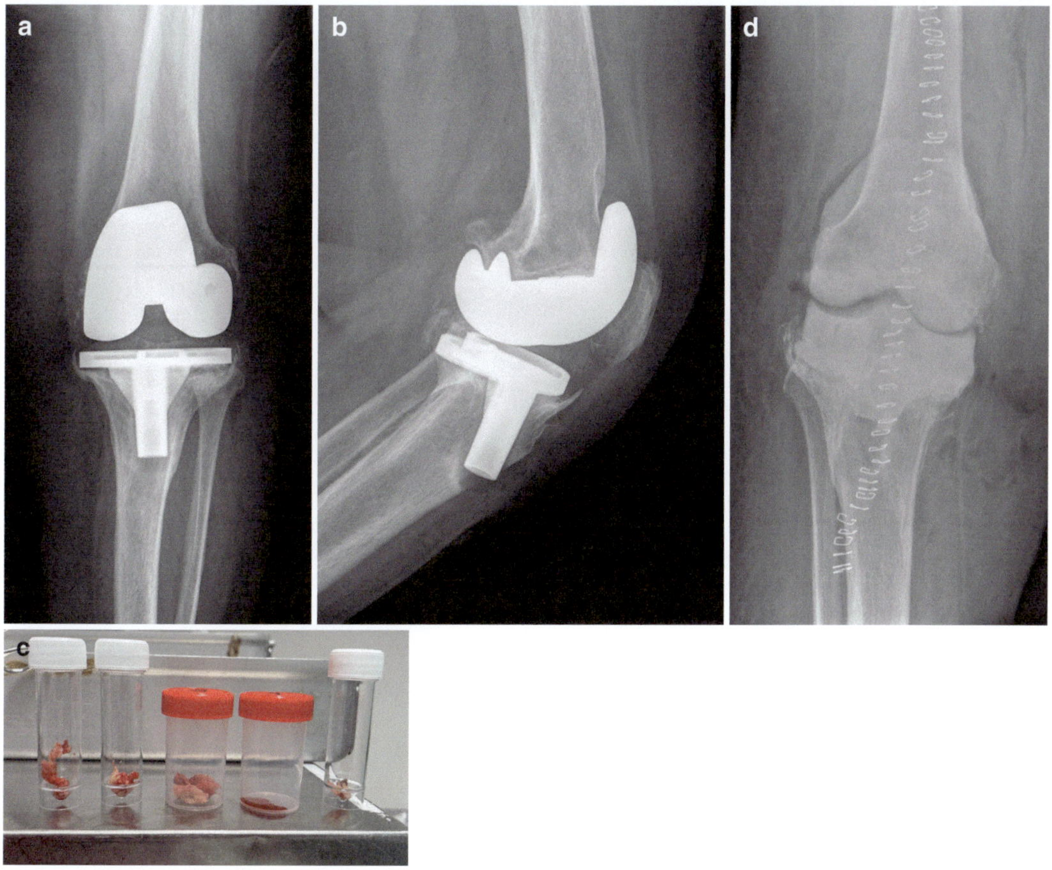

Fig. 14.4 Periprosthetic joint infection (PJI) of a total knee arthroplasty (TKA) that was treated by two-stage revision TKA (rTKA) with a rotating-hinge design: (**a**) anteroposterior (AP) radiograph before the first stage of rTKA; (**b**) lateral radiograph before the first stage of rTKA; (**c**) five samples were taken for culture; (**d**) AP radiograph after the first stage showing hinged spacer; (**e**) lateral radiograph after the first stage showing hinged spacer; (**f**) AP radiograph after the second stage (rotational hinge reconstruction); (**g**) lateral radiograph after the second stage showing the reconstruction carried out by means of a rotating-hinge prosthesis

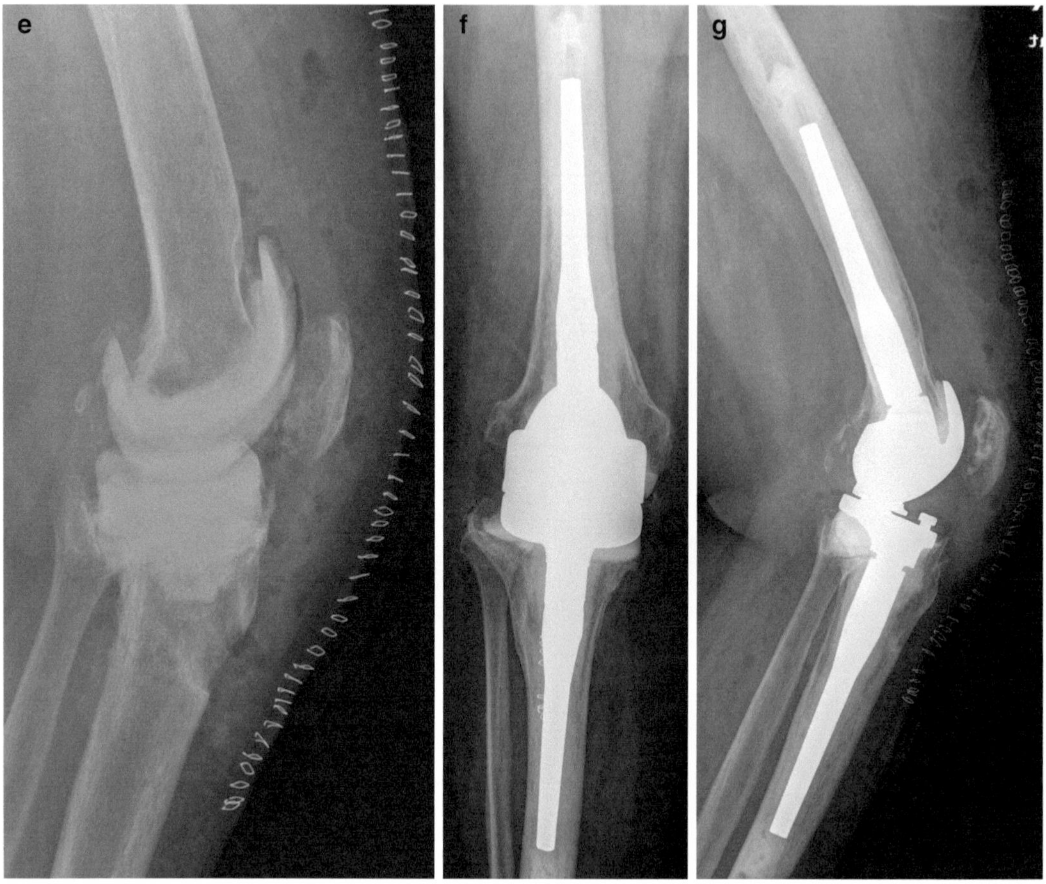

Fig. 14.4 (continued)

of septic loosening of two TKAs with PJI, which were solved by two-stage rTKA using a rotating-hinge design.

14.5 One- or Two-Stage Reimplantation for Infected TKA?

According to Lazic et al. (2021), two-staged revisions are deemed to be the gold standard for revision in chronic PJI with infection eradication rates of over 90%. However, similar infection eradication rates after one-staged revision arthroplasty have been published, raising the question whether the two-staged approach can still be deemed the gold standard [1]. Lazi et al. carried out a literature review to analyze the correlation of one-staged and two-staged rTKAs with recurrent infection rates and functional results. Mean follow-up was at 4.9 years. The mean infection eradication rate after one-staged revision versus two-staged revision in TKA was 87% versus 83%. The functional result measured by the mean Knee Society Score (KSS) of one-staged revision versus two-staged revision in TKA was 80 versus 80 points. One-staged rTKA appeared to have similar infection eradication rates and functional results compared to two-staged rTKA. However, these outcomes should be interpreted with caution, since selection bias may have played a substantial role [1].

In 2021, van den Kieboom et al. stated that removal of infected components and culture-directed antibiotics are important for the successful treatment of chronic PJI. However, 27% of chronic PJI individuals yielded negative culture results. Although culture negativity has been thought of as a contraindication to one-stage revision, information supporting this assertion is limited [20]. In their study, they reported on the clinical results for one-stage and two-stage exchange arthroplasty carried out in individuals with chronic culture-negative PJI. A total of 105 consecutive individuals who experienced revision arthroplasty for chronic culture-negative PJI were retrospectively assessed. One-stage revision arthroplasty was carried out in 30 individuals, while 75 individuals experienced two-stage exchange, with a minimum of 1 year's follow-up. Reinfection, re-revision for septic and aseptic reasons, amputation, readmission, mortality, and length of stay were compared between the two management approaches. The patient demographic characteristics did not differ substantially between the cohorts. At a mean follow-up of 4.2 years, the management failure for reinfection for one-stage and two-stage revision was five (16.7%) and 15 individuals (20%), and for septic re-revision was four (13.3%) and 11 individuals (14.7%), respectively. No substantial differences were found between one-stage and two-stage revision for 30-, 60-, and 90-day readmissions (10% versus 8%; 16.7% versus 9.3%; and 26.7% versus 10.7%), one-year mortality (3.3% versus 4%), and amputation (3.3% versus 1.3%). In this non-randomized study, one-stage revision arthroplasty showed similar results, including reinfection, re-revision, and readmission rates for the management of chronic culture-negative PJI after TKA and THA, compared to two-stage revision. This suggested culture negativity might not be a contraindication to one-stage revision arthroplasty for chronic culture-negative PJI in selected individuals [20].

In 2021, Tuecking et al. stated that controversy continued to surround the proper operative technique of PJI in TKA with single- or two-stage replacement, and that substantial variations were seen in the eradication rates of PJI and in implant survival rates [21]. They performed a retrospective analysis of all rTKA surgeries from 2013 to 2019 and screened with respect to single- or two-stage rTKAs. A total of 63 individuals were included, with 15 individuals experiencing single-stage revision and 48 individuals experiencing two-stage revision. The mean follow-up time was 40.7–43.7 months. Statistically, no difference was encountered between both cohorts in overall survival (54.4% versus 70.1%) and implant survival with respect to reinfection (71.4% versus 82.4%). High reinfection rates were encountered for individuals with difficult-to-treat organisms and low- to semi-constrained implant types, in comparison to constrained implant types. A statistically comparable revision rate for recurrence of infection could be demonstrated for both cohorts, although a tendency to a higher reinfection rate for single-stage change was evident. The revision rate in this study was comparably high, which could be caused by the high comorbidity and high proportion of difficult-to-treat bacteria in individuals at a tertiary center [21]. Table 14.1 summarizes the most important statistical data regarding rTKA.

Table 14.1 Summary of the most important statistical data regarding revision total knee arthroplasty (rTKA)

One-stage rTKA
Razzi et al (2021) [2]: 90.5% of patients were infection-free at a mean follow-up of 7 years, with 9.5% reinfections.
Pellegrini (2021) [6]: 100% of patients were infection-free at a mean follow-up of 6.2 years.
Ji et al (2023) [3]: In varus-valgus constrained (VVC) implants, the overall 5-year revision-free survival was 82.7%, the infection-free survival was 91.1%, and the mechanical failure-free survival was 98.3%.
Ohlmeier et al (2021) [7]: In rotating-hinge arthroplasty, the Kaplan-Meier analysis showed an overall survivorship free from reoperation for any cause of 75% at the mean follow-up of 6 years postoperatively. Survivorship free from any repeat operative procedure for infection was 90% at 6 years.
Liechti et al (2024) [8]: Hinge TKA versus rotating hinge TKA: In the rotating hinge cohort, the mechanical failure rate was more than twice as high as in the pure hinge cohort (13% versus 6%). At a mean follow-up of 6.7 years, 13% had a reinfection and experienced a further surgery. Reinfection rates did not differ between the two cohorts. The use of hinge TKA in the revision of PJI showed favorable 5-year infection-free and all-cause revision-free survival rates of 91% and 77%, respectively.
Two-stage rTKA
Bongers et al (2020) [10]: After a mean follow-up of 7.8 years, infection recurred in 23% of patients: 9% were defined as relapse (same microorganism as index revision) and in 14% another causative was found; 17% experienced re-revision surgery, 11% due to an infection, and 6% for aseptic reasons.
Theil et al (2022) [11]: 24% of patients needed revision surgery for infection. The infection-free survival of rotating hinge revision TKA was 93% at 5 years compared to 50% for distal femoral reconstruction (DFR).
Christiner et al (2022) [12]: In repeat two-stage revision TKA, 70% were failed treatments due to a failure to eradicate infection, further surgical intervention, or death.
Steinicke et al (2023) [14]: In repeat two-stage exchange revision arthroplasty, 78% of patients needed reimplantation. Of those who completed the second-stage surgery, 37% needed additional revision for infection, and 14% experienced amputation. The reinfection-free implant survivorship amounted to 77% after 1 year and 38% after 5 years.
Senel et al (2023) [15]: After a mean follow-up of 4 years, reinfection occurred in 10.4% of patients.
Lee et al (2024) [18]: In 31.8% early septic failures happened within 3 years after reimplantation.
Puetzler et al (2024) [19]: When time to reimplantation (TTR) exceeded 94 days, the adjusted hazard of reinfection was increased 2.8-fold. The reinfection-free rate was 67% after 2 years and 33% after 5 years for a longer TTR compared to 89% and 80% at 2 and 5 years, respectively, for a shorter TTR.
One-stage rTKA versus two-stage rTKA
Lazic et al (2021) [1]: At a mean follow-up of 4.9 years, the mean infection eradication rate after one-staged revisions was 87% versus 83% in two-staged revisions.
van den Kieboom et al (2021) [20]: At a mean follow-up of 4.2 years, the management failure for reinfection for one-stage and two-stage revision was 16.7% and 20%, and for septic re-revision was 13.3% and 14.7%, respectively. No substantial differences were found between one-stage and two-stage revision for 30-, 60-, and 90-day readmissions (10% versus 8%; 16.7% versus 9.3%; and 26.7% versus 10.7%), one-year mortality (3.3% versus 4%), and amputation (3.3% versus 1.3%).
Tuecking et al (2021) [21]: At a mean follow-up of about 40 months, no difference was encountered between one-stage exchange and two-stage exchange in overall survival (54.4% versus 70.1%) and implant survival with respect to reinfection (71.4% versus 82.4%).

14.6 Conclusions

Revision total knee arthroplasty (rTKA) is challenging to carry out in individuals with PJI due to the difficulty of eliminating the infection and potential for bone and ligamentous deficits. There are two basic ways to resolve PJI after TKA: one-stage exchange and two-stage exchange. Individuals with WBC counts of at least 934 and PMN percentage of 52% or more should not experience reimplantation but rather a repeat debridement, as their risk of persistent or recurrent PJI is prohibitively high.

Contraindications to single-stage exchange include systemic sepsis, large osseous or soft-tissue loss, extensor mechanism failure, or if primary wound closure is unlikely to be accomplishable. The reported Kaplan-Meier implant survival rate for all causes of reoperation, including reinfection and aseptic failure, is 95.2% at 1 year, 83.5% at 5 years, and 78.9% at 12 years.

In a meta-analysis all-cause revision surgery rate was 11.8% for one-stage rTKA. One-stage rTKA is a valuable resource to approach PJIs in selected individuals whose infecting microorganism and sensitivity are determined prior to surgery. In order to succeed, strict inclusion criteria should be applied, as only non-immunocompromised individuals with healthy soft tissues with minimal or moderate bone loss are eligible for one-stage rTKA. In varus-valgus constrained (VVC) implants, the overall 5-year revision-free survival was 82.7%, the infection-free survival was 91.1%, and the mechanical failure-free survival was 98.3%. Adverse events occur in 15.2%. With an overall revision rate of about 25% at 6 years and the limited functional results based on the poor OKSs, individuals should be counseled to have modest expectations concerning postoperative pain and function level after one-stage exchange of an infected rotating-hinge arthroplasty. The use of hinge TKA in the revision of PJI showed favorable 5-year infection-free and all-cause revision-free survival rates of 91% and 77%, respectively. Poorer outcomes of the rotating hinge design have been reported.

Treatment of an infection of a TKA by a two-stage revision had acceptable outcomes based on re-revision and reinfection rates in the long run (>5 years), resembling the short-run outcomes (<2 years). Reinfection rates were higher in cases with positive cultures at reimplantation. Megaprosthetic DFR as part of a two-stage exchange for PJI is a salvage treatment that has a high risk for reinfection compared to non-megaprosthetic TKA. Individuals experiencing a repeat two-stage TKA have very poor results. The success rates after repeat two-stage exchange arthroplasty are low. The utilization of dynamic spacers or reimplantation carried out within 10 weeks after the first stage is associated with better ROM results. Besides, the addition of teicoplanin to the cement shortens the duration of antibiotic therapy. Factors such as ESR levels, spacer exchange, and the duration of TTR influence the likelihood of management failure in two-stage exchange arthroplasty for knee PJI. Orthopedic surgeons should be cognizant of acute kidney injury (AKI) and should closely monitor at-risk individuals for AKI following antibiotic-loaded spacer insertion. Male individuals, fungus or mycobacterial infection, and positive culture at reimplantation are independently associated with an increased risk of early septic failure after two-stage exchange rTKA despite normal CRP values before reimplantation.

Comparative studies between one-stage rTKA versus two-stage rTKA have shown that one-stage rTKA had similar infection eradication rates and functional results to two-stage rTKA. However, this information must be interpreted with caution, since selection bias may play a substantial role. One-stage rTKA has shown similar results, including reinfection, re-revision, and readmission rates for the management of chronic culture-negative PJI after TKA, compared to two-stage revision. No difference has been encountered between one-stage rTKA and two-stage rTK in overall survival (54.4% versus 70.1%) and implant survival with respect to reinfection (71.4% versus 82.4%).

References

1. Lazic I, Scheele C, Pohlig F, von Eisenhart-Rothe R, Suren C. Treatment options in PJI – is two-stage still gold standard? J Orthop. 2021;23:180–4. https://doi.org/10.1016/j.jor.2020.12.021.
2. Razii N, Clutton JM, Kakar R, Morgan-Jones R. Single-stage revision for the infected total knee arthroplasty: the Cardiff experience. Bone Joint Open. 2021;2(5):305–13. https://doi.org/10.1302/2633-1462.25.BJO-2020-0185.R1.
3. Ji B, Li G, Zhang X, Wang Y, Mu W, Cao L. Midterm survival of a varus-valgus constrained implant following one-stage revision for periprosthetic joint infection: a single-center study. J Knee Surg. 2023;36(3):284–91. https://doi.org/10.1055/s-0041-1731739.
4. Ascione T, Balato G, Mariconda M, Smeraglia F, Baldini A, De Franco C, et al. Synovial cell count before reimplantation can predict the outcome of patients with periprosthetic knee infections undergoing two-stage exchange. Clin Orthop Relat Res. 2021;479(9):2061–8. https://doi.org/10.1097/CORR.0000000000001788.

5. Peddada KV, Welcome BM, Parker MC, Delman CM, Holland CT, Giordani M, et al. Survivorship and etiologies of failure in single-stage revision arthroplasty for periprosthetic joint infection: a meta-analysis. J Am Acad Orthop Surg Glob Res Rev. 2023;7(5):e22.00218. https://doi.org/10.5435/JAAOSGlobal-D-22-00218.
6. Pellegrini A, Meani E, Macchi V, Legnani C. One-stage revision surgery provides infection eradication and satisfying outcomes for infected knee arthroplasty in selected patients. Expert Rev Anti-Infect Ther. 2021;19(7):945–8. https://doi.org/10.1080/14787210.2021.1851597.
7. Ohlmeier M, Alrustom F, Citak M, Salber J, Gehrke T, Frings J. What is the mid-term survivorship of infected rotating-hinge implants treated with one-stage-exchange? Clin Orthop Relat Res. 2021;479(12):2714–22. https://doi.org/10.1097/CORR.0000000000001868.
8. Liechti EF, Linke P, Gehrke T, Citak M, Lausmann C. Outcomes of rotating versus pure hinge knee arthroplasty in the setting of one-stage exchange for periprosthetic joint infection. Int Orthop. 2024;48(7):1751–9. https://doi.org/10.1007/s00264-024-06139-y.
9. Warth LC, Hadley CJ, Grossman EL. Two-stage treatment for total knee arthroplasty infection utilizing an articulating prefabricated antibiotic spacer. J Arthroplast. 2020;35(3S):S57–62. https://doi.org/10.1016/j.arth.2019.10.049.
10. Bongers J, Jacobs AME, Smulders K, van Hellemondt GG, Goosen JHM. Reinfection and re-revision rates of 113 two-stage revisions in infected TKA. J Bone Joint Infect. 2020;5(3):137–44. https://doi.org/10.7150/jbji.43705.
11. Theil C, Schneider KN, Gosheger G, Schmidt-Braekling T, Ackmann T, Dieckmann R, et al. Revision TKA with a distal femoral replacement is at high risk of reinfection after two-stage exchange for periprosthetic knee joint infection. Knee Surg Sports Traumatol Arthrosc. 2022;30(3):899–906. https://doi.org/10.1007/s00167-021-06474-2.
12. Christiner T, Yates P, Prosser G. Repeat two-stage revision for knee prosthetic joint infection results in very high failure rates. ANZ J Surg. 2022;92(3):487–92. https://doi.org/10.1111/ans.17446.
13. Puetzler J, Schulze M, Gosheger G, Schwarze J, Moellenbeck B, Theil C. Is long time to reimplantation a risk factor for reinfection in two-stage revision for periprosthetic infection? A systematic review of the literature. Front Surg. 2023;10:1113006. https://doi.org/10.3389/fsurg.2023.1113006.
14. Steinicke AC, Schwarze J, Gosheger G, Moellenbeck B, Ackmann T, Theil C. Repeat two-stage exchange arthroplasty for recurrent periprosthetic hip or knee infection: what are the chances for success? Arch Orthop Trauma Surg. 2023;143(4):1731–40. https://doi.org/10.1007/s00402-021-04330-z.
15. Şenel A, Öztürkmen Y, Eren M, Carkci E, Circi E, Kanay E, et al. Factors influencing the clinical outcomes of two-stage re-implantation in patients with periprosthetic joint infection after total knee arthroplasty. Cureus. 2023;15(7):e42566. https://doi.org/10.7759/cureus.42566.
16. Tsai ML, Herng-Shouh Hsu A, Wu CT, Lin PC, Tan TL, Kuo FC. Optimal reimplantation timing in two-stage exchange for periprosthetic joint infection: an observative cohort study in Asian population. BMC Musculoskelet Disord. 2024;25(1):28. https://doi.org/10.1186/s12891-023-07129-8.
17. Thomas TL, Kothari PD, Baker CM, Tarabichi S, Clark SC, Goh GS. High incidence of acute kidney injury following antibiotic-loaded spacer insertion for periprosthetic joint infection: an updated review of the literature. J Arthroplast. 2024;39(2):549–558.e3. https://doi.org/10.1016/j.arth.2023.08.055.
18. Lee WS, Park KK, Cho BW, Park JY, Kim I, Kwon HM. Risk factors for early septic failure after two-stage exchange total knee arthroplasty for treatment of periprosthetic joint infection. J Orthop Traumatol. 2024;25(1):6. https://doi.org/10.1186/s10195-024-00750-w.
19. Puetzler J, Hofschneider M, Gosheger G, Theil C, Schulze M, Schwarze J, et al. Evaluation of time to reimplantation as a risk factor in two-stage revision with static spacers for periprosthetic knee joint infection. J Orthop Traumatol. 2024;25(1):15. https://doi.org/10.1186/s10195-024-00745-7.
20. van den Kieboom J, Tirumala V, Box H, Oganesyan R, Klemt C, Kwon YM. One-stage revision is as effective as two-stage revision for chronic culture-negative periprosthetic joint infection after total hip and knee arthroplasty. Bone Joint J. 2021;103-B(3):515–21. https://doi.org/10.1302/0301-620X.103B.BJJ-2020-1480.R2.
21. Tuecking LR, Silligmann J, Savov P, Omar M, Windhagen H, Ettinger M. Detailed revision risk analysis after single- vs. two-stage revision total knee arthroplasty in periprosthetic joint infection: a retrospective tertiary center analysis. Antibiotics (Basel). 2021;10(10):1177. https://doi.org/10.3390/antibiotics10101177.

Knee Arthrodesis After Failure of Total Knee Arthroplasty due to Infection

15

E. Carlos Rodríguez-Merchán,
Carlos A. Encinas-Ullán,
and Primitivo Gómez-Cardero

15.1 Introduction

According to Hawi et al. (2015), knee arthrodesis is a potential salvage surgical technique for limb preservation after failure of total knee arthroplasty (TKA) due to infection [1]. Periprosthetic joint infection (PJI) is a serious complication of TKA. Control of infection after a failed two-stage TKA is not always feasible, and the resolution of infection might need an above-the-knee amputation or a knee arthrodesis [2]. The purpose of this chapter is to analyze the most recent data on the role of knee arthrodesis after failure of TKA due to infection.

15.2 Knee Arthrodesis or Above-the-Knee Amputation?

In 2015, Rodriguez-Merchan published a review with the aim of determining which treatment method (knee arthrodesis or above-the-knee amputation) yielded better function and ambulatory status for individuals after a failed two-stage revision TKA (rTKA). Knee arthrodesis should be strongly deemed as the method of choice for individuals who have persistently infected TKA after a failed two-stage rTKA. Individuals can walk at least inside the house, and individuals accomplish the activity of daily living independence with successful knee arthrodesis, although walking aids, including a shoe lift, are needed. An intramedullary (IM) nail led to better functional outcomes than an external fixator (EF). The functional result after above-the-knee amputation carried out after TKA is poor. A substantial percentage of individuals never fit with a prosthesis, and those who do seldom obtain functional independence. Only 50% of individuals are able to walk after above-the-knee amputation. Individuals experiencing knee arthrodesis for treating recurrent PJI after TKA have better function and ambulatory status compared to individuals experiencing above-the-knee amputation. Knee arthrodesis must be advised as the treatment of choice for individuals who have persistent infected TKA after a failed two-stage rTKA [2].

15.3 Results of Knee Arthrodesis

In 2020, Yeung et al. [3] published a retrospective and single-surgeon series (level of evidence 4) of 51 failed TKAs due to PJI treated with two-stage knee arthrodesis between 2000 and 2016 with a minimum of 2-year follow-up. Infection was successfully controlled in 48 of 51 individuals

E. C. Rodríguez-Merchán (✉) · C. A. Encinas-Ullán
P. Gómez-Cardero
Department of Orthopedic Surgery, Hospital Universitario La Paz, Madrid, Madrid, Spain

E. C. Rodríguez-Merchán (ed.), *Advances in Periprosthetic Joint Infection*,
https://doi.org/10.1007/978-3-032-02945-4_15

(94.1%); of these, 24 knees (50%) needed no reoperation subsequent to the index knee arthrodesis, whereas the remaining 24 (50%) individuals needed a median of one additional operation. Nonunion, malunion, or delayed union was found in 10 individuals (19.6%). Of the 48 individuals who were successfully treated with knee arthrodesis, 41 individuals (85.4%) remained ambulatory after knee arthrodesis and 9 of these patients (18.8%) did not need assistive devices. Three of 51 individuals (5.9%) progressed to above-the-knee amputation after knee arthrodesis. Individuals experiencing knee arthrodesis for TKA PJI had high rates of infection control and preservation of ambulatory status, with low rates of progression to above-the-knee amputation.

In 2023, Conway et al. assessed whether height, body mass index (BMI), and age impacted patient-reported outcome measures (PROMs) in individuals who experienced knee arthrodesis after rTKA due to PJI [4]. They performed a retrospective review of individuals experiencing arthrodesis for an infected TKA at an orthopedic infection service from 2014 to 2022. Patient demographics and PROMs from 36-Item Short Form Survey (SF-36) and Knee Injury and Osteoarthritis Outcome Score (KOOS) questionnaires were collected. Correlation analysis was carried out to determine if any association between height, BMI, and age was present with the various PROMs and subscores. Forty-four individuals (19 males, 25 females) were included, with a mean follow-up of 2 years. Increases in height (>166 cm), BMI (>30), and age (>62 years) had a statistically significant negative impact on three SF-36 components: health changes, physical functioning ability, and general health components. The results of this study suggested that a knee arthrodesis was an acceptable alternative in individuals with a persistent knee PJI with good functional PROMs and ambulatory status. Individuals with shorter height, lower BMI, and younger age showed overall better results. Knee arthrodesis can be an alternative option for amputation in individuals with an infected TKA and provided good functional results in selected individuals [4].

15.3.1 Intramedullary (IM) Nail

Hawi et al. (2015) assessed the result of single-stage knee arthrodesis utilizing an IM cemented coupled nail without bone-on-bone fusion after failed and infected TKA with extensor mechanism deficiency [1]. Between 2002 and 2012, 27 individuals (ten female, 17 male; mean age 68.8 years) were treated with septic single-stage exchange. Mean follow-up was 67.1 months ($N = 27$) (minimum follow-up 24 months) and for individuals with a minimum follow-up of 5 years, the mean follow-up was 104.9 months ($N = 13$). A subjective patient evaluation [Short Form (SF)-36] was obtained, in addition to the Visual Analogue Scale (VAS). The mean VAS score was 1.44. At final follow-up, four individuals had recurrent infections after arthrodesis (14.8%). Of these, three individuals were treated with a one-stage arthrodesis nail exchange; one of the three individuals had an aseptic loosening with a third single-stage exchange, and one individual experienced knee amputation for uncontrolled sepsis at 108 months. All individuals, including the amputee, indicated that they would choose arthrodesis again. This study indicated that a single-stage knee arthrodesis offered an acceptable salvage procedure after failed and infected TKA [1].

In 2017, Friedrich et al. evaluated clinical and functional outcomes, implant survival, and infection recurrence rates in individuals treated with two-stage arthrodesis after failed rTKA with extensor mechanism deficiencies due to PJI, and tried to identify the factors that affect results after surgery [5]. Thirty-seven individuals with PJI treated with a two-stage exchange and reimplantation of an arthrodesis nail between 2008 and 2014 were included. Systemic and local risk factors were graded preoperatively according to McPherson et al. All individuals were treated according to a structured treatment algorithm. Clinical and functional assessment was carried out utilizing the Oxford Knee Score (OKS) and the VAS. Thirty-two of thirty-seven individuals (86%) were graded as free of infection. Five individuals (13%) had recurrent infection after arthrodesis, with the need for revision surgery (Fig. 15.1). Mean leg-length discrepancy was

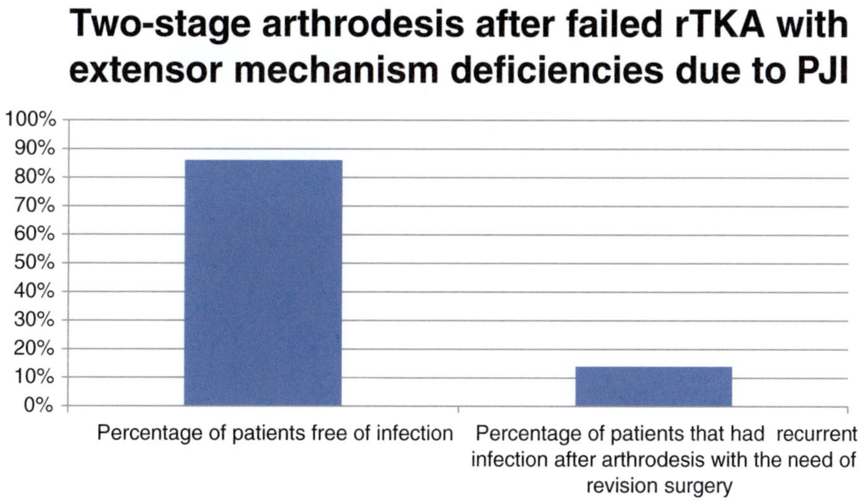

Fig. 15.1 Two-stage arthrodesis after failed revision total knee arthroplasty (rTKA) with extensor mechanism deficiencies due to periprosthetic joint infection (PJI): eradication rate was 86%. However, the rate of recurrent infection after arthrodesis with the need of revision surgery was 13%

2.2 cm. The mean VAS for pain was 3, and the mean OKS was 38. Total implant survival at a 6-year follow-up was 74.3%, as determined by Kaplan-Meier survival curves. Local McPherson Score, as well as the number of revisions, was found to be of substantial influence on the survival rate. The conclusion was that septic failure of rTKA can be effectively treated with two-stage arthrodesis utilizing a modular IM nail, providing a stable and painless limb with satisfactory functional outcomes and acceptable infection eradication rates [5].

In 2023, Coden et al. retrospectively analyzed eight individuals implanted with a modular knee arthrodesis (MKA) at two hospitals between 2016 and 2022 [6]. The mean age was 69.63 years, and 50% of individuals were women. All individuals were indicated for conversion to an MKA as the definitive treatment in the setting of treated chronic PJI after TKA, severe bone loss, and failure of the extensor mechanism not amenable to repair. No individuals needed incision and drainage or exchange of their MKA for PJI at mean 2-year follow-up. One individual needed two revisions for mechanical failure of his implant at 5 and 6.4 years postoperatively. MKA was a viable permanent alternative to AKA for individuals with treated chronic PJI and dysfunctional extensor mechanism after TKA. The procedure restored leg lengths in the setting of severe bone and soft tissue loss, therefore allowing individuals to ambulate independently [6].

Figure 15.2 shows a case of septic loosening of total knee prosthesis (rotational hinge design) in hemophiliac patient that was finally solved by two-stage arthrodesis with IM nail. Figure 15.3 shows a case of septic loosening of total knee prosthesis (rotational hinge design) in a patient who suffered a periprosthetic fracture. The problem was solved by two-stage arthrodesis with IM nail and a femoral metaphyseal cone. Figure 15.4 shows a case of chronic prosthesis infection in the rotational knee hinge solved by two-stage arthrodesis with IM nail.

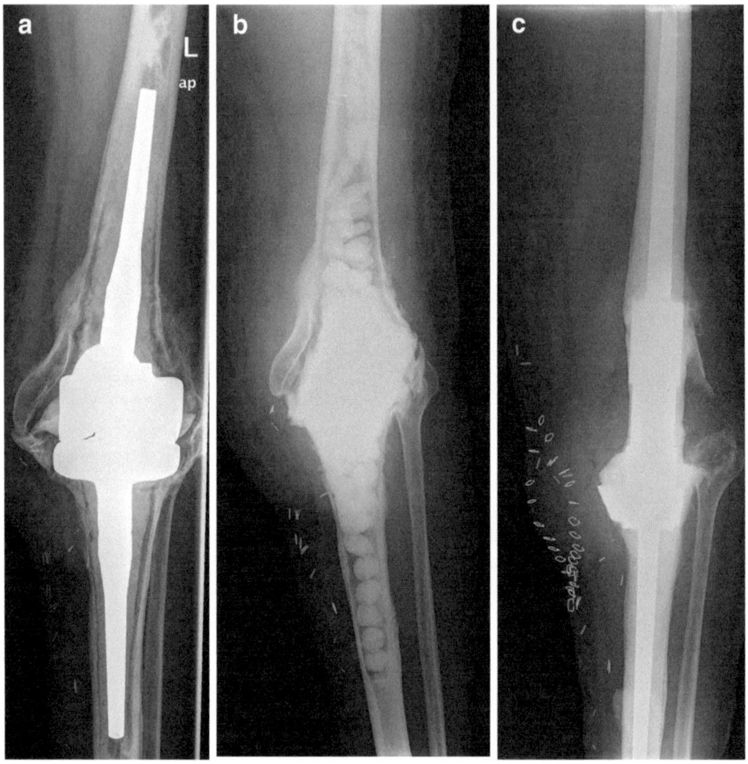

Fig. 15.2 (**a–c**) Septic loosening of total knee prosthesis (rotational hinge design) in hemophiliac patient that was finally solved by two-stage arthrodesis with intramedullary (IM) nail: (**a**) anteroposterior (AP) radiograph before the first surgical stage; (**b**) AP radiograph showing the spacer and antibiotic rosary placed in the first surgical stage; (**c**) AP radiograph showing the arthrodesis nail after the second surgical stage

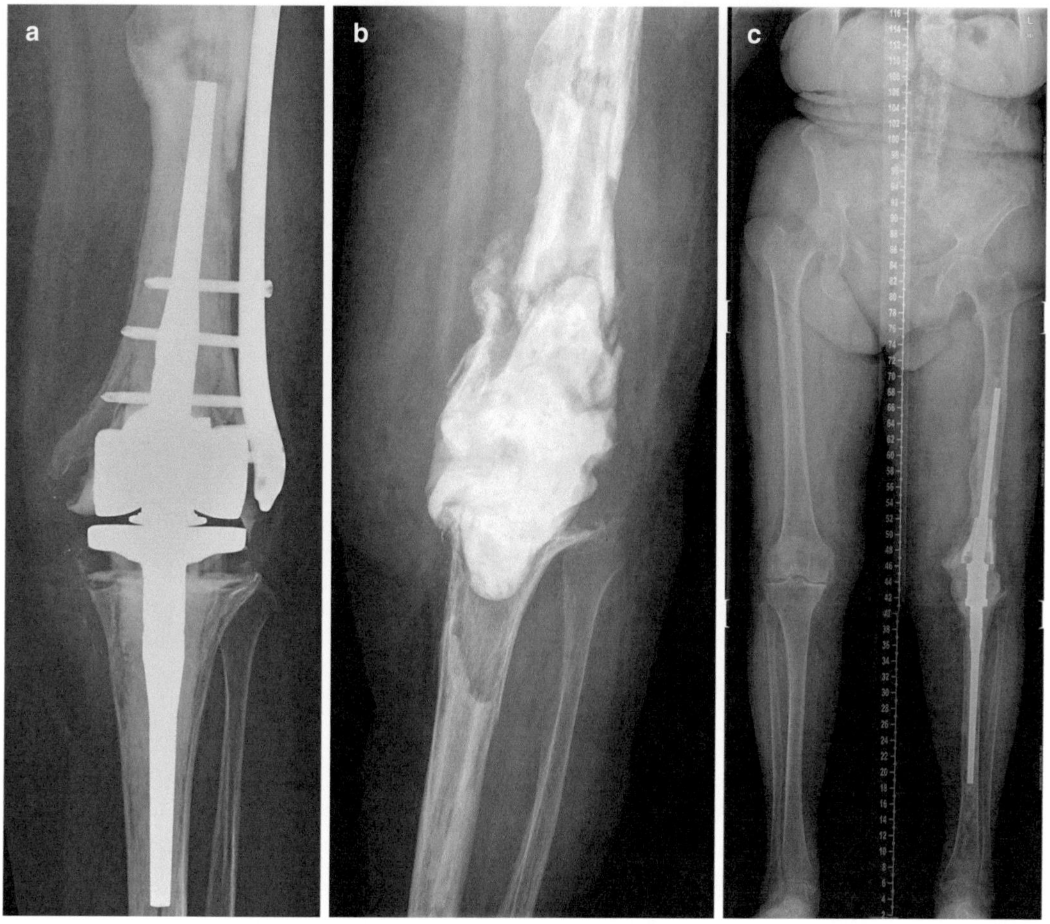

Fig. 15.3 (**a–c**) Septic loosening of total knee prosthesis (rotational hinge design) in a patient who suffered a periprosthetic fracture. The problem was solved by two-stage arthrodesis with intramedullary nail and a femoral metaphyseal cone: (**a**) anteroposterior (AP) radiograph prior to surgery; (**b**) AP radiograph of the nonarticulated spacer with antibiotic (first surgical stage); (**c**) weight-bearing bilateral long-leg standing radiograph showing the arthrodesis nail and metaphyseal cone placed in the femur during the second surgical stage

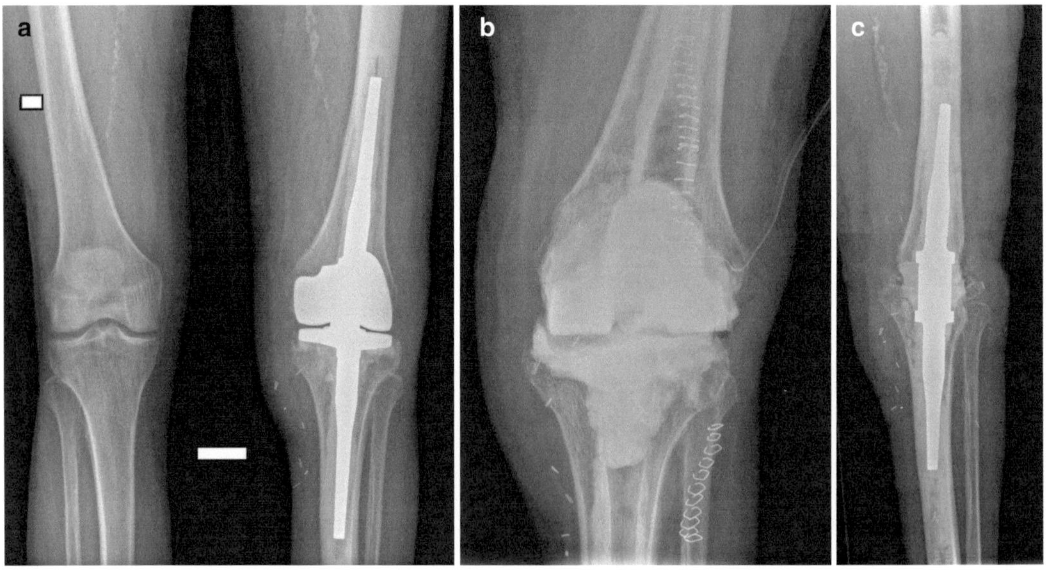

Fig. 15.4 Chronic prosthesis infection in rotational knee hinge solved by two-stage arthrodesis with intramedullary nail: (**a**) anteroposterior (AP) radiograph taken before surgery; (**b**) AP radiograph of the articulated spacer with antibiotics placed in the first surgical stage; (**c**) AP radiograph of the arthrodesis nail implanted in the second surgical stage

15.4 External Fixation Versus IM Nailing for Knee Arthrodesis After Failed Infected TKA

In a systematic review and meta-analysis published in 2018, White et al. compared IM nailing with external fixation for knee arthrodesis after failed infected TKA. Primary outcome was radiographic union. Secondary outcomes included recurrent deep infection, revision arthrodesis, and amputation. IM nailing accomplished a substantially higher rate of radiographic union compared with external fixation at a mean follow-up of 44.22 months. There was no significant difference in the rate of recurrent deep infection or amputation. The rate of revision arthrodesis procedures was significantly lower for IM nailing compared with EF. IM nailing was more effective than EF with respect to several clinically important results. White et al. recommended IM nailing for accomplishing knee arthrodesis as a salvage procedure for infected TKA in the absence of specific indications for EF [7].

In a systematic review and meta-analysis published in 2018, Balato et al. compared reinfection rates following knee arthrodesis for PJI with IM nail or EF. They also compared rates of radiographic union, complication, and reoperation as well as clinical results [8]. The rate of reinfection was 10.6% in IM nail arthrodesis studies. The corresponding reinfection rate for EF was 5.4%. This difference was significant. The utilization of IM nail resulted in more advantages than EF for the frequency of major complications and limb shortening. Other postoperative clinical and radiographic results were similar for both surgical approaches. This study suggested that knee arthrodesis with EF in the specific context of PJI had a reduced risk of reinfection in comparison with the IM nail strategy. The utilization of IM nail was more effective for the complication rate and shortening of the affected limb [8].

In 2021, Suda et al. compared IM nail arthrodesis and EF arthrodesis [9]. In a single-center retrospective setting, clinical and radiographic assessment of consecutive individuals after knee arthrodesis using IM nail and EF for infected knee joints was carried out. All individuals were assessed clinically, with x-ray and questionnaire, including analysis of any complications at latest follow-up of a minimum of 1 year postoperatively. Suda et al. included 152 individuals (75 females, 77 males) in this study. The mean age of the individuals at surgery was 63.6 years. The minimum follow-up was 1 year (mean 3.1 years). Arthrodesis with EF (83 individuals, 52.2%) demonstrated less blood loss and fewer perioperative complications (1.6%) but a high rate of postoperative pin-track infections (35.5%), loose pins (12.7%), and pin fractures (4.8%), and were therefore risk factors for instability and nonunion (30.9%). Revision rate was 22.6% for arthrodesis with EF, and the primary union rate was 65.6%. IM nail arthrodesis (69 individuals, 43.4%) demonstrated a similar reinfection rate to EF (16.1% and 15.9%, respectively) but a substantially lower revision rate (5.4%). Eighty percent of individuals with IM nail arthrodesis demonstrated very good patient-related outcomes regarding pain, function, and daily life activities in the questionnaire. In spite of similar outcomes regarding patient satisfaction and everyday competences in questionnaires, IM nail arthrodesis of the knee was superior to the EF, as it resulted in fewer complications, a lower revision rate, and better union rates/loosening [9].

15.5 Comparison of Two-Stage Revision Arthroplasty and IM Nail Arthrodesis in Patients with Failed Infected TKA

In a study with level 3 of evidence published in 2018, Gathen et al. presented a comparison of results in individuals with failed infected TKA treated with two-stage rTKA or knee arthrodesis and evaluated clinical and functional outcomes, implant survival, and infection recurrence [10]. The hypothesis was that an arthrodesis might result in beneficial effects on patients' outcomes. Clinical data of 81 individuals with PJI of the knee joint were analyzed retrospectively. Between 2008 and 2014, a total of 36 individuals had been treated with a two-stage exchange procedure and reimplantation of a modular IM arthrodesis nail and 45 individuals with rTKA. Individuals were treated according to the same structured treatment algorithm. Clinical and functional assessment was carried out utilizing the OKS and the VAS. The mean follow-up was 32.9 months. The rate of individuals definitely free of infection at last follow-up in the arthrodesis cohort was 32 of 36 (88.9%) and 36 of 45 (80%) in the revision TKA cohort. Mean VAS for pain in the arthrodesis cohort was 3.1 compared to 3.2 in the revision TKA cohort. The OKS in the arthrodesis cohort was 38.7 and 36.5 in individuals with rTKA. The rate of revisions in the rTKA cohort was 2.8 compared to 1.2 in the arthrodesis cohort. The conclusion was that a knee arthrodesis is a limb salvage procedure that demonstrated no substantial benefits on the considered outcome factors compared to rTKA but was associated with a substantially lower revision rate. A knee arthrodesis should be deemed as an alternative in selected individuals [10].

15.6 Knee Arthrodesis Using a Modular IM Nail Versus Hinged TKA

In 2021, Gramlich et al. compared the results of knee arthrodesis versus hinged total TKA in individuals suffering from PJI [11]. One hundred four individuals with PJI were treated utilizing a two-stage rTKA of failed TKA. In cases of non-reconstructible bone loss or loss of extensor mechanism, a modular IM arthrodesis nail was utilized for reimplantation [Knee Arthrodesis Module (KAM); $N = 52$]. The control cohort was retrospectively matched and treated utilizing a hinged revision TKA [Rotating Hinge Knee (RHK); $N = 52$]. PJI remission rates, functional outcomes [Western Ontario and McMaster *Universities* (WOMAC) Arthritis Index, Knee Society Score (KSS)], quality of life [Short-Form (SF)-12], and comorbidities and pain were assessed. Mean age was 72.5 years. Charlson

Comorbidity Index was higher in the KAM group (3.3 versus 2.8). PJI remission rate was 89.4% (88.5% versus 90.4%, respectively). In cases of reinfection, implant retention was mostly possible in the RHK cohort (7.7%), whereas amputations were mostly carried out in the KAM cohort (9.6%). Substantial pain improvement (VAS 7.9–2.8) was accomplished in both cohorts. Walking distance was substantially diminished in the KAM cohort versus the RHK cohort (504 versus 1064 m). WOMAC and KSS function scores were substantially diminished in the KAM cohort (25 versus 40 and 35 versus 64). Only a moderate reduction in quality of life was found in the KAM cohort (SF-12 physical: 34 versus 40; SF-12 mental: 51 versus 56), respectively. Arthrodesis utilizing a modular IM nail seemed to be an alternative for limb salvage, pain alleviation, and preservation of quality of life and everyday mobility, when rTKA is not an alternative [11].

15.7 Floating Knee Arthrodesis

In 2024, Ortega-Yago et al. analyzed the outcomes of floating knee arthrodesis in individuals who had a history of knee PJI [12]. The analysis consisted of determining reinfection rates, functional outcomes, and the survival of arthrodesis. There were 48 individuals who experienced a cemented floating knee arthrodesis in cases of PJI retrospectively included in the study, having been operated on between 2012 and 2020. In addition to being assessed clinically, analytically, and radiographically, the individuals were evaluated functionally by means of a newly created scale. At a mean follow-up of 4 years, seven individuals suffered reinfection (14.6%). The recurrence of infection was not found to be substantially affected by sex, age, or the type of surgery previously experienced, nor was the McPherson Host Grade found to have a substantial effect. Individuals who had a McPherson Limb Grade 3 were more likely to suffer reinfection than those with a McPherson Limb Grade 2. There were 26 individuals (54%) fully assessed and scored on the Knee Arthrodesis Functional Scale (BAOR). For 11 individuals (42%), the outcomes were assessed as excellent, for 11 (42%) acceptable, for 3 (12%) low, and for 1 (4%) poor (Fig. 15.5). The arthrodesis nail was an effective and safe procedure for individuals who had a recurrent PJI, providing an effective option when the criteria for a new rTKA were not met [12].

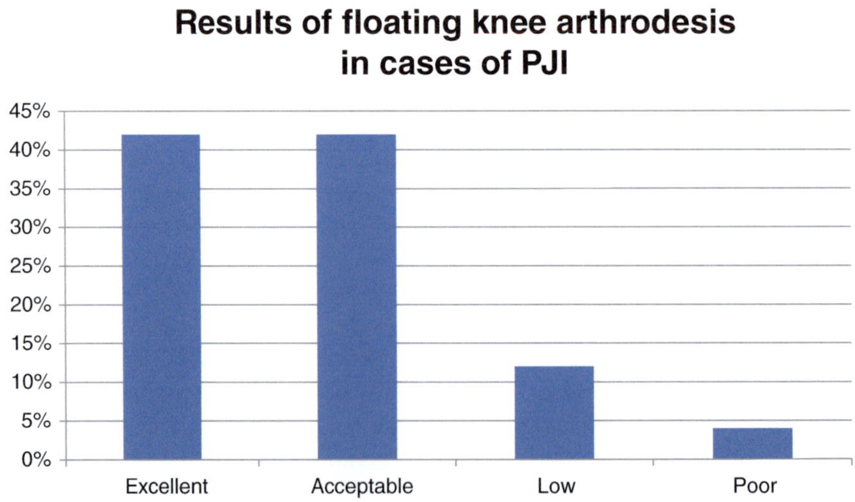

Fig. 15.5 Results of floating knee arthrodesis in cases of periprosthetic joint infection (PJI): 42% excellent, 42% acceptable, 12% low, 4% poor

15.8 Conclusions

Knee arthrodesis must be advised as the treatment of choice for individuals who have persistently infected TKA after a failed two-stage rTKA. Individuals experiencing knee arthrodesis for TKA PJI had high rates of infection control and preservation of ambulatory status, with low rates of progression to above-the-knee amputation. IM nailing accomplishes a substantially higher rate of radiographic union compared with EF. The rate of revision arthrodesis procedures is significantly lower for IM nailing compared with EF. IM nailing is more effective than EF with respect to several clinically important results. Arthrodesis utilizing a modular IM nail seems to be an alternative for limb salvage, pain alleviation, and preservation of quality of life and everyday mobility, when rTKA is not an alternative.

References

1. Hawi N, Kendoff D, Citak M, Gehrke T, Haasper C. Septic single-stage knee arthrodesis after failed total knee arthroplasty using a cemented coupled nail. Bone Joint J. 2015;97-B(5):649–53. https://doi.org/10.1302/0301-620X.97B5.34902.
2. Rodriguez-Merchan EC. Knee fusion or above-the-knee amputation after failed two-stage reimplantation total knee arthroplasty. Arch Bone Jt Surg. 2015;3(4):241–3. PMID: 26550586.
3. Yeung CM, Lichstein PM, Varady NH, Maguire JH, Chen AF, Estok DM 2nd. Knee arthrodesis is a durable option for the salvage of infected total knee arthroplasty. J Arthroplast. 2020;35(11):3261–8. https://doi.org/10.1016/j.arth.2020.06.034.
4. Conway JD, Annasamudram A, Abalkhail T, Tom JH, Farley RP, Gesheff M, et al. Functional outcomes of knee arthrodesis for infected total knee arthroplasty. Cureus. 2023;15(10):e46397. https://doi.org/10.7759/cureus.46397.
5. Friedrich MJ, Schmolders J, Wimmer MD, Strauss AC, Ploeger MM, Wirtz DC, et al. Two-stage knee arthrodesis with a modular intramedullary nail due to septic failure of revision total knee arthroplasty with extensor mechanism deficiency. Knee. 2017;24(5):1240–6. https://doi.org/10.1016/j.knee.2017.05.019.
6. Coden G, Bartashevskyy M, Berliner Z, Niu R, Freccero D, Bono J, et al. Modular knee arthrodesis as definitive treatment for periprosthetic infection, bone loss, and failure of the extensor mechanism after total knee arthroplasty. Arthroplast Today. 2023;25:101261. https://doi.org/10.1016/j.artd.2023.101261.
7. White CJ, Palmer AJR, Rodriguez-Merchan EC. External fixation vs intramedullary nailing for knee arthrodesis after failed infected total knee arthroplasty: a systematic review and meta-analysis. J Arthroplast. 2018;33(4):1288–95. https://doi.org/10.1016/j.arth.2017.10.055.
8. Balato G, Rizzo M, Ascione T, Smeraglia F, Mariconda M. Re-infection rates and clinical outcomes following arthrodesis with intramedullary nail and external fixator for infected knee prosthesis: a systematic review and meta-analysis. BMC Musculoskelet Disord. 2018;19(1):361. https://doi.org/10.1186/s12891-018-2283-4.
9. Suda AJ, Brachtendorf X, Tinelli M, Wagokh R, Abou-Nouar G, Bischel OE. Low complication rate and better results for intramedullary nail – arthrodesis for infected knee joints compared to external fixator-a series of one hundred fifty two patients. Int Orthop. 2021;45(7):1735–44. https://doi.org/10.1007/s00264-021-05054-w.
10. Gathen M, Wimmer MD, Ploeger MM, Weinhold L, Schmid M, Wirtz DC, et al. Comparison of two-stage revision arthroplasty and intramedullary arthrodesis in patients with failed infected knee arthroplasty. Arch Orthop Trauma Surg. 2018;138(10):1443–52. https://doi.org/10.1007/s00402-018-3007-9.
11. Gramlich Y, Steinkohl D, Kremer M, Kemmerer M, Hoffmann R, Klug A. Modular knee arthrodesis secures limb, mobility, improves quality of life, and leads to high infection control in periprosthetic knee infection, when revision knee arthroplasty is not an option. Arch Orthop Trauma Surg. 2021;141(8):1349–60. https://doi.org/10.1007/s00402-021-03907-y.
12. Ortega-Yago A, Pedraza-Corbi A, Argüelles-Linares F, Baeza-Oliete J. Floating knee arthrodesis after prosthetic knee infection: a report of 48 cases. J Arthroplast. 2024;39(2):494–500. https://doi.org/10.1016/j.arth.2023.08.011.

Periprosthetic Joint Infection in Total Ankle Arthroplasty

16

E. Carlos Rodríguez-Merchán and Inmaculada Moracia-Ochagavía

16.1 Introduction

Periprosthetic joint infection (PJI) after total ankle arthroplasty (TAA) is a challenging complication, which frequently needs open debridement, antibiotics, and implant retention (DAIR) with or without polyethylene (PE) exchange, revision surgery, implantation of a cement spacer, conversion to arthrodesis, or even amputation. The best treatment for ankle PJI is not well established [1].

In 2022, Pfahl et al. stated that there was little valid information available on treating infected TAA. In a single-center, retrospective evaluation from 20 patients with PJI of the ankle, they compared the bacteria isolated by preoperative arthrocentesis and intraoperative cultures to the pathogens of knee PJI [2]. Long-run failure rates of irrigation and debridement (I&D) and polyethylene exchange, revision arthroplasty, and arthrodesis were analyzed. The most frequent bacteria were *Staphylococcus aureus* and coagulase-negative staphylococci. There was no substantial difference when comparing the causing pathogens of PJI of the ankle with the knee. After a follow-up of 4.2 years, the long-run failure rate after I&D and PE exchange was 40%, and the revision rate was 9%. Pfahl et al. concluded that the pathogenesis of PJI of the ankle and knee appeared to be comparable. Regarding management alternatives, they encountered that standardized techniques for PJIs of the knee had their limitations regarding infected TAA [2].

According to Zunarelli et al. (2023), PJI after TAA is a serious complication, frequently needing further surgery, including revision arthroplasty, conversion to ankle arthrodesis, or even amputation. In a systematic review, they analyzed the evidence on the treatment of TAA PJI. A total of 298 PJIs were retrieved [3]. The mean incidence of PJI was 3.8%. Moreover, 53 (17.8%) were acute PJIs, whereas most of them (156, 52.3%) were late PJIs. Most of the studies were heterogeneous regarding the treatment protocols utilized, with a two-stage revision TAA (rTAA) carried out in most of the cases (107, 35.9%). While the prevalence of ankle PJI remained low, it was potentially one of the most devastating complications of TAA. This review highlighted the lack of strong literature regarding TAA infections, thus highlighting a need for multicentric studies with homogeneous data regarding the management of ankle PJI to better understand results [3].

According to Dickinson et al. (2024) in recent years, TAA has gained extensive recognition as a surgical treatment for end-stage ankle osteoarthritis. This change was due to remarkable improvements in implant design, surgical instru-

E. C. Rodríguez-Merchán (✉) · I. Moracia-Ochagavía
Department of Orthopedic Surgery, Hospital Universitario La Paz, Madrid, Madrid, Spain

E. C. Rodríguez-Merchán (ed.), *Advances in Periprosthetic Joint Infection*,
https://doi.org/10.1007/978-3-032-02945-4_16

mentation, technique, and surgeon expertise, leading to high levels of patient satisfaction comparable to ankle arthrodesis. Besides, indications for TAA have expanded to include advanced deformities that were beforehand deemed inappropriate for the procedure, making ankle arthrodesis the only alternative. In spite of these advancements, TAA still has a higher complication rate compared to other ankle surgeries. The complex anatomy of the ankle, coupled with limited soft tissue, presents substantial challenges in treating complications associated with TAA [4]. The purpose of this chapter is to analyze the most recent data on PJI in TAA.

16.2 Diagnostic Criteria of PJI in TAA

In 2023, Izzo et al. tried to define which were the criteria utilized to diagnose PJI after TAA. In a systematic review, they found that ankle pain with swelling and unexplained increased local temperature were the most frequent clinical findings leading to a suspicion of PJI [5]. In 100% of cases, the diagnosis was confirmed through synovial fluid analysis associated with positive blood tests. In all the revision surgeries, intraoperative cultures (at least 3) were carried out. In 109 ankles (90%), there was a microbiological isolation. Out of these, 38 (35%) were single-organism infections by coagulase-negative *Staphylococcus* and 37 (34%) were single-organism infections by *Staphylococcus aureus*. The conclusion was that there was a lack of diagnostic criteria specific to PJI after TAA. Clinical and laboratory tests, adapted from the knowledge of total knee and total hip arthroplasty, were generally adopted in the field of TAA. The quality of evidence for studies included in this review was poor [5].

16.3 Clinical Efficacy of Diverse Treatment Approaches for Infected Ankle Prostheses

In 2020, Kunutsor et al. published a systematic review and meta-analysis to compare the clinical efficacy of diverse treatment approaches for infected ankle prostheses. The reinfection rates for DAIR with or without PE exchange, one-stage revision, two-stage revision, cement spacer, and arthrodesis were 39.8%, 0%, 0%, 0.2%, and 13.6%, respectively (Table 16.1). Rates of amputation for DAIR with or without polyethylene exchange and cement spacer were 5.6% and 22.2%, respectively. One- and two-stage revision approaches appeared to be associated with the lowest reinfection rates, but these findings were based on limited information (Fig. 16.1). Arthrodesis and open DAIR with or without PE exchange seemed to be commonly utilized in treating infected ankle prostheses, but were associated with poor infection control (Fig. 16.2) [1].

Table 16.1 Reinfection rates of different surgical techniques for the treatment of periprosthetic joint infection (PJI) in total ankle arthroplasty (TAA)

Surgical technique	Reinfection rate (%)
Open debridement, antibiotics, and implant retention (DAIR) with or without polyethylene (PE) exchange	39.8
One-stage revision TAA (rTAA)	0
Two-stage revision TAA (rTAA)	0
Cement spacer	0.2
Ankle arthrodesis	13.6

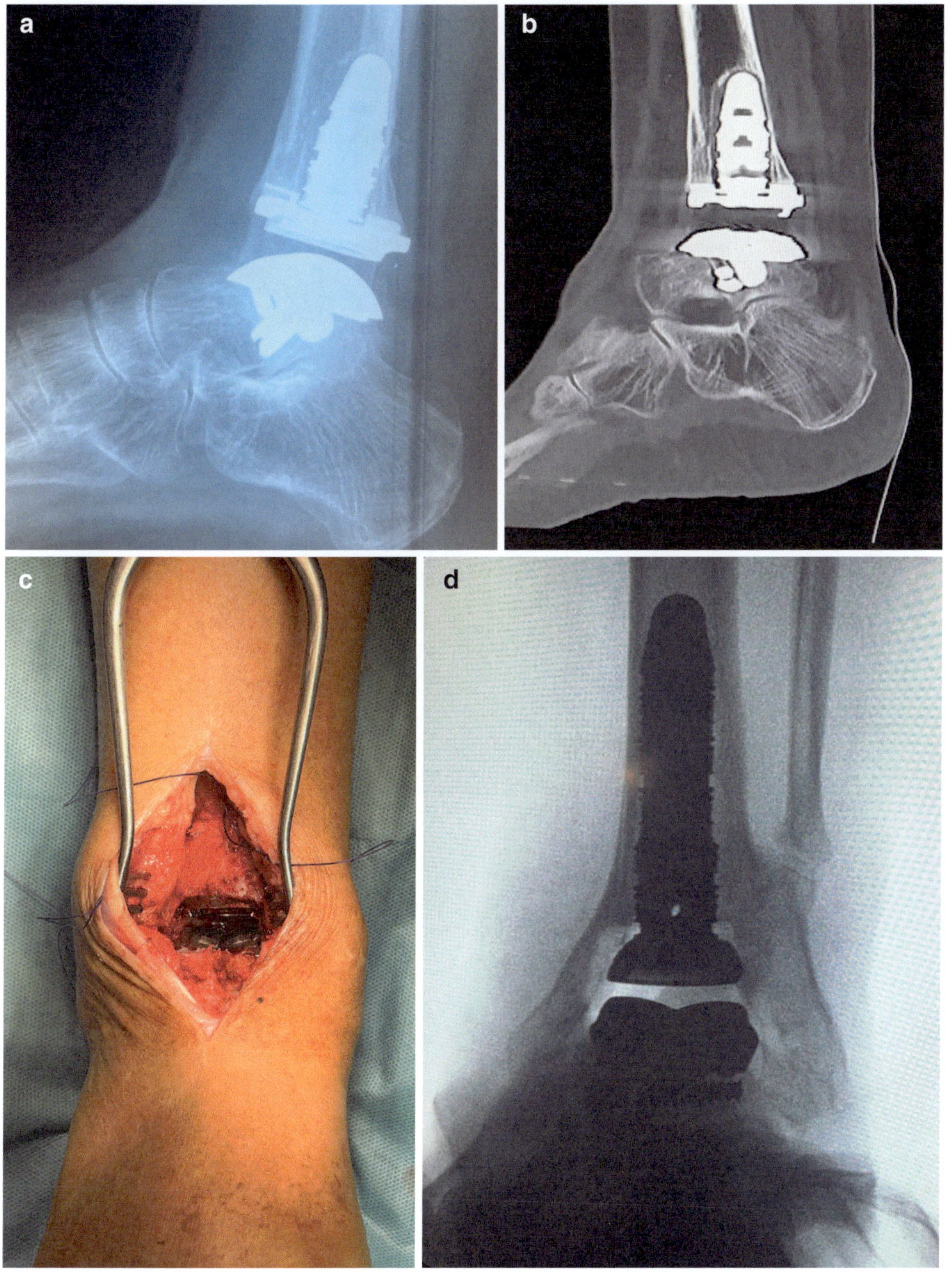

Fig. 16.1 (**a**–**e**) Patient with ankle prosthesis of 10 years of evolution who presented pain, increased local temperature, and episodes of fever. Laboratory tests showed a progressive increase in C-reactive protein (CRP) and erythrocyte sedimentation rate (ESR): (**a**) Lateral ankle X-ray showed loosening of the tibial component of the ankle prosthesis and mobilization of the tibial stem with thinning of the posterior cortex; (**b**) sagittal computed tomography (CT) scan, which showed loosening around the tibial stem of the ankle prosthesis, with displacement toward the posterior cortex and thinning of the latter; (**c**) surgery was performed to replace the ankle prosthesis in one stage; intraoperative imaging of the loosened prosthesis showed no macroscopic signs of joint infection; removal of the prosthesis was performed, plus debridement and lavage; samples were taken for culture and empirical antibiotherapy was started after surgery; (**d**, **e**) anteroposterior (**d**) and lateral (**e**) images after implantation of the new ankle prosthesis, with increased length of the intramedullary (IM) stem; the culture results were positive for *Staphylococcus hominis* and *Enterococcus faecalis*, so specific antibiotic treatment was started with levofloxacin 750 mg and rifampicin 600 mg for 6 weeks

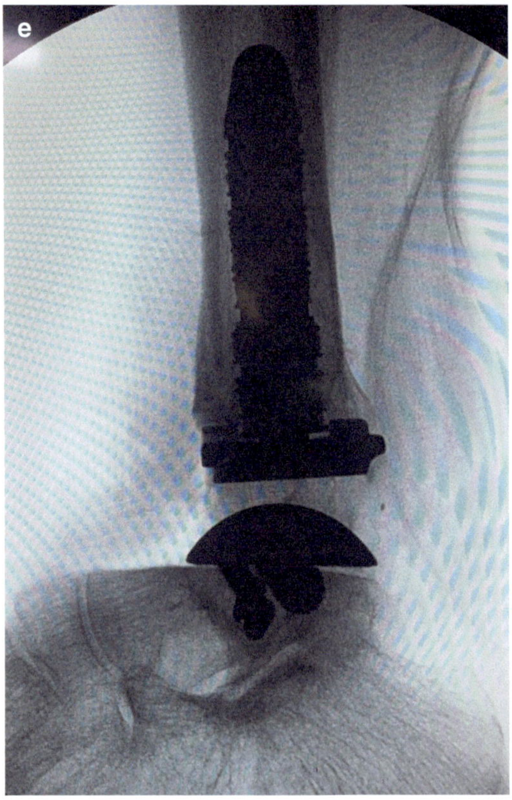

Fig. 16.1 (continued)

Fig. 16.2 (**a**–**f**) Septic loosening of ankle prosthesis; surgical intervention was performed to remove the prosthesis, bone and soft tissue debridement, and placement of a cement spacer with vancomycin, which was maintained for 6 weeks; specific antibiotic treatment was also carried out for 8 weeks until the normalization of the analytical parameters: (**a**) anteroposterior (AP) ankle radiograph showing loosening and mobilization of the talar component of the ankle prosthesis; (**b**, **c**) ankle and subtalar arthrodesis with tricortical posterior iliac crest autograft contribution (12 weeks after removal of the primary prosthesis); (**d**) posterior iliac crest tricortical graft block; (**e**) intraoperative image of the ankle showing complete consolidation of the ankle arthrodesis after removal of the osteosynthesis material; (**f**) intraoperative radioscopic image showing complete consolidation of the ankle and subtalar arthrodesis after removal of the osteosynthesis material

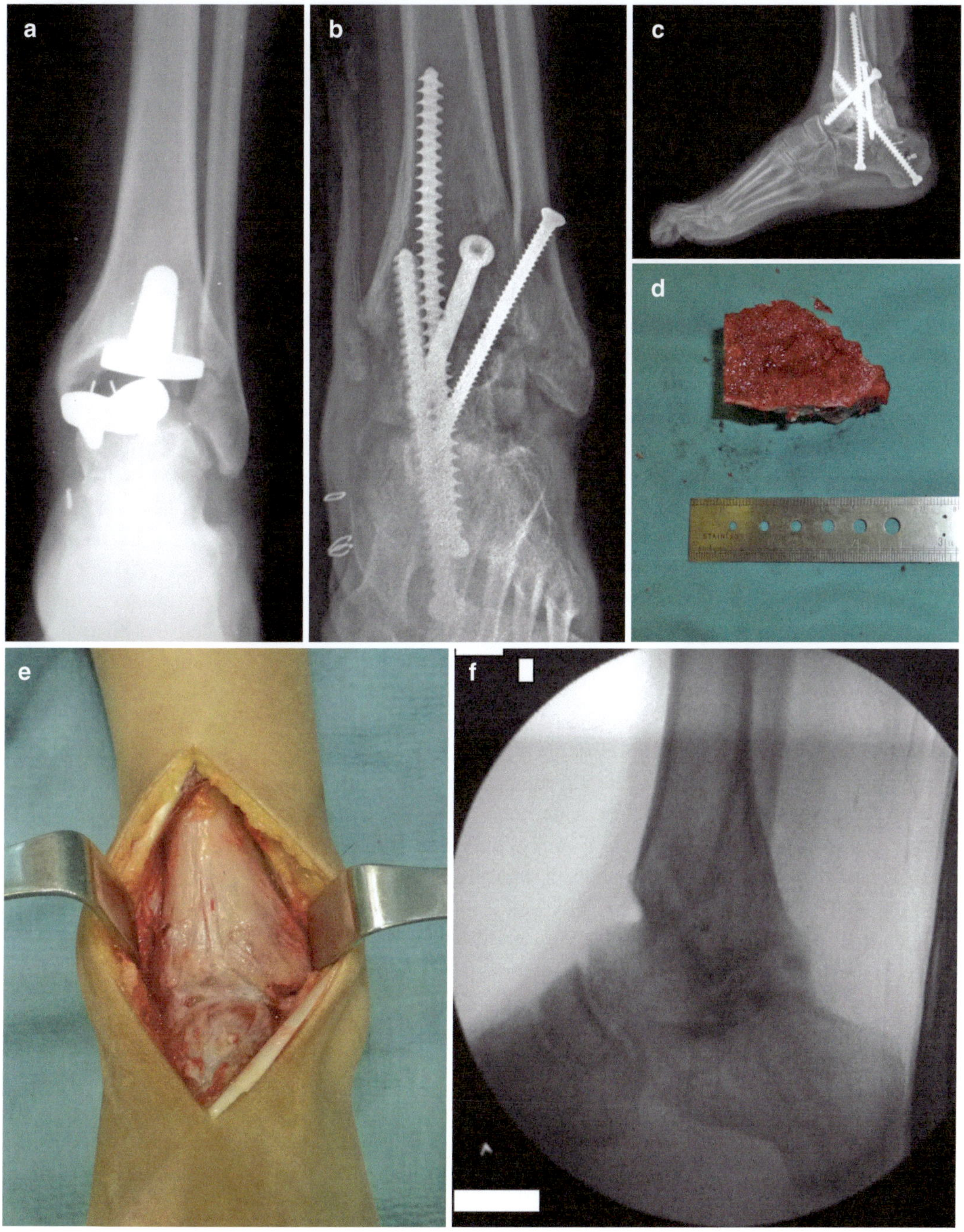
a
b
c
d
e
f

16.4 Current Trends in TAA

According to Ha et al. (2024), ankle arthritis can result in substantial pain and restriction in range of motion [6]. TAA is a motion-preserving surgical alternative utilized as an alternative to total ankle arthrodesis to treat end-stage ankle osteoarthritis. There are several generations of TAR techniques based on component design, implant material, and surgical technique. With more recent TAA implants, an attempt is made to minimize bone resection and mirror the native anatomy. There are more than 20 implant devices currently available. Implant survivorship varies among prosthesis types and generations, with improved results published with utilization of the more recent third- and fourth-generation ankle implants. Pre- and postoperative evaluations of TAA are primarily carried out by utilizing weight-bearing radiography, with weight-bearing computerized tomography (CT) emerging as an additional imaging tool. Preoperative evaluations include those of the tibiotalar angle, offset, and adjacent areas of arthritis needing additional surgical procedures. Ultrasonography (US), nuclear medicine studies, and magnetic resonance imaging (MRI) can be utilized to troubleshoot complications. Effective radiologic evaluation requires an understanding of the component design and corresponding normal perioperative imaging features of ankle implants, as well as recognition of frequent and device-specific complications. General complications seen at radiography include aseptic loosening, osteolysis, hardware subsidence, periprosthetic fracture, infection, gutter impingement, heterotopic ossification, and syndesmotic nonunion [6].

16.5 The Use of Surgical Sterile Helmet System (SHS) Does Not Affect the Frequency of Postoperative SSI or PJI After TAA

In 2022, So et al. compared the infection rates between patients who underwent TAA with a surgical team wearing a sterile helmet system (SHS) versus without SHS [7]. A retrospective chart review of individuals experiencing primary TAA with the surgeon wearing SHS (cohort 1) or standard surgical attire (cohort 2) was performed. The primary outcome was postoperative surgical site infection (SSI) and PJI. They identified 109 individuals in cohort 1 and 151 individuals in cohort 2. The rate of SSI was 12.8% in cohort 1 and 14.6% in cohort 2. The rate of PJI was 0.92% in cohort 1 and 2.6% in cohort 2. There was no difference in revision rates between the two cohorts. This study suggested that SHS did not seem to protect against postoperative SSI or PJI after TAA. Conversely, So et al. did not encounter a higher infection rate compared to standard surgical attire in spite of some in-vitro studies suggesting SHS as a source of wound contamination. The use of SHS did not seem to affect the frequency of postoperative SSI or PJI [7].

16.6 The Mayo Score Could Predict PJI Risk After TAA

In a study with level 2 of evidence, Zhang et al. (2023) stated that evaluating patient's risk of infection was essential for the prevention of PJI after TAA. The Mayo Prosthetic Joint Infection

Risk Score (Mayo Score) is based on data from total hip and knee arthroplasty and had not been validated for application in TAA [8]. A total of 405 consecutive TAA cases were followed for 6 months for PJI. There were 10 cases of PJI (2.5%) among the 405 cases within 6 months after TAA. Of the 405 individuals, the Mayo Scores ranged between −4 and 13. The average Mayo Score was 2.5 in the non-PJI individuals and 7.7 in the PJI individuals. Logistic regression showed that the probability of PJI increased with higher Mayo Scores. All but one PJI individual had a Mayo Score >5. The sensitivity and specificity were 90% and 84.3%, respectively, when a Mayo Score >5 was utilized as a criterion for high risk of PJI. This study showed that the Mayo Score could similarly predict PJI risk after TAA as in total hip and knee arthroplasty. Mayo Score >5 could be a criterion for identifying high-risk individuals for PJI, although further validation with a large number of PJI cases is required [8].

16.7 Risk Factors for PJI Following TAA

In 2020, Smyth et al. stated that recognizing preoperative patient characteristics that correlate with an increased risk of PJI following TAA was of great interest to orthopedic surgeons, as this might help with adequate patient selection [9]. They published a systematic review of the literature in order to identify risk factors that were associated with PJI following TAA. They found that the following preoperative patient characteristics correlated with an increased risk of PJI following TAA: inflammatory arthritis, prior ankle surgery, age less than 65 years, body mass index (BMI) less than 19, peripheral vascular disease, chronic lung disease, hypothyroidism, and low preoperative AOFAS (American Orthopedic Foot and Ankle Society) hindfoot scores (Fig. 16.3). There was conflicting evidence in the literature regarding the effect of obesity, tobacco use, diabetes, and duration of surgery (Fig. 16.4) [9].

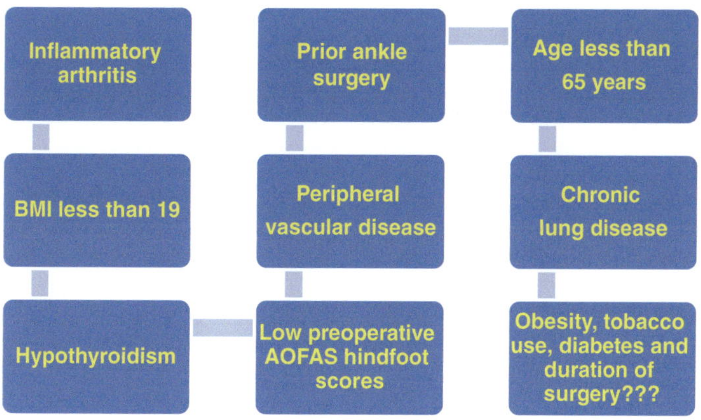

Fig. 16.3 Preoperative patient characteristics correlated with an increased risk of periprosthetic joint infection (PJI) following total ankle arthroplasty (TAA). There is conflicting evidence in the literature regarding the effect of obesity, tobacco use, diabetes, and duration of surgery. BMI = body mass index; AOFAs = American Orthopedic Foot and Ankle Society

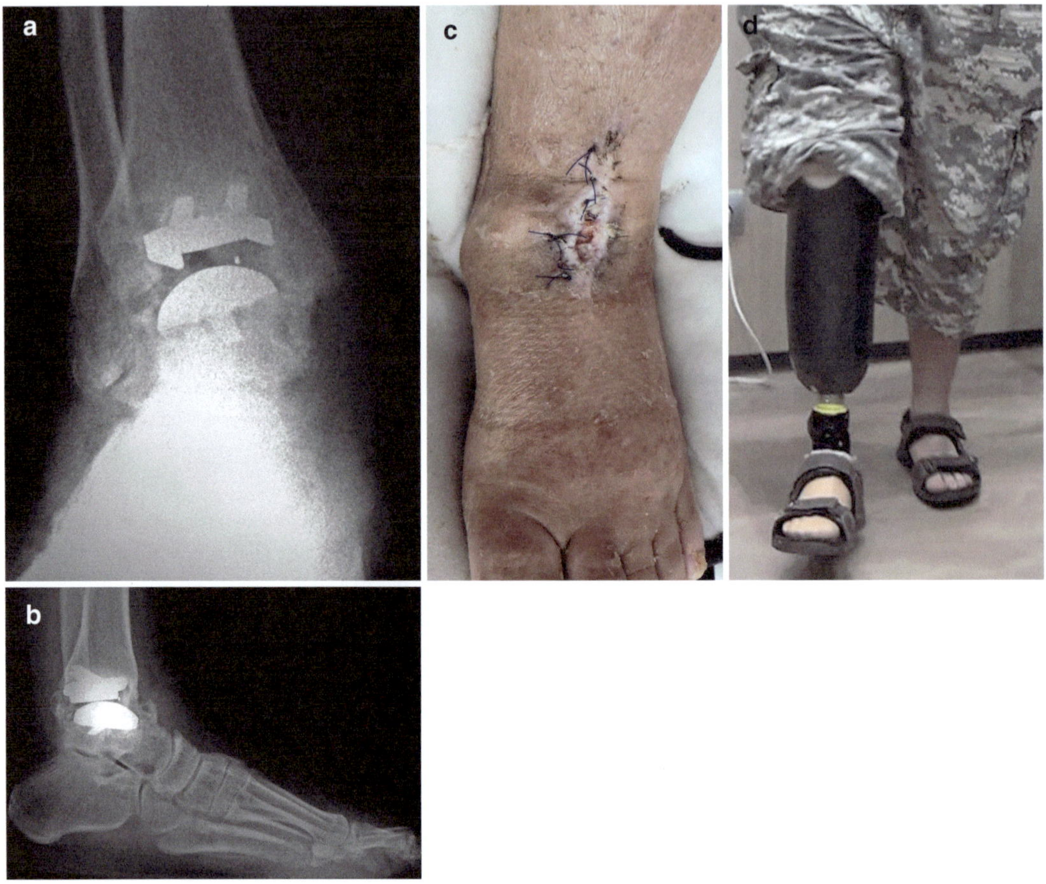

Fig. 16.4 (**a–d**) Patient with septic loosening of ankle prosthesis; given the systemic involvement, emergency treatment was required for removal of the prosthesis, debridement, taking samples for culture, and placement of a cement spacer with antibiotic. The patient's personal history included type 2 diabetes mellitus, rheumatoid arthritis and active smoking; after surgery, specific intravenous antifungal treatment was started due to positive cultures for *Candida fungus*: (**a**, **b**) anteroposterior (AP) and lateral radiographs of the ankle showed loosening and subsidence of the tibial and talar prosthetic components; (**c**) dehiscence of the surgical wound with exposure of tendon structures, macerated and devitalized edges; fungal infection persisted in cultures, without improvement of clinical and analytical parameters; (**d**) infracondylar amputation and orthoprosthetic fitting were performed; after 9 months of different antifungal treatment options and reiterative surgical debridement, the infection persisted, so it was decided, in agreement with the patient, to perform an infracondylar amputation

16.8 Complications, Reoperations, and Patient-Reported Outcomes Following a Two-Stage Revision TAA for Chronic PJIs

According to Conti et al. (2022) as TAA becomes more frequent, chronic PJIs will be found more commonly [10]. In a study with level 4 of evidence they investigated postoperative clinical results at a minimum of 2 years following a two-stage rTAA for chronic PJI. Individuals who experienced a two-stage rTAA for a chronic PJI (>4 weeks after a primary TAA) between January 2010 and December 2019 were analyzed. Chronic PJI was defined as a sinus tract that directly communicated with the prosthesis or the same organism identified in $\geq$2 synovial fluid samples. Twelve individuals were eligible to be included in the study. One individual died prior to 2-year follow-up, which left 11 individuals available for analysis. All 11 individuals experienced reimplantation. At a median of 3 years after the second stage of their revision arthroplasty, the median Foot and Ankle Ability Measure (FAAM) Activities of Daily Living and Sports scores were 60.7 and 31.3, respectively. At final follow-up, 10 individuals (90.9%) were ambulating with a TAA in place. Seven individuals (63.6%) needed a reoperation, including one individual who experienced a below-knee amputation. This study suggested that a two-stage rTAA might be an alternative for individuals with a chronic PJI. However, individuals who experienced a two-stage rTAA for a chronic PJI had lower than previously reported 2-year FAAM scores and a high rate of reoperation [10].

16.9 Time to Revision After PJI in TAA

In 2023, Miner et al. stated that while not a frequent complication after TAA, PJI presented a substantial risk of implant failure [11]. In a systematic review, they assessed time to revision after PJI in individuals who had experienced TAA. The prevalence of PJI was 1.12% ($N = 34$). Miner et al. encountered that the average time to revision due to PJI was 30.7 months, or approximately 2.6 years after the index TAA procedure. By literature definitions, the majority of cases (91.2%, $N = 31$) were beyond the "acute" PJI phase. The population was divided into two cohorts for further analysis of chronic infections. PJIs before the median were classified as "early" and those after as "late" chronic. The majority of cases (61.8%) were late chronic with an average time to revision of 44.3 months. A smaller number were early chronic (29.4%) with revision within 10.8 months. Miner et al. suggested modifying the current PJI classification to include early chronic and late chronic subgroups so that the orthopedic surgeon is better prepared to prudently diagnose and treat PJIs [11].

16.10 Diabetes Mellitus and TAA Complications

In a study with level 3 of evidence published in 2024 by Helbing et al., they stated that while previous studies had demonstrated diabetes as a risk factor predisposing individuals to postoperative complications, not all literature supports this association following TAA [12]. In their study, Helbing et al. tried to determine if diabetes influences mid-run results following TAA. An insurance database was used to identify individuals experiencing TAA for ankle arthritis with a concurrent diagnosis of diabetes based on Current Procedural Terminology (CPT) and International Classification of Diseases, Ninth Revision (ICD-9) and Tenth Revision (ICD-10), diagnosis and procedure codes from 2010 to 2021. The postoperative results of all-cause revision, PJI, septic revision, and aseptic revision were compared between individuals with and without diabetes with a minimum 2-year follow-up using Kaplan-Meier and multivariate Cox proportional hazards analyses. Patient demographics, comorbidities, and the Charlson Comorbidity Index were analyzed via univariate and multivariate analysis. The study population included 8317 individuals, 345 (4.1%) of whom had a concurrent diabetes diagnosis, who experienced TAA. After multivariate Cox proportional hazards analysis, the 5-year cumulative incidence of being coded as having PJI was 7.3% in individuals with known diabetes compared to 3.9% in individuals without known diabetes, with a 95% increased risk. Individuals with diabetes also showed a 5-year cumulative incidence of septic revision of 1.4% compared to 0.4% in those without, with a 363% increased risk. However, there was no difference in the 5-year cumulative incidence of all-cause revision TAA, with 4.6% in individuals with diabetes and 4.3% in those without. In this database, the 5-year risk of PJI and septic revision was higher among individuals with diabetes compared to those without, but the cumulative incidence of all-cause rTAA was not different between cohorts [12].

In a study with level 3 of evidence (2024), Wu et al. stated that diabetes increased the risk of infection due to compromised immunity and impaired wound-healing mechanisms. However, there was limited research on how diabetic management, inclusive of medications and glucose control, might influence infection risks post-TAA [13]. In their study, Wu et al. tried to demonstrate the impact of diabetic management on the occurrence of PJI following TAA. Individuals with diabetes who developed an intraarticular infection following TAA were propensity score matched (1:3) to diabetic individuals who did not. PJI was diagnosed based on Musculoskeletal Infection Society (MSIS) criteria. Of the 1863 individuals who experienced TAA, 177 individuals had a diagnosis of diabetes. The infection rate in individuals with diabetes (2.8%) was higher than the total cohort rate (0.8%). Five individuals with diabetes developed a PJI at an average of 2.2 months postoperatively. This group (N = 5) was compared to propensity score-matched controls (N = 15). There was no substantial difference in diabetic medication utilization. Individuals who developed PJI had higher rates of uncontrolled diabetes (60% versus 6.7%) and average hemoglobin A1c levels (7.02% versus 6.29%) compared to controls. The findings of this study suggested that the elevated risk of PJI found in patients with diabetes subsequent to TAA might be attributed not solely to the presence of diabetes, but to inadequate glycemic control. Successfully managing blood glucose levels is mandatory for accomplishing favorable results following TAA [13].

16.11 Early Results of the Exactech Vantage Fixed-Bearing TAA

In 2023, Henry et al. stated that the Vantage Total Ankle System was a fourth-generation low-profile fixed-bearing implant that had been available since 2016 [14]. In their study, they aimed to describe their early experience with this implant. This was a single-center retrospective review of individuals who experienced primary TAA with a Vantage implant between November 2017 and February 2020, with a minimum of 2 years' follow-up. Four surgeons contributed individuals. There were 168 patients (171 ankles) included with a mean follow-up of 2.81 years and mean age of 63 years. Of the ten ankles with implant failure (5.8%), six had loosening of the tibial component. In the remaining four failed implants, one was due to PJI, one was due to loosening of the talar component, and two were due to loosening of both the tibial and talar components. Seven individuals experienced reoperation: irrigation and debridement for superficial infection ($N = 4$); bone grafting for cysts (N = 2); and open reduction internal fixation ($N = 1$). Asymptomatic peri-implant lucency/subsidence occurred in 20.1% of ankles, with the majority involving the tibial component ($N = 25$). There were statistically significant improvements in patient-related outcome measures (PROMs) in all domains. Short-run outcomes of this implant showed early survival comparable to the published survivorship of similar low-profile, non-stemmed implants. Radiological lucency happened more frequently at the tibial component, and revisions happened primarily due to loosening of the tibial component. However, further research is required to assess longer-run survivorship [14].

16.12 Conclusions

PJI after TAA is a challenging complication, which frequently needs open DAIR with or without PE exchange, revision surgery, implantation of a cement spacer, conversion to arthrodesis, or even amputation. The best treatment for ankle PJI is not well established.

The following preoperative patient characteristics correlate with an increased risk of PJI following TAA: inflammatory arthritis, prior ankle surgery, age less than 65 years, BMI less than 19, peripheral vascular disease, chronic lung disease, hypothyroidism, and low preoperative AOFAS hindfoot scores. There is conflicting evidence in the literature regarding the effect of obesity, tobacco use, diabetes, and duration of surgery.

The reported mean incidence of PJI is 3.8% (17.8% acute PJIs, 52.3% late PJIs). A two-stage approach is carried out in most of the cases (35.9%). After a follow-up of 4.2 years, the reported long-run failure rate after I&D and polyethylene exchange is 40%, and of revision is 9%. In a study, the reinfection rates for open DAIR with or without PE exchange, one-stage rTAA, two-stage rTAA, cement spacer, and ankle arthrodesis were 39.8%, 0%, 0%, 0.2%, and 13.6%, respectively. Rates of amputation for open DAIR with or without PE exchange and cement spacer were 5.6% and 22.2%, respectively. It has been reported that at 3-year follow-up after two-stage rTAA for a chronic PJI (>4 weeks after a primary TAA), 90.9% of patients were ambulating with a TAA in place, but 63.6% needed a reoperation, including one individual who experienced a below-knee amputation.

The use of sterile helmet system (SHS) did not seem to affect the frequency of postoperative SSI or PJI.

The Mayo Prosthetic Joint Infection Risk Score (Mayo Score) >5 could be a criterion for identifying high-risk individuals for PJI, although further validation with a large number of PJI cases is required.

References

1. Kunutsor SK, Barrett MC, Whitehouse MR, Blom AW. Clinical effectiveness of treatment strategies for prosthetic joint infection following total ankle replacement: a systematic review and meta-analysis. J Foot Ankle Surg. 2020;59(2):367–72. https://doi.org/10.1053/j.jfas.2019.04.016.
2. Pfahl K, Röser A, Gottschalk O, Hörterer H, Mehlhorn A, Dolp PA, et al. Common bacteria and treatment options for the acute and chronic infection of the total ankle arthroplasty. Foot Ankle Surg. 2022;28(7):1008–13. https://doi.org/10.1016/j.fas.2022.02.010.
3. Zunarelli R, Fiore M, Lonardo G, Pace A, Persiani V, De Paolis M, et al. Total ankle replacement infections: a systematic review of the literature. J Clin Med. 2023;12(24):7711. https://doi.org/10.3390/jcm12247711.
4. Dickinson JD, Collman DR, Russel LH, Choung DJ. Navigating the challenges of total ankle replacement: deformity correction and infection considerations. Clin Podiatr Med Surg. 2024;41(1):119–39. https://doi.org/10.1016/j.cpm.2023.06.004.
5. Izzo A, Di Gennaro D, Sgadari A, Coviello A, Marasco D, Balato G, et al. Periprosthetic joint infection in total ankle replacement: which are the current diagnostic criteria? Acta Biomed. 2023;94(4):e2023105. https://doi.org/10.23750/abm.v94i4.14082.
6. Ha J, Jones G, Staub J, Aynardi M, French C, Petscavage-Thomas J. Current trends in total ankle replacement. Radiographics. 2024;44(1):e230111. https://doi.org/10.1148/rg.230111.
7. So E, Juels CA, Seidenstricker C, Walker R, Scott RT. Postoperative infection rates after total ankle arthroplasty: a comparison with and without the use of a surgical helmet system. J Foot Ankle Surg. 2022;61(4):802–6. https://doi.org/10.1053/j.jfas.2021.11.021.
8. Zhang Z, Chien BY, Noori N, Day J, Robertson C, Schon L. Application of the Mayo periprosthetic joint infection risk score for total ankle arthroplasty. Foot Ankle Int. 2023;44(5):451–8. https://doi.org/10.1177/10711007231157697.
9. Smyth NA, Kennedy JG, Parvizi J, Schon LC, Aiyer AA. Risk factors for periprosthetic joint infection following total ankle replacement. Foot Ankle Surg. 2020;26(5):591–5. https://doi.org/10.1016/j.fas.2019.07.015.
10. Conti MS, Irwin TA, Ford SE, Jones CP, Anderson RB, Davis WH. Complications, reoperations, and patient-reported outcomes following a 2-stage revision total ankle arthroplasty for chronic periprosthetic joint infections. Foot Ankle Int. 2022;43(12):1614–21. https://doi.org/10.1177/10711007221133398.
11. Miner SA, Martucci JA, Brigido SA, DiDomenico L. Time to revision after periprosthetic joint infection in total ankle arthroplasty: a systematic review. J Foot Ankle Surg. 2023;62(1):186–90. https://doi.org/10.1053/j.jfas.2022.09.001.
12. Helbing J, Farley B, Gu A, Zhao AY, Siram G, Stein B, et al. Diabetes mellitus and total ankle arthroplasty complications. Foot Ankle Int. 2024;45(4):320–7. https://doi.org/10.1177/10711007241226929.
13. Wu KA, Anastasio AT, Krez AN, O'Neill C, Adams SB, DeOrio JK, et al. Diabetic management and infection risk in total ankle arthroplasty. Foot Ankle Surg. 2024;30(7):552–6. https://doi.org/10.1016/j.fas.2024.04.008.
14. Henry JK, Shaffrey I, Wishman M, Palma Munita J, Zhu J, Cody E, et al. Early outcomes of the Exactech Vantage fixed-bearing total ankle replacement. Bone Joint J. 2023;105-B(10):1099–107. https://doi.org/10.1302/0301-620X.105B10.BJJ-2023-0173.R2.

17 Flap Coverage in Patients with Periprosthetic Joint Infections

Mónica Rubio-Yanchuck, Jorge Bonastre-Juliá, and Francisco Leyva-Rodríguez

17.1 Introduction

Periprosthetic joint infection (PJI) is one of the most serious complications in orthopedic surgery, with a significant impact on patient morbidity and healthcare costs. Its incidence is estimated to be 1%–2% in primary arthroplasties and may exceed 10% in revision arthroplasties with a history of previous infection [1]. Its management requires a multidisciplinary approach combining infection control strategies, bone reconstruction, and soft tissue coverage.

Treatment of PJI depends on several factors, including the time course of the infection, the type of microorganism involved, the condition of the host, and the integrity of the surrounding soft tissues. Success requires a combination of strategies, including aggressive surgical debridement, administration of specific antibiotics and, in cases of soft tissue involvement, flap reconstruction. Flap coverage becomes a mainstay in eradicating infection and preserving the joint, especially when there are extensive defects and exposure of prosthetic components or spacers to antibiotics. The purpose of this chapter is to review the options for flap coverage in the setting of PJI, addressing specific strategies for the hip, knee, ankle, and shoulder.

17.2 Pathophysiology and PJI Coverage Considerations

PJIs are the result of bacterial contamination of the implant, leading to the formation of biofilms that protect the microorganisms from the host immune response and the effects of systemic antibiotics. This biofilm is one of the main reasons why PJIs are difficult to eradicate and in many cases require implant removal as part of definitive treatment [2]. There are different factors that influence soft tissue coverage in this context:

1. Bacterial colonization and biofilm formation: Microorganisms such as *Staphylococcus aureus* and *Staphylococcus epidermidis* and gram-negative bacilli can adhere to prosthetic surfaces and form biofilms that are resistant to conventional antibiotic treatment [3]. The persistence of the biofilm hinders the penetration of antibiotics and causes the recurrence of infection despite multiple eradication attempts. All of this can lead to implant removal for definitive control of the infection.
2. Effect on vascularization of surrounding tissues: Infection induces a chronic inflamma-

M. Rubio-Yanchuck · J. Bonastre-Juliá
F. Leyva-Rodríguez (✉)
Department of Plastic and Reconstructive Surgery, Hospital Universitario La Paz, Madrid, Spain
e-mail: francisco.leyva@salud.madrid.org

E. C. Rodríguez-Merchán (ed.), *Advances in Periprosthetic Joint Infection*,
https://doi.org/10.1007/978-3-032-02945-4_17

tory response that compromises soft tissue perfusion, increasing the risk of necrosis and wound dehiscence. Similarly, previous surgery, radiation therapy (in patients with a history of oncology), or systemic diseases such as diabetes mellitus may exacerbate the deterioration of local vascularization and predispose to failure of primary coverage [4].

3. Risk factors for conventional treatment failure: Immunosuppression, smoking, malnutrition, as well as diabetes mellitus and peripheral vascular disease are associated with an increased likelihood of postoperative complications, including wound dehiscence and reinfection [5]. In addition, extensive defects after aggressive debridement may make primary coverage difficult without the need for flaps.
4. The importance of flap coverage in reconstruction: Well-vascularized flaps not only provide mechanical coverage over the prosthesis or spacer, but also improve local perfusion and delivery of systemic antibiotics [6].

17.3 General Strategies for Flap Coverage in PJI

The efficacy of flap coverage in PJI is contingent upon meticulous planning and the judicious selection of the reconstructive technique. The primary objective is to provide a well-vascularized tissue that covers the defect, thereby reducing dead space and facilitating the delivery of systemic antibiotics [7].

17.3.1 Fundamental Principles in Flap Selection

- Eradication of infection prior to definitive reconstruction: Aggressive debridement is recommended to remove necrotic tissue and reduce bacterial load prior to reconstruction [8]. In many cases, the placement of a spacer with antibiotics is required prior to the reimplantation of the definitive prosthesis [9].
- Choice of flap according to the location and type of defect: For deep defects with significant dead space, muscle flaps are preferred because of their ability to fill cavities and improve local perfusion [7]. For superficial defects, fasciocutaneous flaps are a more suitable option, as they provide stable coverage with less morbidity at the donor site.
- Preservation of joint functionality: The use of flaps that limit joint mobility should be avoided, especially in the knee and ankle, where flexion restriction may affect postoperative rehabilitation [10]. In the shoulder and hip, the priority is to restore stable coverage without compromising the muscle strength needed for support and mobility [11].
- Optimization of patient conditions: Malnutrition, smoking, and immunosuppression adversely affect healing and increase the risk of postoperative complications. It is recommended to optimize albumin levels, correct anemia, and stop smoking at least 4–6 weeks before reconstructive surgery [12].

17.3.2 Choice of Flap Type

The choice of the type of flap depends on the location of the defect and its extension, as well as the quality of the recipient bed. We can classify them as follows:

- According to their vascularization: pedicled versus free flaps

  Pedicled flaps conserve their blood supply through a vascular pedicle that remains connected to their anatomical origin. They are mainly used when the defect is within the rotational territory of the flap. In extensive defects or in situations where pedicled flaps are not feasible, the use of free flaps is an indispensable option in the coverage of PJI. The choice of the ideal free flap depends on multiple factors, including the availability of recipient vessels, the quality of the recipient bed, the volume of tissue required, and the morbidity of the donor site (Table 17.1).

Table 17.1 Comparison between pedicled flaps and free flaps

Feature	Pedicle flaps	Free flaps
Irrigation	Maintain their original vascular connection	They are disconnected and require microsurgical anastomosis
Surgical complexity	Minor, no microsurgery required	High, requires vascular anastomosis
Surgical time	Shorter	Longer
Main indication	Defects close to the donor site	Extensive defects or in areas without adequate local tissues
Risk of flap failure	Low	High if there is thrombosis of the anastomosis
Flexibility in reconstruction	Limited by the pedicle	High, allows adaptation to any location
Postoperative management	Less intensive	Requires strict microvascular monitoring

- By composition: Muscular versus fasciocutaneous flaps: Muscular flaps have an excellent capacity to fill dead spaces and are therefore often used in defects with great tissue loss or in areas with active infection due to their potential to improve bacterial eradication by increasing local perfusion. Fasciocutaneous flaps, on the other hand, provide a thinner, more flexible, and resistant coverage, with less morbidity at the donor site. The choice between muscle and fasciocutaneous flaps has been extensively studied, and the available evidence indicates that there are no significant differences between the two types of flaps [13]. While muscle flaps have historically been preferred because of their ability to improve local perfusion and control bacterial load, recent studies have shown that fasciocutaneous flaps can achieve similar success rates in terms of effective coverage and eradication of infection. Therefore, the decision should be based on the availability of tissue, the surgeon's experience, and the functional and aesthetic needs of the patient.

17.4 Coverage Techniques According to the Affected Joint

Each joint presents specific challenges in terms of soft tissue reconstruction. Coverage strategies for the hip, knee, ankle, and shoulder are detailed below.

17.4.1 Hip Flap Coverage

The hip region is a complex area for reconstruction due to the depth of defects and proximity to important neurovascular structures. PJIs in this joint often generate extensive defects after resection of devitalized tissue, leaving the proximal femur or acetabulum exposed, which complicates reconstruction. In addition, patient mobility and the need to preserve functionality make the use of certain bulky flaps difficult [14]. This region is surrounded by many muscles, which makes the option of regional flap coverage more feasible. There are different coverage options in this region (Table 17.2):

- Muscle flaps: These flaps are frequently employed in the coverage of hip defects due to their high vascularity and ability to fill the cavity. Some options include the following:
  - Rectus femoris flap: Useful option in small to moderate defects of the anterior and lateral hip region. Its pedicle, based on the lateral femoral circumflex artery, allows an

Table 17.2 Advantages and disadvantages of hip flap coverage

Type of flap	Advantages	Disadvantages
Muscular (rectus femoris, gluteus maximus)	High perfusion, dead space filling, promotes eradication of infection	Donor site morbidity, possible muscle weakness
Fasciocutaneous (ALT, gluteal perforator)	Stable coverage, less functional impact	Reduced ability to fill dead space

ALT anterolateral thigh

adequate arc of rotation and provides well-vascularized coverage without significantly affecting patient function [5].
- Vastus lateralis flap: Also based on the lateral femoral circumflex artery, it is used in anterior and lateral hip defects, where it provides important filling to the cavity if necessary [14, 15] (Fig. 17.1).
- Gluteus maximus flap: This flap based on the inferior gluteal artery is a good option in posterior and lateral defects, with good volume to fill dead space [16].
- Tensor fascia lata flap: Generally musculocutaneous flap based on the lateral femoral circumflex artery. It is useful in lateral and anterolateral hip defects. Its reliable pedicle and versatility make it ideal to adapt to irregular surfaces, although it may have volume limitations if the defect is very extensive [17].
- Rectus abdominis flap: Based on the deep inferior epigastric artery, it is used in the reconstruction of hip and pelvic defects, providing volume filler for dead spaces as well as stable coverage [18].

- Fasciocutaneous flaps: These flaps are considered in shallower defects or when muscle function must be preserved.
  - Anterolateral thigh flap (ALT): Based on the lateral femoral circumflex artery, it is one of the best options for defects in this location. Its versatility allows it to be used as a pedicled or free flap, adapting it to the size of the defect [19].
  - Gluteal perforator flap: Provides fasciocutaneous coverage without compromising the gluteus maximus muscle, reducing donor site morbidity [20].

17.4.2 Knee Flap Coverage

The knee presents specific challenges in defect coverage due to the limited availability of surrounding soft tissue and the proximity of critical neurovascular structures. Resection of devital-

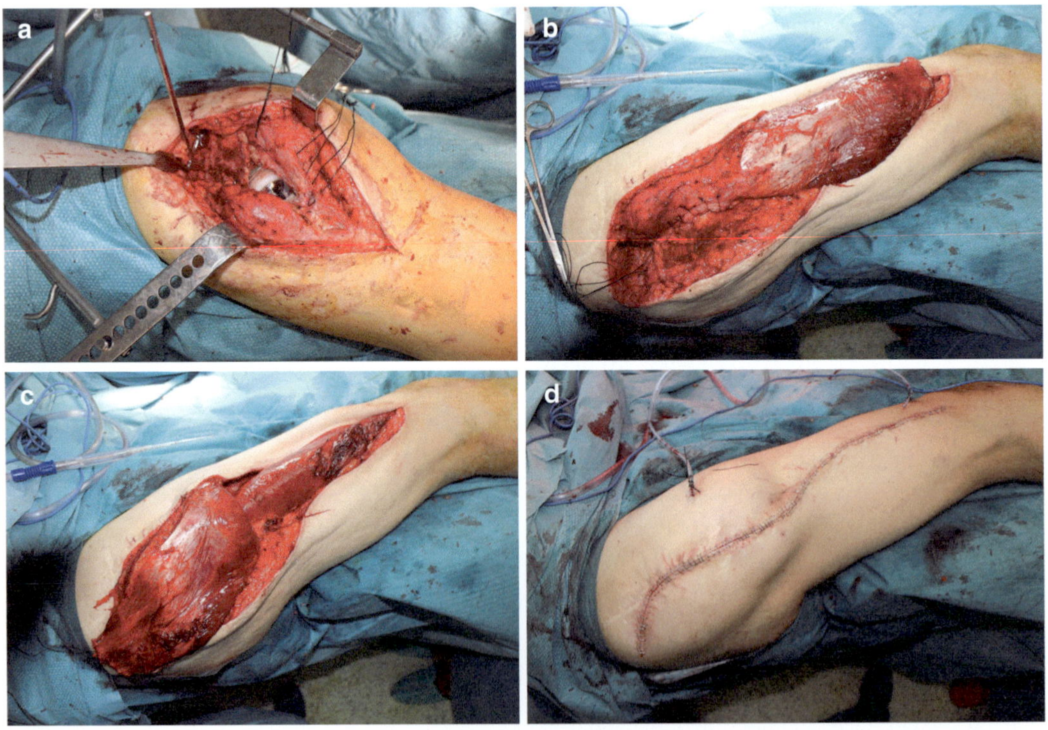

Fig. 17.1 (**a–d**) Hip prosthesis infection (**a**); vastus lateralis flap dissection (**b**); flipped lateral vastus flap for dead space padding and hip joint coverage (**c**); final result with closed surgical wound (**d**)

ized tissue in PJIs may expose the prosthesis or generate extensive defects, increasing the risk of treatment failure if adequate coverage is not achieved. It is also one of the most challenging joints in terms of coverage, as its mobility must be preserved to avoid postoperative stiffness. We can find different options for knee coverage:

- Muscle flaps:
  - Gastrocnemius flap (medial or lateral): This is the first-line option in defects with prosthetic exposure. Based on the sural arteries, it provides robust coverage without affecting joint function [21] (Fig. 17.2).

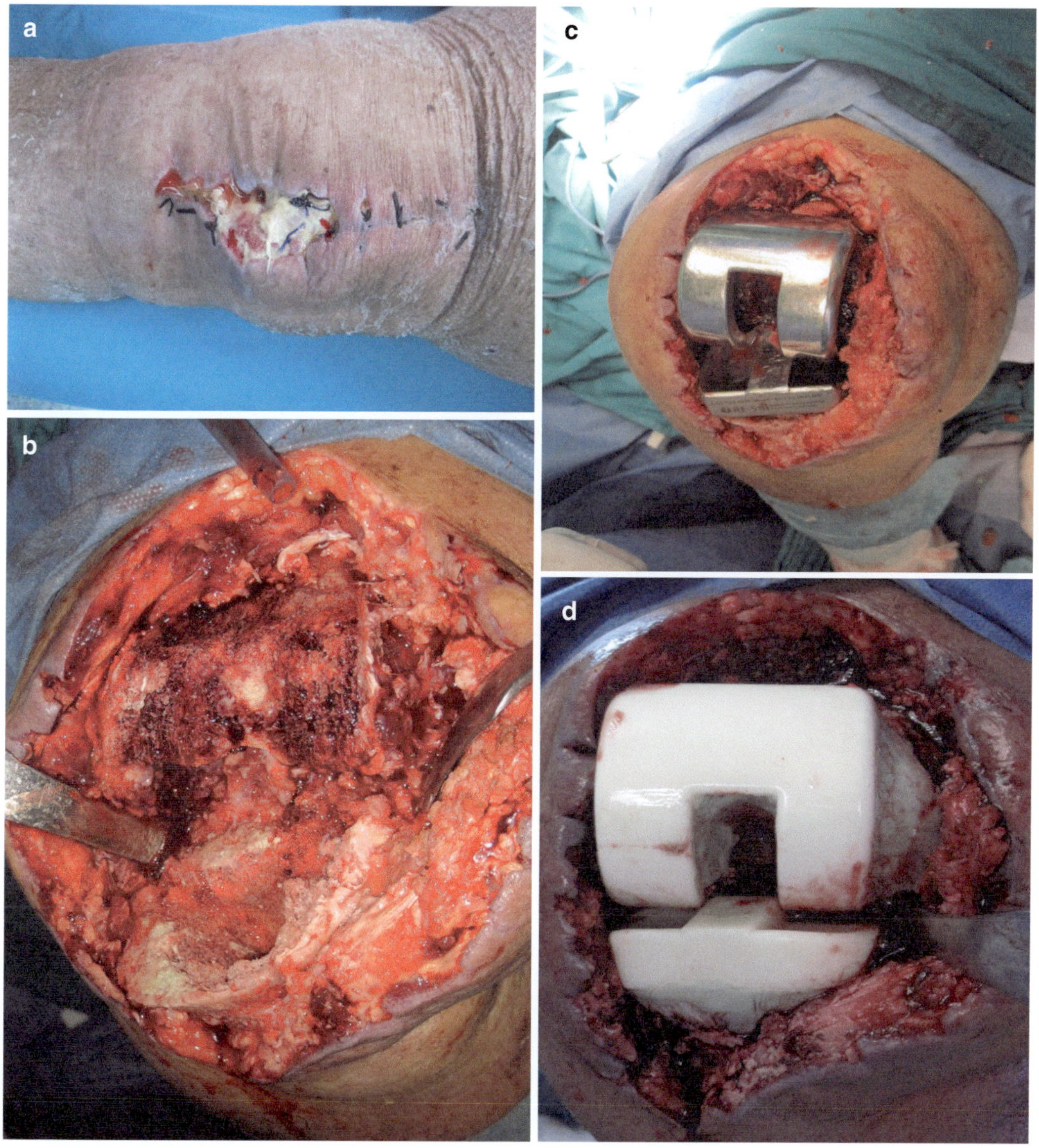

Fig. 17.2 Infected knee prosthesis with surgical wound dehiscence (**a**); after knee prosthesis removal and debridement of of devitalized tissues (**b**) an antibiotic-loaded articulated spacer was implanted (**c, d**); then, medial gastrocnemius flap dissection was performed (**e**); incisions in the fascia of the muscle were carried out to extend the length of the muscle (**f**); then, the spacer was covered with the flap and with partial thickness skin graft taken from the ipsilateral thigh (**g**)

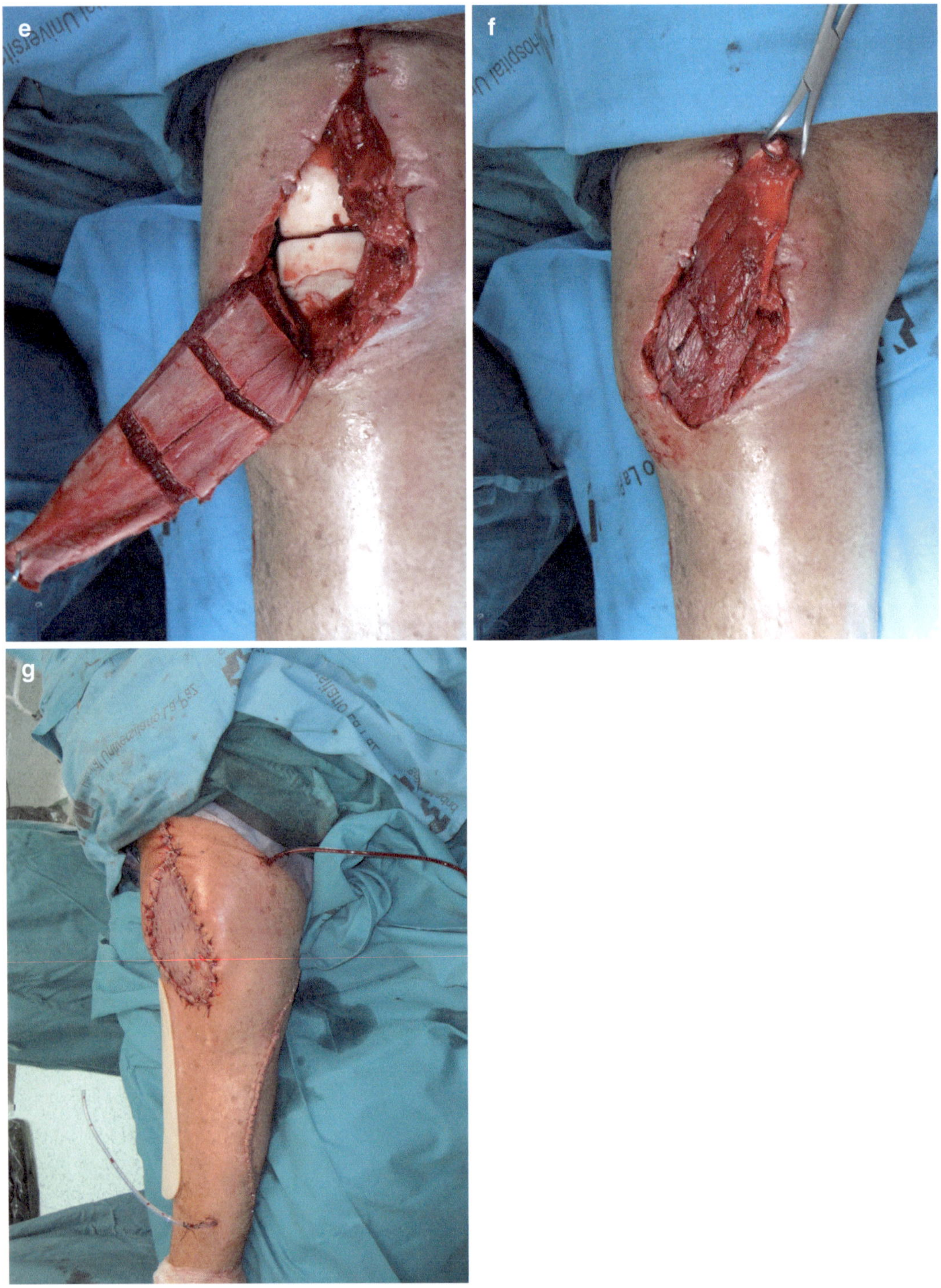

Fig. 17.2 (continued)

  - Soleus flap: Indicated for more distal defects in the proximal region of the leg. It is usually used half of the muscle (hemisoleus flap) so as not to sacrifice its function [22].
  - Medial or lateral vastus flap: For proximal knee defects.
- Fasciocutaneous flaps:
  - ALT flap: Designed for retrograde flow, it is useful for large defects when more proximal or extensive coverage than that offered by the gastrocnemius is required [23]. Free-form is the most commonly used when the size of the defect requires it or when it cannot be based on its distal pedicle.
  - Saphenous or anteromedial thigh flap: Its main use is to cover medial knee defects [24].
  - Lateral supragenicular flap: Based on the superolateral genicular artery, it is used for anterior and lateral knee defects [25].
  - Anterograde flow sural flap: Irrigated by the middle superficial sural artery, a branch of the cutaneous perforator that originates in the popliteal fossa of the popliteal artery, it can cover defects of up to 8 × 17 cm [26].

17.4.3 Ankle Flap Coverage

The ankle is a joint with little soft tissue coverage, which increases the risk of exposure of the osteosynthetic material. In this location, we can find the following local coverage options:

- Muscle flaps: Usually rarely used due to the lack of local muscles with adequate pedicles.
  - Extensor digitorum brevis flap: Based on the lateral tarsal artery, it is a useful option for dorsal ankle defects, although its volume is limited [27].
  - Flexor hallucis longus flap: Mainly used for Achilles tendon reconstruction, it can also be used in cases of ankle coverage defects. As in the previous case, its volume is limited [28].
  - Peroneus brevis flap: Based on the perforating branches of the peroneal artery, it is a valid option for small defects in the lateral region of the ankle [29].
- Fasciocutaneous flaps:
  - Reverse sural flap: This is one of the most commonly used options for ankle coverage due to its ability to reach practically all areas of the ankle [30] (Fig. 17.3).
  - Supramalleolar flap: Used for anteromedial defects, it is based on perforators of the anterior tibial artery [31].

However, given the scarcity of soft tissue in this location and therefore the limited availability of regional pedicled flaps, the use of free flaps is a fundamental strategy in the reconstruction of defects resulting from PJI of the ankle. In this context, the most commonly used flaps include the ALT (Fig. 17.4), for its versatility and pedicle length, and the latissimus dorsi flap, ideal for wide defects. Other useful flaps in this location are the gracilis and serratus or the SCIP (superficial circumflex iliac perforator) flap.

17.4.4 Shoulder Flap Coverage

The shoulder is a well-vascularized region, but resection of infected tissue in PJIs can result in extensive defects that expose the prosthesis or critical structures such as the humeral head and great vessels. Shoulder mobility also presents challenges for flap stability. Different flap options are available for coverage:

- Muscle flaps:
  - Pectoralis major flap: This is the most commonly used flap in the coverage of anterior and anteromedial defects of the shoulder. Its main pedicle comes from the thoracoacromial artery and allows a reliable coverage [32].
  - Pectoralis minor flap: Can also be used for coverage of the anterior shoulder region, with less morbidity in terms of sequelae than the pectoralis major flap [33].

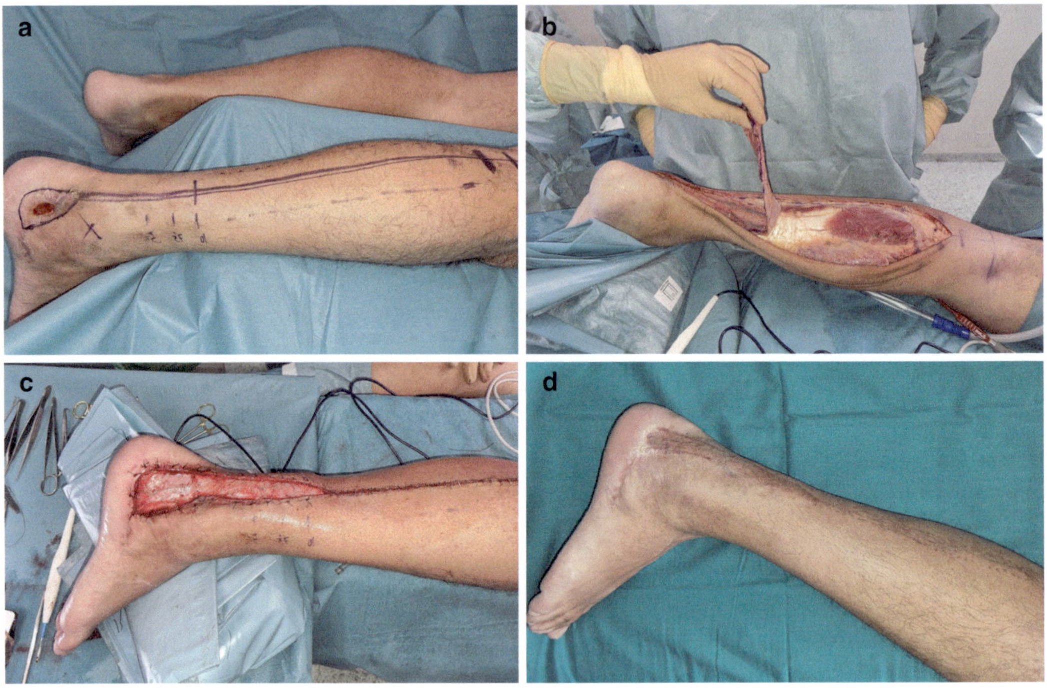

Fig. 17.3 (**a**-**d**) Chronic infection and fistula in the posterolateral region of the ankle (**a**); adipofascial sural flap disssection was performed (**b**); the defect was covered with the sural flap (**c**); at 3 months postoperative the result was excellent

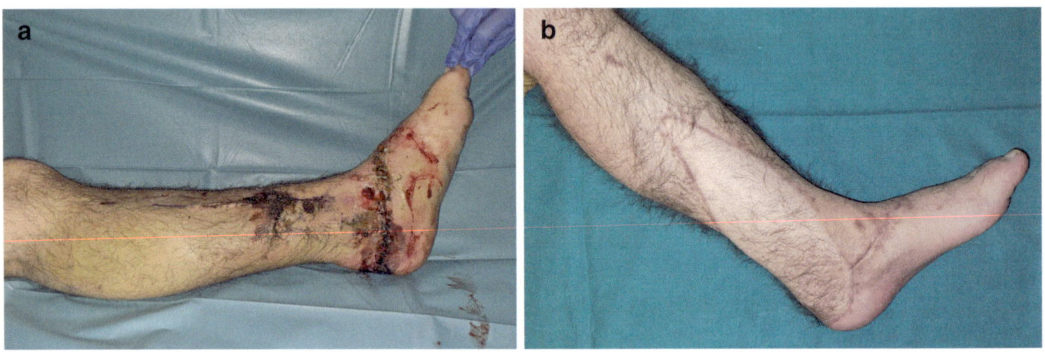

Fig. 17.4 (**a**, **b**) Soft tissue defect of the ankle solved using anterolateral thigh (ALT) free flap coverage (**a**); the final result was excellent (**b**)

  - Trapezius flap: Useful in posterior defects of the shoulder and scapula. Its pedicle depends on the transverse cervical artery [34].
  - Latissimus dorsi flap: Its wide arc of rotation and its size make it a frequently used flap in large defects of this joint [32].
- Fasciocutaneous flaps:
  - Supraclavicular flap: Based on perforators of the transverse cervical artery, it is useful in anterolateral shoulder defects [35].
  - Pectoralis flap: Based on perforators of the second, third, and fourth intercostal spaces. It is used for small defects in the anterior aspect of the shoulder [32].

- Occipito-cervico-thoracic perforator flaps are based on the perforators of the transverse cervical artery and its branches, including the superficial cervical artery. Its wide arc of rotation allows this flap to be used for coverage of the superior and posterior shoulder region [36].
- Distal trapezius flap: Based on the dorsal artery of the scapula, it is a musculocutaneous flap that allows coverage of losses of substance of the most apical area of the shoulder. If it is based on the descending branch of the transverse cervical artery, its arc of rotation increases and can reach the acromial and acromioclavicular area [37].
- Scapular and parascapular flaps: Based on a branch of the scapular circumflex artery, it emerges from the triangular space to the posterior area of the shoulder. With an arc of rotation of 90° it can cover the anterior surface of the shoulder [38].
- Lateral brachial flap: Allows coverage of defects in the anterior and lateral area of the shoulder. It is based on the perforators of the posterior branch of the radial collateral artery [39].

Given the abundance of regional flaps in this location, as with the hip joint, the use of free flaps is rarer than in other locations, being relegated to very large defects or lack of local resources [32].

17.5 Outcomes and Prognosis of Flap Coverage in PJIs

Flap coverage in PJIs has proven to be an effective strategy to preserve the joint, improve quality of life, and reduce the need for amputation. Success rates in terms of flap viability range from 85% to 95%, with a risk of partial or total necrosis of 5% to 15%, depending on the type of flap used and patient conditions [13, 40–43]. No significant differences have been found between muscle and fasciocutaneous flaps in the eradication of infection, provided that surgical debridement is adequate and antibiotic treatment is optimized [13]. Infection resolution rates vary between 75% and 90%, depending on the type of microorganism involved and the host response [6]. In addition, the use of flaps has significantly reduced the amputation rate, with studies reporting figures of 5%–20% compared to 40%–50% in patients without flap reconstruction [6]. Functional recovery after coverage depends on the stability of the prosthesis and the degree of scar fibrosis, which can affect mobility and the load supported by the joint. Factors such as the patient's age, the presence of comorbidities, the time of surgery, and the type of flap used directly influence the prognosis [44]. Free flaps offer greater reconstructive versatility, but require careful evaluation of the recipient vessels to minimize the risk of microvascular failure. In general, flap coverage, when performed properly and in a timely manner, improves functional outcomes and reduces the risk of major complications, consolidating as a fundamental strategy in the management of periprosthetic infections.

17.6 Conclusions

Flap coverage in PJIs is a surgical challenge that requires careful planning and appropriate flap selection based on the affected joint, the size of the defect, and the presence of active infection. Muscle flaps have proven to be reliable options due to their ability to provide well-vascularized tissue, which aids in the eradication of infection and coverage of exposed prosthetic materials. However, fasciocutaneous flaps, such as the sural flap at the ankle or the supraclavicular flap at the shoulder, offer advantages such as less donor site morbidity and a better cosmetic result. The choice between pedicled and free flaps depends on the availability of local tissues and the extent of the defect. In extensive defects, free flaps, such as the ALT or latissimus dorsi, are indispensable for effective coverage. Ultimately, the success of flap coverage in PJIs depends on a multidisciplinary approach, combining reconstructive surgery, infection control, and functional rehabilitation to improve long-term patient outcomes.

References

1. Tande AJ, Patel R. Prosthetic joint infection. Clin Microbiol Rev. 2014;27(2):302–45. https://doi.org/10.1128/CMR.00111-13.
2. Zimmerli W, Trampuz A, Ochsner PE. Prosthetic-joint infections. N Engl J Med. 2004;351(16):1645–54. https://doi.org/10.1056/NEJMra040181.
3. Kramer TS, Gastmeier P, Remschmidt C. Prosthetic joint infections. Lancet Infect Dis. 2018;18(12):1308. https://doi.org/10.1016/S1473-3099(18)30670-4.
4. Haddad FS, Ngu A, Negus JJ. Prosthetic joint infections and cost analysis? Adv Exp Med Biol. 2017;971:93–100. https://doi.org/10.1007/5584_2016_155.
5. Parvizi J, Tan TL, Goswami K, Higuera C, Della Valle C, Chen AF, et al. The 2018 definition of periprosthetic hip and knee infection: an evidence-based and validated criteria. J Arthroplast. 2018;33(5):1309–1314.e2. https://doi.org/10.1016/j.arth.2018.02.078.
6. Casey WJ 3rd, Rebecca AM, Krochmal DJ, Kim HY, Hemminger BJ, Clarke HD, et al. Prophylactic flap reconstruction of the knee prior to total knee arthroplasty in high-risk patients. Ann Plast Surg. 2011;66(4):381–7. https://doi.org/10.1097/SAP.0b013e3181e37c04.
7. Parvizi J, Gehrke T, Chen AF. Proceedings of the international consensus on periprosthetic joint infection. Bone Joint J. 2013;95-B(11):1450–2. https://doi.org/10.1302/0301-620X.95B11.33135.
8. Plate JF, Zuskov A, Seyler TM. Use of adjunct antiseptic agents in periprosthetic joint infections. J Am Acad Orthop Surg. 2021;29(23):e1151–8. https://doi.org/10.5435/JAAOS-D-21-00154.
9. Siqueira MBP, Saleh A, Klika AK, O'Rourke C, Schmitt S, Higuera CA, et al. Chronic suppression of periprosthetic joint infections with oral antibiotics increases infection-free survivorship. J Bone Joint Surg. 2015;97(15):1220–32. https://doi.org/10.2106/JBJS.N.00999.
10. Yuan K, Zhang F, Lineaweaver WC, Chen X, Li Z, Yan H. The coverage of soft-tissue defects around the foot and ankle using free or local flaps. Ann Plast Surg. 2021;86(6):668–73. https://doi.org/10.1097/SAP.0000000000002811.
11. Fernando N, Yacovelli S, Parvizi J. Periprosthetic infection in the setting of periprosthetic total hip fractures: evaluation and management. J Am Acad Orthop Surg. 2022;30(20):957–64. https://doi.org/10.5435/JAAOS-D-21-00083.
12. Zmistowski B, Karam JA, Durinka JB, Casper DS, Parvizi J. Periprosthetic joint infection increases the risk of one-year mortality. J Bone Joint Surg. 2013;95(24):2177–84. https://doi.org/10.2106/JBJS.L.00789.
13. Buono P, Castus P, Dubois-Ferrière V, Rüegg EM, Uçkay I, Assal M, et al. Muscular versus non-muscular free flaps for soft tissue coverage of chronic tibial osteomyelitis. World J Plast Surg. 2018;7(3):294–300. https://doi.org/10.29252/wjps.7.3.294.
14. Rovere G, De Mauro D, D'Orio M, Fulchignoni C, Matrangolo MR, Perisano C, et al. Use of muscular flaps for the treatment of hip prosthetic joint infection: a systematic review. BMC Musculoskelet Disord. 2021;22(Suppl 2):1059. https://doi.org/10.1186/s12891-021-04945-8.
15. Suda AJ, Heppert V. Vastus lateralis muscle flap for infected hips after resection arthroplasty. J Bone Joint Surg Br. 2010;92-B(12):1654–8. https://doi.org/10.1302/0301-620X.92B12.25212.
16. Ricciardi BF, Henderson PW, McLawhorn AS, Westrich GH, Bostrom MP, Gayle LB. Gluteus maximus advancement flap procedure for reconstruction of posterior soft tissue deficiency in revision total hip arthroplasty. Orthopedics. 2017;40(3):e495–500. https://doi.org/10.3928/01477447-20170308-06.
17. Paletta CE, Freedman B, Shehadi SI. The VY tensor fasciae latae musculocutaneous flap. Plast Reconstr Surg. 1989;83(5):852–7. https://doi.org/10.1097/00006534-198905000-00012.
18. Windle BH, Stroup RT, Beckenstein MS. The inferiorly based rectus abdominis island flap for the treatment of complex hip wounds. Plast Reconstr Surg. 1996;98(1):99–102. https://doi.org/10.1097/00006534-199607000-00016.
19. Saint-Cyr M, Schaverien M, Wong C, Nagarkar P, Arbique G, Brown S, et al. The extended anterolateral thigh flap: anatomical basis and clinical experience. Plast Reconstr Surg. 2009;123(4):1245–55. https://doi.org/10.1097/PRS.0b013e31819e2718.
20. Hurwitz DJ, Walton RL. Closure of chronic wounds of the perineal and sacral regions using the gluteal thigh flap. Ann Plast Surg. 1982;8(5):375–86. https://doi.org/10.1097/00000637-198205000-00004.
21. Theil C, Stock ME, Gosheger G, Moellenbeck B, Schwarze J, Schmidt-Braekling T. Gastrocnemius muscle flaps for soft tissue coverage in periprosthetic knee joint infection. J Arthroplast. 2020;35(12):3730–6. https://doi.org/10.1016/j.arth.2020.06.074.
22. Ahmad I, Akhtar S, Rashidi E, Khurram MF. Hemisoleus muscle flap in the reconstruction of exposed bones in the lower limb. J Wound Care. 2013;22(11):635–42. https://doi.org/10.12968/jowc.2013.22.11.635.
23. Pan S-C, Yu J-C, Shieh S-J, Lee J-W, Huang B-M, Chiu H-Y. Distally based anterolateral thigh flap: an anatomic and clinical study. Plast Reconstr Surg. 2004;114(7):1768–75. https://doi.org/10.1097/01.prs.0000142416.91524.4c.
24. Acland RD, Schusterman M, Godina M, Eder E, Taylor GI, Carlisle I. The saphenous neurovascular free flap. Plast Reconstr Surg. 1981;67(6):763–74. https://doi.org/10.1097/00006534-198106000-00009.
25. Pozzobon LR, Helito CP, Guimarães TM, Gobbi RG, Pécora JR, Camanho GL. Rotation flaps for

coverage after total knee arthroplasty. Acta Ortop Bras. 2013;21(4):219–122. https://doi.org/10.1590/S1413-78522013000400007.
26. Lin C-H, Hsieh Y-H, Lin C-H. The medial sural artery perforator flap in lower extremity reconstruction. Clin Plast Surg. 2021;48(2):249–57. https://doi.org/10.1016/j.cps.2021.01.003.
27. Houdek MT, Wagner ER, Pensy RA, Eglseder WA. Extensor digitorum brevis flap for the coverage of ankle and dorsal foot wounds: a technical trick. J Orthop Trauma. 2016;30(12):e404–8. https://doi.org/10.1097/BOT.0000000000000650.
28. Periasamy M, Muthukumar V, Ahamed PIF, Ahammed VA, Venkatramani H, Sabapathy SR. Single-stage flexor hallucis longus transfer and gracilis free flap cover for failed Achilles tendon repair with soft tissue defect. J Plast Reconstr Aesthet Surg. 2023;77:236–43. https://doi.org/10.1016/j.bjps.2022.11.028.
29. Neiman R, Finkemeier CG, Swentik AG. Distally based peroneus brevis Rotation flap. J Orthop Trauma. 2020;34(Suppl 2):S44–5. https://doi.org/10.1097/BOT.0000000000001823.
30. Noaman HH, Mohamed MA, Faisal A, Soroor YO. Different surgical procedures for reconstruction of soft-tissue defects around the ankle. Injury. 2022;53(7):2657–65. https://doi.org/10.1016/j.injury.2022.03.066.
31. Nguyen TN, Trong Mai T, Cao T, Thai TT. Lateral supramalleolar flap for soft-tissue coverage of ankle and foot defects. J Plast Surg Hand Surg. 2023;57(1–6):459–65. https://doi.org/10.1080/2000656X.2022.2152826.
32. Auquit-Auckbur I, Coquerel-Beghin D, Vanaret J. Coverage losses of substance in the shoulder. Ann Chir Plast Esthet. 2020;65(5–6):570–88. https://doi.org/10.1016/j.anplas.2020.06.008.
33. Palmer RS, Miller TA. Anterior shoulder reconstruction with pectoralis minor muscle flap. Plast Reconstr Surg. 1988;81(3):437–9. https://doi.org/10.1097/00006534-198803000-00022.
34. Motamed S, Davami B, Daghagheleh H. Trapezius musculocutaneous flap in severe shoulder and neck burn. Burns. 2004;30(5):476–80. https://doi.org/10.1016/j.burns.2004.02.006.
35. Sheriff HO, Mahmood KA, Hamawandi N, Mirza AJ, Hawas J, Moreno EG, et al. The supraclavicular artery perforator flap: a comparative study of imaging techniques used in preoperative mapping. J Reconstr Microsurg. 2018;34(7):499–508. https://doi.org/10.1055/s-0038-1639577.
36. Ogawa R, Hyakusoku H, Murakami M, Gao J-H. Clinical and basic research on occipito-cervico-dorsal flaps: including a study of the anatomical territories of dorsal trunk vessels. Plast Reconstr Surg. 2004;113(7):1923–33. https://doi.org/10.1097/01.prs.0000122204.39434.12.
37. Rasheed MZ, Tan B-K, Tan K-C. The extended lower trapezius flap for the reconstruction of shoulder tip defects. Ann Plast Surg. 2009;63(2):184–7. https://doi.org/10.1097/SAP.0b013e318189a9a7.
38. Kim PS, Lewis VL Jr. Use of a pedicled parascapular flap for anterior shoulder and arm reconstruction. Plast Reconstr Surg. 1985;76(6):942–4. https://doi.org/10.1097/00006534-198512000-00029.
39. Jordan SW, Wayne JD, Dumanian GA. The pedicled lateral arm flap for oncologic reconstruction near the shoulder. Ann Plast Surg. 2015;74(1):30–3. https://doi.org/10.1097/SAP.0b013e3182853f0b.
40. Nahabedian MY, Orlando JC, Delanois RE, Mont MA, Hungerford DS. Salvage procedures for complex soft tissue defects of the knee. Clin Orthop Relat Res. 1998;356:119–24. https://doi.org/10.1097/00003086-199811000-00017.
41. Rao AJ, Kempton SJ, Erickson BJ, Levine BR, Rao VK. Soft tissue reconstruction and flap coverage for revision total knee arthroplasty. J Arthroplast. 2016;31(7):1529–38. https://doi.org/10.1016/j.arth.2015.12.054.
42. Panni AS, Vasso M, Cerciello S, Salgarello M. Wound complications in total knee arthroplasty. Which flap is to be used? With or without retention of prosthesis? Knee Surg Sports Traumatol Arthrosc. 2011;19(7):1060–8. https://doi.org/10.1007/s00167-010-1328-5.
43. Gad B, Styron J, Goergy M, Klika A, Barsoum W, Higuera C. Patient factors associated with failure of flap coverage used during revision total knee arthroplasty. J Knee Surg. 2018;31(8):723–9. https://doi.org/10.1055/s-0037-1607060.
44. Economides JM, DeFazio MV, Golshani K, Cinque M, Anghel EL, Attinger CE, et al. Systematic Review and Comparative Meta-Analysis of Outcomes Following Pedicled Muscle versus Fasciocutaneous Flap Coverage for Complex Periprosthetic Wounds in Patients with Total Knee Arthroplasty. Arch Plast Surg. 2017;44(2):124–35. Available from: http://www.thieme-connect.de/DOI/DOI?10.5999/aps.2017.44.2.124.

MIX
Papier aus verantwortungsvollen Quellen
Paper from responsible sources
FSC® C105338

If you have any concerns about our products,
you can contact us on
ProductSafety@springernature.com

In case Publisher is established outside the EU,
the EU authorized representative is:
Springer Nature Customer Service Center GmbH
Europaplatz 3, 69115 Heidelberg, Germany

Printed by Libri Plureos GmbH
in Hamburg, Germany